THEORETICAL AND APPLIED ASPECTS OF HEALTH PSYCHOLOGY

THEORETICAL AND APPLIED ASPECTS OF HEALTH PSYCHOLOGY

Edited by

L.R. Schmidt
University of Trier, FRG

P. Schwenkmezger
University of Trier, FRG

J. Weinman
Guy's Hospital, London, UK

and

S. Maes
Tilburg University, The Netherlands

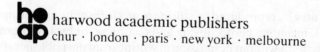
harwood academic publishers
chur · london · paris · new york · melbourne

Harwood Academic Publishers

Post Office Box 197
London WC2E 9PX
United Kingdom

58, rue Lhomond
75005 Paris
France

Post Office Box 786
Cooper Station
New York, New York 10276
United States of America

Private Bag 8
Camberwell Virginia 3124
Australia

Library of Congress Cataloging-in-Publication Data

Theoretical and applied aspects of health psychology / edited by L.R.
  Schmidt ... [et al.].
      p.   cm.
  Includes index.
  ISBN 3-7186-5053-3
  1. Clinical health psychology.   I. Schmidt, Lothar R.
  [DNLM: 1. Behavioral Medicine.   2. Disease--psychology.   3. Health
Behavior.   4. Psychology, Medical.]
R726.7.T44   1990
616' .0019--dc20
DNLM/DLC
for Library of Congress   90-5100
                                                                      CIP

CONTENTS

PREFACE

This book emerged mainly from the "International Congress on Health Psychology", which was held at the University of Trier, 26 – 28 May 1988. However, instead of publishing the entire proceedings of this conference, we selectively chose presentations with regard to their impact on the rapidly growing field of health psychology.

Our focus, as outlined in the introductory chapter, is on recent developments in health psychology, emphasizing health models, health education and primary prevention. Nevertheless, this volume also includes contributions about coping with severe and chronic illness and about secondary and tertiary prevention.

Every manuscript was reviewed by two different reviewers, including the editors as well as specialists for the specific topics. Some manuscripts had to be rejected, most of them were revised intensively. We thank all the reviewers for their valuable suggestions, and also thank them on behalf of the authors. On behalf of the many authors who are not native speakers of English, we would like to take this opportunity to express our deep appreciation of the work of Dipl.-Psych. Martha Keating, Wuppertal, who not only corrected the chapters with regard to spelling and grammar but reviewed and reformulated parts of them to make them more understandable.

We want to thank our secretaries Helga Linder and Lore Merkt, who not only wrote our own manuscripts and reviews but also rewrote entire manuscripts and parts of chapters, especially the references of other authors. Gabriele Dlugosch was of invaluable help as an expert on health psychology, especially as regards developments in the USA. Furthermore, we are grateful to Birgit Albs, Dorothea Hinrichs and Muna El-Giamal for their assistance in checking and correcting the manuscripts.

Last but not least, we are appreciative of the German Research Foundation, the Minister of Education of the State of Rheinland-Pfalz, and the Society of the Friends of the University of Trier, whose financial support enabled us to organize the "International Congress on Health Psychology."

Lothar Schmidt
Peter Schwenkmezger

LIST OF CONTRIBUTORS

Augustiny, K-F.
Department of Psychiatry, University of Bern, Murtenstrasse 21, 3010 Bern, Switzerland

Bisping, R.
Institute of Medical Psychology, University of Düsseldorf, Moorenstrasse 5, 4000 Düsseldorf, FRG

Blaser, A.
Department of Psychiatry, University of Bern, Murtenstrasse 21, 3010 Bern, Switzerland

Bode, U.
Department of Paediatric Haematology/Oncology, University of Bonn, Adenauer Allee 119, 5300 Bonn 1, FRG

Breteler, R. H. M.
Department of Clinical Psychology and Personality, University of Nijmegen, PO Box 9104, HE Nijmegen, The Netherlands

Bruggemans, E.
Health Psychology Section, Tilburg University, PO Box 90153, 5000 LE Tilburg, The Netherlands

Couzijn, A. L.
Department of Clinical and Health Psychology, University of Utrecht, Heidelberglaan 1, 3508 TC Utrecht, The Netherlands

De Backer, G.
Dienst voor Hygiene en Sociale Geneeskunde, Rijksuniversiteit Gent, Henri Dunantlaan 2, 9000 Gent, Belgium

Diebschlag, U.
Department of Psychology, University of Trier, PO Box 3825, 5500 Trier, FRG

Diekstra, R. F. W.
Division of Mental Health, World Health Organization, 1211 Geneva 27, Switzerland

Dlugosch, G. E.
Department of Psychology, University of Trier, PO Box 3825, 5500 Trier, FRG

Dramaix, M.
ESP, Erasmus Campus, Free University of Brussels, Route de Lennik 808, 1070 Brussels, Belgium

Dvorak, J.
Department of Psychiatry, University of Bern, Murtenstrasse 1, 3010 Bern, Switzerland

Eiser, C.
Department of Psychology, Washington Singer Laboratories, University of Exeter, Exeter EX4 4QG, UK

Fehm-Wolfdorf, G.
Department of Medical Psychology, University of Ulm, Am Hochstrasse 8, 7900 Ulm, FRG

Ferring, D.
Department of Psychology, University of Trier, PO Box 3825, 5500 Trier, FRG

Filipp, S.-H.
Department of Psychology, University of Trier, PO Box 3825, 5500 Trier, FRG

Fitzpatrick, R.
Wuffield College, Oxford University, Oxford OX1 1NF, UK

Freudenberg, E.
Department of Psychology, University of Trier, PO Box 3825, 5500 Trier, FRG

Fuhrimann, P.
Department of Psychiatry, University of Bern, Murtenstrasse 21, 3010 Bern, Switzerland

Gilbert, P.
Psychology Unit, Royal Free Hospital, School of Medicine, Pond Street, London NW3 2QG, UK

Hardt, J.
Department of Psychology, University of Mainz, PO Box 3980, 6500 Mainz 1, FRG

Heim, E.
Department of Psychiatry, University of Bern, Murtenstrasse 21, 3010 Bern, Switzerland

Hellhammer, D.
Department of Psychology, University of Trier, PO Box 3825, 5500 Trier, FRG

Humphris, G. M.
Department of Psychology, Fazakerley Hospital, Liverpool L9 7AL, UK

Idänpään-Heikkilä, U.
The Jorvi Hospital, 02740 Espoo, Finalnd

Jabaaij, L.
General and Theoretical Psychology Section, Tilburg University, PO Box 90153, 5000 LE Tilburg, The Netherlands

Jansen, M. A.
Department of Clinical, Health and Personality Psychology, University of Leiden, The Netherlands

Jeninga, A.
Insitute for Research in Extramural Medicine, Free University of Amsterdam, PO Box 7161, 1007 MC Amsterdam, The Netherlands

Johnston, M.
University of London, Psychology Unit, Royal Free Hospital, School of Medicine, Pond Street, London NW3 2QG, UK

Jonkers, R.
Dutch Health Education Center, PO Box 5104, 3502 JC Utrecht, The Netherlands

Julkunen, J.
Rehabilitation Foundation, Pakarituvantie 4, 00410 Helsinki, Finland

Kemmer, F. W.
Department of Nutrition and Metabolism, University of Düsseldorf, Universitätsstrasse 1, 4000 Düsseldorf, FRG

Kittel, F. M. T.
ESP, Erasmus Campus, Free University of Brussels, Route de Lennik 808, 1070 Brussels, Belgium

Klauer, T.
Department of Psychology, University of Trier, PO Box 3825, 5500 Trier, FRG

Kleemann, P. P.
Department of Medicine, Clinic for Anaesthesiology, University of Mainz, PO Box 3960, 6500 Mainz 1, FRG

Kok, G.
University of Limburg, PO Box 616, 6200 MD Maastricht, The Netherlands

Kornitzer, M.
ESP, Erasmus Campus, Free University of Brussels, Route de Lennik 808, 1070 Brussels, Belgium

Krohne, H. W.
Department of Psychology, University of Mainz PO Box 3980, 6500 Mainz 1, FRG

Lamb, R.
Academic Department of Psychiatry UCMSM, University of London, Middlesex Hospital, Mortimer Street, London W1N 8AA, UK

Landsiedel, W.
Department of Psychology, University of Trier, PO Box 3825, 5500 Trier, FRG

Lang, J.
Department of Psychology, University of Trier, PO Box 3825, 5500 Trier, FRG

Lehnert, H.
Department of Internal Medicine, University of Mainz, PO Box 3980, 6500 Mainz 1, FRG

Leppin, A.
Department of Psychology, WE 7, Free University of Berlin, Habelschwerdter Allee 45, 1000 Berlin 33, FRG

Liedekerken, P.
Dutch Health Education Center, PO Box 5104, 3502 JC Utrecht, The Netherlands

Maes, S.
Health Psychology Section, Tilburg University, PO Box 90153, 5000 LE Tilburg, The Netherlands (Now: Health Psychology Section, University of Leiden, Wassenaarseweg 52, 2300 RB Leiden, The Netherlands)

Marteau, T.
Psychology Unit, Royal Free Hospital, School of Medicine, Pond Street London
NW3 2QG, UK

Menges, L.
Department of Medical Psychology, Free University of Amsterdam, PO Box 7161,
1007 MC Amsterdam, The Netherlands

Mertens, N. H. M.
Faculty of Social Sciences, PO Box 80.1, 140, 3508 TC Utrecht, The Netherlands

Moleman, P.
Department of Biological Psychiatry, University Hospital, Dijkzigt, Molenwater-
plein 40, 3015 GD Rotterdam, The Netherlands

Murison, R.
Department of Physiological Psychology, University of Bergen, Arstadveien 21,
5000 Bergen, Norway

Murza, G.
c/o IDIS - Institute für Dokumentation und Information, Sozialmedizin und
öffentliches Gesundheitswesen, Westerfeldstrasse 35–37, 4800 Bielefeld, FRG

Netter, P.
Department of Psychology, University of Giessen, Otto-Behaghelstrasse 10, 6300
Giessen, FRG

Newman, S.
Academic Department of Psychiatry UCMSM, niversity of London, Middlesex Hospital, Mortimer Street, London W1N 8AA, UK

Noeker, M.
Department of Paediatric Haematology/Oncology, University of Bonn, Adenauer
Allee 119, 5300 Bonn 1, FRG

Partridge, C.
Psychology Unit, Royal Free Hospital, School of Medicine, Pond Street, London
NW3 2QG, UK

Pennings-van der Eerden, L. J. M.
Department of General Health Care and Epidemiology, Faculty of Medicine, State
University of Utrecht, Bijhouwerstraat 6, 3511 ZC Utrecht, The Netherlands

Petermann, F.
Department of Psychology, University of Bonn, Römerstrasse 164, 5300 Bonn 1,
FRG

Raaheim, A.
Research Center for Occupational Health and Safety, Department of Social and
Organizational Psychology, University of Bergen, Öisteinsgt, 3, Norway

Ratliff-Crain, J.
Department of Medical Psychology, Uniformed Services, University of the Health
Sciences, 4301 Jones Bridge Road, Bethesda, MD 20814–4799, USA

Rombouts, R.
Department of Clinical Psychiatry, University of Groningen, PO Box 30.001, 9700 Groningen, The Netherlands

Ros, W. J. G.
Department of Clinical and Health Psychology, University of Utrecht, Heidelberglaan 1, 3508 TC Utrecht, The Netherlands

Rosenman, R. H.
SRF International, 333 Ravenswood Avenue, Menlo Park, CA 94025, USA

Saarinen, T.
Rehabilitation Foundation, Pakarituvantie 4, Helsinki, Finland

Schmidt, L. R.
Department of Psychology, University of Trier, PO Box 3825, 5500 Trier, FRG

Schwarz, P.
Department of Medical Psychology, University of Ulm, Am Hochsträss 8, 7900 Ulm, FRG

Schwarzer, R.
Department of Psychology, Free University of Berlin, Habelschwerdter Allee 45, 1000 Berlin 33, FRG

Schwenkmezger, P.
Department of Psychology, University of Trier, PO Box 3825, 5500 Trier, FRG

Seiffge-Krenke, I.
Department of Psychology, University of Bonn, Römerstrasse 164, 5300 Bonn 1, FRG

Seydel, E.
Department of Psychology, University of Twente, PO Box 217, 7500 AE Enschede, The Netherlands

Shipley, M.
Department of Rheumatology UCMSM, University of London, Middlesex Hospital, Mortimer Street, London W1N 8AA, UK

Spector, N. H.
Division of Fundamental Neurosciences, NINDS, The National Insitutes of Health, Federal Building, Room 916, Bethesda, MD 20892, USA

Steingrüber, H.-J.
Department of Medical Psychology, University of Düsseldorf, Universitätstrasse 1, 4000 Düsseldorf, FRG

Steptoe, A.
Department of Psychology, St George's Hospital Medical School, University of London, Cranmer Terrace, London SW17 0RE, UK

Taal, E.
Department of Psychology, University of Twente, PO Box 217, 7500 AE Enschede, The Netherlands

Theisen, A.
Department of Medical Psychology, Clinic for Anaesthesiology, University of Mainz, PO Box 3960, 6500 Mainz 1, FRG

Tschaggelar, W.
Department of Psychiatry, University of Bern, Murtenstrasse 21, 3010 Bern, Switzerland

Valach, L.
Department of Psychiatry, University of Bern, Murtenstrasse 21, 3010 Bern, Switzerland

Vinck, J.
Limburg University Centre, University Campus, 3610 Diepenbeek, Belgium

Vingerhoets, A.
Department of Medical Psychology and Institute for Research in Extramural Medicine, Free University of Amsterdam, PO Box 7161, 1007 MC Amsterdam, The Netherlands

Voigt, K.-H.
Institute for Physiology, University of Marburg, Deutschhausstrasse 1–2, 3550 Marburg, FRG

Weinman, J.
Unit of Psychology, Guy's Hospital Medical School, University of London, London SE1 9RT, UK

Weishaupt, I.
Department of Psychology, University of Trier, PO Box 3825, 5500 Trier, FRG

Wiegman, O.
Department of Psychology, University of Twente, PO Box 217, 7500 AE Enschede, The Netherlands

Winnubst, J. A. M.
Department of Clinical and Health Psychology, University of Utrecht, Heidelberglaan 1, 3508 TC Utrecht

Zenz, H.
Department for Medical Psychology, University of Ulm, Am Hochsträss 8, 7900 Ulm, FRG

Section 1

Models and Concepts of Health and Illness

The Scope of Health Psychology

Lothar R. Schmidt, Peter Schwenkmezger and
Gabriele E.Dlugosch

This brief overview cannot deal with all the many aspects of the very broad field of health psychology. We cannot, for example, go into the variety of definitions of health and descriptions of health psychology and space does not permit a detailed differentiation between health psychology and other disciplines such as behavioral medicine, medical psychology, clinical health psychology, health education, and health promotion on the basis of concepts, contents and methodology. In three sections, we shall (1) define goals and motives of health psychology, (2) describe health models, health behavior models and health promotion/health education models, and (3) discuss several aspects of assessment and practical applications in health psychology. Although health psychology does of course include the area of mental health, we shall mainly limit our review to physical health and illness, because psychological health research has different accentuations.

The following discussion is most relevant for highly developed countries. In developing countries, health psychology is confronted with very different issues – for instance, the health risks resulting from infectious diseases or the almost constant threat of death by starvation, as well as the existence of completely different conditions for health education and compliance.

Defining the Goals and Motives

Over the past decade there has been a large international movement toward health and health behavior; the clearest indication of this trend is manifested in the World Health Organization's program "Health for All by the Year 2000". This call was taken up enthusiastically by many countries throughout the world and many health initiatives were begun. In the field of psychology, too, research and practice have focused more and more on issues of health and its impairment; this is attested to by the growing number of publications on this subject, the establishment of specialized societies, new health divisions in established societies, new journals such as Health Psychology and Psychology & Health, a special section in the catalogue of the Annual Review of Psychology (Krantz, Grunberg & Baum, 1985; Rodin & Salovey, 1989), scientific congresses, and many psychological programs for health education and primary prevention. The establishment of the "European Health Psychology Society" in Trier in 1988 was aimed at giving a new impetus to the field of health psychology in Europe.

Nevertheless, the term "health psychology" is often used in a very vague sense. At conferences and in publications health psychology sometimes covers the same topics as "behavioral medicine" or "medical psychology"; secondary and tertiary prevention are often more emphasized than primary prevention or health education. However, it is a concept that can signal an emphasis on health rather than illness, one that is able to stimulate new approaches beyond the field of medicine and that, as a "program", can help to coordinate and channel developments.

Earlier discussions in health psychology concentrated mostly on the individuals concerned, their families and immediate social support systems. Likewise, the individual is the center of Matarazzo's often-quoted definition (1980, p. 815):

"Health psychology is the aggregate of the specific educational, scientific, and professional contributions of the discipline of psychology to the promotion and maintenance of health, the prevention and treatment of illness, and the identification of etiologic and diagnostic correlates of health, illness, and related dysfunction."

Bloom (1988) claims this to be a comprehensive description of health psychology, namely all contributions psychologists can make to promoting health. This description defines health as broadly as possible, encompassing both health *and* illness, physical *and* mental health, specific types or forms of illness as well as the general feeling of well-being or of "not feeling well". Health psychology is not limited to research and theory construction; it also covers applications, the areas of prevention, counseling and treatment. Health is not only oriented toward the individual; it also includes an analysis of the social environment as well as the ecological and economic systems.

According to Sartorius' (1989) definition, health can be considered "a state of balance between the individual, his inner self and the world around him." If one agrees in principle with this statement (each of its components would of course require a precise, operationalized definition), it becomes obvious that health movements or programs can have quite different goals, targets and motives.

Goals of Health Psychology

At first glance, it appears easy to define the goals of health psychology. There is widespread agreement that the main purpose of health psychology is to reduce risks to physical and mental health. Taking a somewhat closer look at the defined goals presented by some of the more important representatives of health psychology, it becomes apparent that these goals differ in their complexity and are particularly dependent on the underlying theoretical orientation. In the following, we will illustrate this with some examples.

One way health behavior can be analyzed is on the basis of learning theory. Miller (1984), for example, proposes that health and illness behavior are learned through reinforcement contingencies. Each specific behavior is regarded as a learned habit resulting from a particular learning history or mechanisms of model learning. With such a model, the goal of health psychology is to change the reinforcement pattern so as to encourage the acquisition of health-promoting or illness-avoiding behavior. Behavioral medicine largely follows this type of model.

A much more general goal is named by Matarazzo (1984 a,b). According to him, the task of health psychology is to identify risk factors for the most frequently-occurring diseases, pathogens and immunogens, and their interactions, to explain them and to initiate appropriate behavior changes. Particular emphasis is placed on the individual's responsibility for health. The general goal of health psychology in this framework is to change specific, health-damaging life styles. Matarazzo feels that change processes can be initiated more quickly when the goal is defined concretely and objectively. Specific goals for behavior change include, according to Harris (1980), changes in the areas of preventive health services, health protection and health promotion. These can in turn be classified into five sub-goals (see Table 1).

Table 1 Specific goals of health psychology (according to Harris, 1980)

Health Promotion

- Smoking and health

- Misuse of alcohol and drugs

- Nutrition

- Physical fitness and exercise

- Control of stress and violent behavior

Health Protection

- Control of toxic agents

- Occupational safety and health

- Accident prevention and injury control

- Fluoridation and dental health

- Surveillance and control of infectious diseases

Preventive Health Services

- Control of high blood pressure

- Family planning

- Pregnancy and infant health

- Immunization

- Sexually transmitted diseases

As in most highly-developed countries during the last century, there has been an extreme shift in the United States in the illness spectrum, along with a change in risks for most prevalent illnesses and causes of death. According to Bloom (1988) one can assume that about half of the deaths in the United States today depend to a great extent upon health risk behaviors and life styles. Comparative mortality statistics (cf., Junge, 1986) can provide interesting and important information for different countries and their specific risks.

Lütjen and Frey (1987) also stress health psychology's connections to social psychological factors, thus extending the spectrum to include conditions associated with work and living, the social environment, life events and psychosocial aspects of treatment (e.g. the physician-patient relationship, compliance, issues regarding hospitalization).

This brings us to the area of holistic approaches, a perspective that extends far beyond the individual and his immediate surroundings, taking long-neglected *ecological* aspects and dangers into account. These also play a role in psychological models, to the extent that they can be influenced by individual behavior. Lately, psychological and health educational aspects of this approach have been mentioned more and more often in publications (cf., Winett, 1985; von Cube & Storch, 1988; Stark, 1989a).

Historical health movements – in ancient Greece and Rome, in China, in Arabic countries and in Europe during the Middle Ages – have always emphasized the importance of a balance with the environment (cf., Schipperges, 1982). These ancient approaches can give us an insight into our current ideas about health psychology, helping to illuminate the relationship between health trends and "Zeitgeist", religions and political systems. For this reason, many approaches that have been used in the United States should not be applied to Europe without reflection: We have to deal with completely different life spaces, where both quality of life and health standards sharply differ from their American counterparts.

The holistic approach requires a system-oriented view in health psychology and, as a result, the analysis of the interdependency between health-related measures. This is also true for the analysis of risk factors. Every inventory of health psychology goals mentions the identification and change of risk factors or risk behavior. Health psychological research should not, however, be limited to questions of identification; it must also analyze how these risk factors work and how they interact. This field of health research is still very much in need of improvement (cf. Ridder, 1987).

The assessment of risk factors is very difficult, primarily because the way they work and their interactions are often unknown or not taken into account in experimental designs. It is relatively easy to prove the pathogenic effects of cigarette smoking and excessive alcohol consumption, but the health consequences of other risk behaviors are much more debatable. For example, the health-promoting effects of exercise have been discussed often, but so has its risk potential (Clearing-Sky, 1988). A similar situation exists for particular foods or diets. The need for a systems-oriented approach to health psychology becomes even more evident when very complex questions are made the subject of health psychology. For example, increased use of automobiles has resulted in more individual freedom and thus an increase in life quality, but these advantages are gained at the cost of individual risks and enormous damage to the environment.

This brings us to the normative question of goals in health psychology. Although almost no one denies the importance of identifying the actual harmful potential of risk behaviors, the demand to cease performing a particular behavior elicits questions concerning restrictions in the quality of life. A normative discussion also includes the analysis of inconsistent social standards, for example, the question why the use of certain drugs such as alcohol and pills are tolerated in our society or even encouraged, whereas their misuse or the use of "illegal" drugs is strictly sanctioned. Questions concerning the evaluation of the quality of life, current abstinence or use compared to future consequences, etc. also fall in this area as well as changes in the appraisals that occur over the course of a lifetime. In addition to adolescence, old age – during which certain diseases or illnesses become more prevalent – should also be considered. Moreover, one has to regard the conditions under which life expectancy as such should be extended: Simply helping a person linger on in weakness, helplessness or dementia cannot be the goal for health psychology interventions.

Although health activities are wholeheartedly endorsed, we have to be careful not to promote a naive "healthism" which ignores human "nature" and cultural standards. Diekstra and Jansen (1988) describe healthism as "... establishing an ideal of a healthy, socially fully-integrated, psychologically well-balanced individual as a social norm. Before and after the year 2000 physical and emotional suffering, loneliness, poverty and misery, illness and dying will remain part of the human condition." Ullman (1988) has warned against blaming people too strongly for their own illnesses. "This is a New Age form of machismowellness macho." It seems to be correct to suggest that "You may not be responsible for being sick, but you *are* responsible for doing something about it."

Let's return to the question of risk factors. Equations of risks and health stabilizers can help us to analyze and operationalize the field systematically. According to Becker (1982), the following equation depicts the individual probability for a mental disorder occuring within a particular time period:

$$WPF = f \frac{\text{constitutional vulnerabilities; intensity and duration of stressors}}{\text{degree of mental health; protective environmental conditions}}$$

In principle this equation can be applied to all diseases; in this case the amount of health as a general trait would be entered into the denominator.

The constructs in this equation must of course be clearly specified and operationalized. The evaluation of stimuli as stressors as well as coping with stressors are to a large extent dependent upon subjective, interindividual functions that vary greatly. According to Becker, constitutional vulnerabilities are inherited or acquired somatic conditions that make an individual susceptible to disease. The degree of mental health, in Becker's view, is a function of complex constructs such as regulation competencies, self-actualization and search for meaning.

In psychological research there is no general consensus about "critical" situations and coping with them or about potential moderating or intervening (personality) variables (cf., Becker, 1986; Beutel, 1988; Rodin & Salovey, 1989) and their operationalization. What is urgently needed is high-quality basic research in health psychology that takes methods and findings from developmental psychology, differential psychology and social psychology into account. Even general psychology should be included, not only for the development and consideration of action theories (cf., Boesch, 1976) but also for the assessment of central psychological functions, especially motives and emotions, selecting both multivariate and multimodal measurement techniques.

Motives and Motivation in Health Psychology

There are many different types of motivational questions in health psychology-for example, motivation for health-related behavior or the motives behind professional attention to health psychology. Both aspects can be differentiated on the individual, economic and sociological level. The question of motivation for health-related behavior is more concerned with the individual and his social environment, whereas economic and ecological motives have to be taken into account for the question of the professional practice of health psychology.

Individual motives for health-relevant behavior have many levels and cannot be subsumed under one particular motive. Concepts with a unidimensional health motive can neither be found in health psychology nor motivational psychology textbooks. Although from the phylogenetic viewpoint primary motives such as hunger, thirst, pain or sexuality have a homeostatic, life-preserving function, they are hardly sufficient for analyzing motivation for health relevant behavior. Since health *behavior* must be regarded as multidimensional, health-related motives can only be described in broader motive systems, along with their hierarchical structure, significance and interaction with situational factors.

The task of analyzing the significance of different conflicting motives for health-related living seems complex enough already. We would like to illustrate this point with a relatively simple example, i.e., smoking. We describe this case as relatively simple because the health-damaging effects of smoking are well-known and undisputed and they have a relatively high probability of actually occuring. This knowledge, however, has little effect on the behavioral level. With adolescents, group pressure, power and social motives, possibly also curiosity, risk and stimulation-seeking motives make the potentially harmful behavior more attractive in the present than its avoidance. Emotional states that can occur both as antecedent conditions (fear or anger states as causes for smoking, drug use or inappropriate eating) and as consequences (drug use, smoking or eating can lead to relaxation) also have motivational effects.

Health-relevant motives alone, without a corresponding reinforcement system, are certainly ineffective; this aspect was discussed by Miller (1984) with regard to health behavior. In our case, one can assume that satisfaction of social, power or curiosity motives are more immediately effective behaviorally than any damage to health which has an uncertain probability of occurring, mostly after a long time period in the future. In this context the importance of theories on delay of gratification are to be mentioned (Fuchs, Hahn, Jerusalem, Leppin, Mittag & Schwarzer, 1989; Miller, 1984). These theories (Mischel, 1974; Utz, 1979) follow the research paradigm of a rejection of short-term material reward in favor of higher profits in the long term. However, with health-related behavior the only probable gain is the absence of impairment, a view that adolescents will hardly regard as a higher material benefit.

The future orientation of health-supportive behavior implies a further motivational consequence. Health-injurious behavior such as smoking mostly only becomes relevant when it is maintained over a long period of time. Current behavior can thus be overshadowed by a wide variety of arguments like minimizing ("It's only for a little while"), avoidance and denial ("I won't necessarily be affected by any harmful consequences"), attribution ("Effects on health don't necessarily occur because of smoking"), self-efficacy expectancies and intentions for future action ("I can stop any time").

As we mentioned earlier, the example of smoking is relatively clear, since the long-term negative consequences are known and generally accepted. The relationships become much more complicated in the case of health behavior like endurance training, where positive effects on health are expected but not completely proven, the mechanisms of its effects are disputed and the benefits of which are overshadowed in part by negative consequences (risk of injury to muscles, tendons and joints). The motivational analysis becomes even more complex when other incentives for health-supporting behavior are taken into account such as energy, fitness, feeling good about body and mind, or attractiveness. As long as these lead to a health-conscious life style, they can have a motivating effect. It does, however, become problematic when secondary motives begin to dominate and stand in the way of attaining the goal of a healthy life style. When the goal discrepancy between current state and ideal is too large, secondary consequences can also have a demotivating effect, for example when the present state makes the slimness ideal seem almost unreachable. Moreover, this type of incentive is also subject to fashion trends, and raises the question of how standards regarded as ideal come to be and how appropriate they are.

Fuchs et al. (1989) recently pointed out that motives are necessary but not yet sufficient conditions for health-related *behavior*, and have to be extended to include the question of carrying out resolutions, i.e. the volition aspect. This might be possible when a health-related behavior or life style is integrated into a broad self-concept that has an action-initiating effect.

Consideration should also be given to the interdependency of health-relevant behaviors, or health on the one hand and dispositions or behavior styles on the other. In the context of stress research the anxiety construct has received the most attention (for a summary, see Endler, 1988) and several hypotheses suggest that coping styles such as repression and sensitization are related to having preventive medical checkups. Anger, anger expression and hostility seem to go along with cardiovascular disorders and hypertension (for a summary, see Schwenkmezger, 1990). Other hypotheses deal with risk and sensation-seeking behavior (Schwenkmezger, 1977; Zuckerman, 1988). The concept of hardiness with its aspects of commitment, control and challenge has also been discussed with regard to health-relevant behavior (Kobasa, 1982), as have aspects of general and illness-specific control beliefs (Wallston & Wallston, 1982). Various different relationships have also been reported between indices of the strength of specific motive dimensions and health indices (Jemmott, 1987; McClelland, 1989). Finally, several findings show that higher-order values have a prognostic significance for preventive health behavior (Kristiansen, 1985; Lau, Hartman & Ware, 1986).

With regard to the question of *economic* motives, interest is focused on cost-benefit analyses. According to Rodin and Salovey (1989), illness costs 400 billion dollars per year in the United States today, which corresponds to 11% of the gross national product. For that reason, there is increasing awareness in the United States about the need for a "health care revolution" or the "medical-industrial complex" (cf. Kiesler & Morton, 1988).

In the Federal Republic of Germany, with a population of 60 million, in 1987 13 million hospital cases were counted, with a total of 213 million days spent in hospitals (Presse- und Informationsamt der Bundesregierung, 1989).

Many countries are trying to find ways to cut these costs. Psychologically relevant efforts are concerned among other things with questions of primary prevention. In the Federal Republic of Germany Bengel (1989) has developed a model showing how including psychologists in the field of health counseling, which is largely dominated by physicians, can lead to a reduction in medical care costs. Generally, one should ask to which extent costs could be reduced by the integration of psychologists into the curative treatment process; yet, for estimates no exact cost-benefit analyses exist (cf., Yates, 1984).

Another aspect is represented by the idea that it might be possible to "reward" healthy behavior. This does, however, present an almost insoluble dilemma of apportioning responsibility and costs for sick people (cf. Ullman, 1988). In this regard it is worth mentioning Carlton's (1985) statement that most health problems are beyond the ability of the individual to resolve. With regard to sociopolitical aspects, one must decide how important the field of health and illness should be compared to other social goals (cf. Braun, Martini & Minger, 1989). A careful comparative analysis of the very different European health and social systems could provide knowledge that might also be important from an economic point of view.

With all economic reflections one should consider not only the current structure but also the changes in age distribution that will occur in many countries in the near future. There will be more and more elderly and very old people, who represent a high risk for relatively expensive chronic diseases and for professional care; at the same time there will be increasingly fewer young people, who are particularly economical for the health system.

Our discussion turns finally to *socio-ecological motives,* which supported the trend toward health psychology. Causes lie in theoretical essays, for example by Sartorius (1989) who defines health as a homeostatic balance between the inner self and the surrounding world. This results, however, in a very wide range of motives and goals of health psychology. Questions of healthy living — which can be found, for example, in architectural psychology (Evans & Cohen, 1987) — fall into this category, as well as analyses of injury and mortality risks to adolescents in certain residential areas of countries. For example, in some American cities, the greatest risks to adolescents' health in addition to accidents are found in drug use, suicide or in being the victim of violent crimes (cf., Boyd & Moscicki, 1986; Millstein, 1989). Studies on the risk-reducing design of work places (Goldsmith, 1986) are representative for the ecological perspective, as are studies on the perception of health-related threat potentials of environmental risks (water and air pollution, acid rain, holes in the ozone layer or destruction of the forests and countryside).

Models in Health Psychology

In health psychology literature, three types of health models are often subsumed under the term "health model". (For a detailed analysis of *disease* models, see Netter's chapter in this book.) Although these three types of models are not totally distinctive and overlap to some degree, they differ greatly in their main focus of explanation. Therefore, one should always specify whether one is dealing with (1) health models, (2) health behavior models or (3) health promotion/health education models.

In this section we shall give examples of each of these models and describe and evaluate the few integrative approaches. Because a definition or discussion of what constitutes a model is beyond the scope of this chapter, we shall include any concept that has been named a model by its authors.

Health Models

The use of this general term should be restricted to models which attempt to predict the *health status* of a person or an environment. One basic problem inherent in this approach is the measurement of "health", which is both a subjective and an objective state encompassing physiological, psychological, social and ecological factors. In an extreme definition, Stone (1979) describes health as an "unmeasurable state of a complex, continuously adapting organism", while Sek (1987) calls for the development of models of *healthy environments* or "normal life fields" and for concrete, empirically-based indices of health.

In view of these difficulties, it is not surprising that "true" health models are rare.

One is Antonovsky's (1979; see also Becker, 1982) *"Salutogenesis"* which proposes criteria for locating a person on the "health ease/dis-ease" continuum. A person's "health profile", which portrays how healthy he or she is, depends upon his or her "sense of coherence" (SOC), which in turn is positively influenced by "general resistance resources" (GRRs). Health-promoting experiences are those which are consistent and balanced and which permit participation in the decision-making process — factors that should be taken into account in planning health promotion programs.

Subjective or lay models of health have been studied to find out what people think about health and how it is maintained or enhanced in order to be able to restructure distorted images or misconceptions about health-related behaviors, and to tailor health-promotion efforts and increase their efficiency.

In an interview study conducted by Herzlich (1973) in France, the respondents viewed health as "given", consisting of biological or medical aspects as well as personal, social and cultural aspects; disease, on the other hand, was described as being *caused* by the environment, developing in interaction with the person and as a result of moving away from nature.

Diaz-Guerrero (1984) compared the subjective meaning of health across cultures and found some important differences in folklore attitudes toward health that need to be considered when planning effective health promotion programs.

According to Buchmann, Karrer and Meier (1985), cognitive — both etiological and preventive — health concepts (classified as the individual model, the social model or the professional model) and evaluative concepts (which emphasize instrumental versus existential value) depends upon an individual's societal norms, life goals, social positions and environmental conditions. They influence how the health care system is perceived, evaluated and used as well as the nature of coping with health and disease.

In their study of a representative American population, Yankelovitch, Skelly and White (1979) found a global awareness of health risk factors but only little awareness of the specific relative values of each of these risks.

The last concepts to be mentioned here are the *ecological models of health*. In a "synoptic-conceptual view" Hoyman (1975) describes the determinants of health and its dimensions (physical fitness, mental health, social well-being and spiritual faith) as "ecologic-epidemiologic interaction of genetic, environmental, experimental and individual factors."

Ecological and sociological (e.g. Kosa & Robertson, 1969; Voigt, 1978) perspectives are combined in *social-ecological health models*. Based on the concept of an "ecology of the body" (Wenzel, 1986), health is described as a dynamic process that is part of the personal and social development. A person cannot be healthy unless he or she is socially integrated, maintains constructive social relationships, is able to adapt to stressful life circumstances, to express personal needs and to find meaning in life. This is a holistic view of health where health is regarded as physiological, psychological and social, with special emphasis on societal and environmental structures and the individual's subjective adaptation to them (see also Dana & Hoffmann, 1987). A person is described as being part of a network consisting of other individuals and systems that permit the development of health-enhancing resources and abilities. The task of prevention is to design an adequate living space rather than to change individual behavior. Risk behavior — for example, cigarette smoking or alcohol consumption (cf., Franzkowiak, 1986) — is interpreted with regard to its social and cultural functions. The meaning that risk behavior has for an individual is influenced by its potential for stress reduction, social integration, symbolic opposition and escape from social pressures.

The social-ecological concept has also been used as a framework for describing the incidence of a disorder within certain populations, so that preventive action may be taken. Elias (1987), in his modification of Albee's (1983) work (cf., Stark, 1989), demonstrates this in the following equation:

$$\text{Likelihood of the incidence of a disorder within a population} = \frac{(1)\text{ stressors} + (2)\text{ environmental risk factors}}{(3)\text{ possibilities for social learning} + (4)\text{ social support resources} + (5)\text{ opportunity to experience community}}$$

The social-ecological concept can be considered a comprehensive approach with a high explanatory value that needs further testing of its applications within the areas of health promotion and health education.

Health Behavior Models

An almost overwhelming amount of work has been done by health psychology researchers in predicting health behaviors rather than health per se. Health behaviors (for a typology see Kolbe, 1988; see also Matarazzo et al., 1984) are mostly analyzed as targets for intervention or as antecedents or causes of a person's health status, a linkage that can be determined on the basis of direct psychophysiological effects, health-related habits and behaviors, or reactions to health and illness (see Krantz, Grunberg & Baum, 1985). Kolbe (1988) depicts the two relationships of interest in behavioral epidemiology as follows:

$$\text{Behavioral determinants} \underset{R_2}{\longmapsto} \text{Behavior} \underset{R_1}{\overset{1}{\longmapsto}} \text{Health/disease}$$

He stresses the great complexity of the relationship between behaviors and health or diseases (R_1).

In Gochman's (1988) view, health behaviors should be analyzed as general personal and social phenomena resulting from various personal and social processes, thereby increasing "the chance of generating basic, conceptually derived, rigorous, systematic scientific investigations".

As *determinants of health behaviors* a wide range of personal, family, social, institutional and cultural variables have been investigated and found to be more or less predictive of different, mostly rather specific, health behavior outcomes (e.g., Gochman, 1988; Kressin, 1987). Problems with this kind of research arise from the lack of generalizability of findings and the need for an integration into one comprehensive model. Major efforts in this direction have been made by cognitive approaches in the area of health behavior models.

Cognitive Health Behavior Models

Cognitive approaches to health behavior models are based on the view of a person as a rational being whose cognitions are the key factor in conscious decision processes and behavior changes.

The *Health Belief Model* is one of the most commonly cited of such models; it has been tested in various ways, been reformulated several times and "referred to in virtually every dissertation related to health behavior" (Green, 1974). The original version (Rosenstock, 1966) explained and predicted the likelihood of a person's engaging in specific *medical* preventive behaviors (e.g. immunizations, screening procedures) in terms of perception of susceptibility to a particular condition, its seriousness and the availability of behaviors for preventing or treating it.

Changes over the years in conceptualization and measurement methods have transformed this rather simple model into a more complex one which takes into account the influence of social and environmental factors, cues for action and perceived benefits of or impediments to a certain behavior. It is currently being used to predict a multitude of health actions (see Kirscht, 1988) but, in order to be able to determine whether and where its applications will result in reliable predictions, it needs to be specified in terms of the dimensions of the predicted behavior (habitual versus non-habitual; repetitive versus one-time-only; initiating versus discontinuing), the development and temporal course of particular types of beliefs, the effect of modifying beliefs and the relationship between perceived benefits and costs to the health behavior outcome.

The Health Belief Model has been used as the basis for a variety of other models – for example, Langlie's (1977) Social Network Model which includes a social support dimension, or the Preventive Behavior Model (Bausell, 1986) that describes a preventive life-style (operationalized by and assessed with the "Prevention Index" (Bausell, 1985, 1986) as dependent upon the interplay between primary determinants (i.e. efficacy, vulnerability, barriers to action, health value, desire to control health, predisposing personality, love of life), secondary determinants (demographic, cognitive, affective) and cues to action (external, internal or self-initiated).

Locus of Control Models

Models based on the locus of control construct and applied specifically to the area of health state that the degree to which a person perceives him- or herself as being in control over events in his or her life (internal locus of control) and not subject to control by external agencies or others (external locus of control) has a great influence on the probability that he or she will engage in health-related behaviors (Seeman & Seeman, 1983; Wallston & Wallston, 1978).

The most intensive studies on this approach have focused on a psychometric or measurement-constructive perspective. Health Locus of Control Scales have been developed (Lau & Ware, 1981; Lohaus & Schmitt, 1989; Wallston, Wallston & DeVellis, 1978) and proven more or less successful in predicting various health behaviors (e.g., Lau, 1988). Future research should take into account the multidimensionality of health behaviors, distinguish between control beliefs and the actual *desire* for control, investigate the *value* a person puts on health and the *stability* of health locus of control beliefs.

Some evidence exists that behavioral change programs that "fit" clients' control beliefs or preferences are more effective than those that do not. Lau (1988) asks health professionals and the mass media to use this knowledge in order to design successful interventions and maximize compliance.

Advantageous to this approach is the availability of psychometrically adequate and valid measures of health locus of control orientation. However, this concept alone may be too narrow for a full understanding of human health behaviors.

Behavioral Intention Models

Less widely employed and less well known are models based on the theory that a person's attitude toward an action, related moral beliefs and perceptions of relevant social norms determine his or her intention to engage in that particular action.

According to the *Theory of Reasoned Action (REACT)* by Ajzen and Fishbein (1980), *subjective norms* – influenced by normative beliefs and individual motivation – and *attitudes* – determined by beliefs and values concerning a specific outcome – result in behavioral *intentions* which in turn lead to health-related behaviors.

Failure to find consistent support for this model set in motion a controversial "attitude-behavior discussion". The lack of evidence for a direct linkage can be explained in part by the use of global measures of attitudes to specific health behaviors. Specific health behaviors can be predicted more accurately from specific attitudes and from an attitude measure that is affective (enjoyable, pleasant, emotional) rather than evaluative (desirable, useful, "good for you")(cf., Ajzen & Timko, 1986).

The specificity of predictors and outcome has been regarded both as a great advantage and as the concept's weakest point. By including an individual's physiological arousal and facilitating conditions as model components, the *Theory of Social Behavior* (Triandis, 1977) was designed to predict both specific actions and alternative actions or "non-action". Behavioral intentions, which are a function of social factors, the individual's affect towards the behavior and the value he or she places on the perceived consequences of the behavior are considered to be major predictors only if the predicted behavior is not "habitual" or automatic. In that case, *habit* plays a more important role than intention. There is still a need for multimethod measurement and convergent operations in order to distinguish between the constructs in this model, and further testing and comparison with similar models (such as Ajzen & Fishbeins's REACT) would be desirable.

The *Protection Motivation Theory* (Wurtele & Maddux, 1987) combines the Health Belief Model and Locus of Control models into a model of *health decision*. In their study of exercise behavior, they found cognitive appraisal processes (especially *perceived self-efficacy*) to be significant predictors of *intentions* to exercise; these in turn were predictive of *self-reported exercise behavior* (for other personal choice behavior models see Horn, 1976; Milio, 1976).

Fuchs *et al*. (1989) mean to improve present cognitive models with their *social-cognitive health behavior theory*, which focuses on the cognitive, motivational and emotional conditions – represented in self-schemata – for initiating and maintaining health-related behavior in social situations. However, this promising approach still has to be tested.

Health behavior research has mainly focused on "inducing changes in individuals or on generating knowledge that ultimately increases the likelihood of such individual change" (Gochman, 1988). However, efforts should also be aimed at encouraging professional and political changes and taking into account social, political and structural aspects, in addition to improving conceptual clarity, methodological complexity and *integrative approaches*.

The first steps in this direction have been made by Cummings, Becker and Maile (1980), who derived the following six factors in their analysis of 14 models and 99 variables used to explain health behavior: (1) accessibility of health services; (2) attitudes toward health care; (3) threat of illness; (4) knowledge about disease; (5) social interactions, social norms, social structure; and (6) demographic characteristics.

In comparing the Health Belief Model, Social Learning Theory, Ajzen and Fishbein's REACT model and Triandis' Theory of Social Behavior, Wallston and Wallston (1984) come to the conclusion that attitude, vulnerability/threat, norms, motivation, habit and facilitating conditions are the "general labels" for critical variables that would be included in an integrative health behavior model. Conceptual differentiation and clarification, however, are most urgently needed.

One of the few models explaining *health status and health-related behavior* is the "integrative conceptual framework" by Moos (1979), in which the relationship between these two outcome variables has to be elaborated before either can be reliably predicted. This is also the weakest point in the "person-environment-interaction systems model" by Kar (1986). Kar describes health *behavior* as "a function of direct, additive, and interaction effects of specific action intentions, social support from significant others, accessibility of services, autonomy of decisions, and action situation" (see Figure 1).

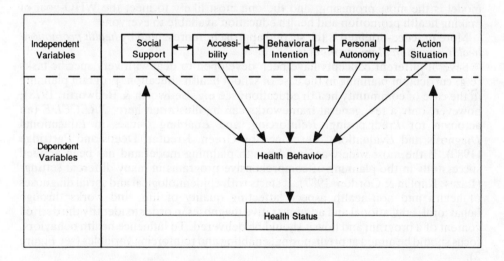

Figure 1. The person-environment-interaction systems model.
Notes: Exogenous variables from four subsystems (socio-economic; environmental; political; biological) affect all variables in the model (endogenous variables). The variables defined by the model (endogenous variables) include independent and dependent variables. Adapted from S. B. Kar (1986).

Oliver (1974) considers the general problem of rational-choice models to be that they are limited to organizing what health professionals think about rather than *explaining* a person's health behavior. We certainly need more data concerning the relationship between a person's health behaviors and his or her actual health status. Prospective studies should be planned to monitor "healthy" people and people with "healthy life styles" over a long period of time. Moreover, we also need to investigate what motives lead people to initiate and maintain health behavior, the kinds of conflicts involved, and the general coping mechanisms relevant to a person's health status (Gochman, 1988). Finally, we need more knowledge about the origins and the development of health behavior in the family, and how it is affected by social relationships, social and cultural values, norms and institutions.

Health Promotion/Health Education Models

Since health promotion/health education models (health education here is considered to be one component of health promotion; for definitions see e.g. Kolbe, 1988) can only be regarded as "health models" in a very broad sense, they will be mentioned briefly with just a few examples.

In general, two approaches can be identified. The first approach provides us with a rationale for professional health promotion activities by using them as "*applied health models*".

Under this aspect, Erben (1983) distinguishes four kinds of health education models: the *biomedical*, the *(social-) psychological*, the *sociological* and the *social-ecological model of health education*. According to Erben, the social-ecological model is the most promising, and the one most likely to meet the WHO-goal of making health promotion and health education available to everyone.

More practice-oriented is the second approach, represented by *health promotion/ health education planning models*.

Several different concepts have been developed to deal with very specific tasks (e.g. curriculum planning in the case of school health education, program planning in the case of community health education; see e.g. Bedworth & Bedworth, 1978); however, only a few general frameworks can be illustrated here. *PRECEDE* (an acronym for *P*redisposing, *R*einforcing, and *E*nabling *C*auses in *E*ducational *D*iagnosis and *E*valuation), developed by Green, Kreuter, Deeds and Partridge (1980), is the most widely-accepted health planning model and has been applied successfully in the planning of comprehensive programs in many different settings (Lazes, Kaplan & Gordon, 1987). It starts with epidemiological and social diagnoses of health and non-health aspects affecting quality of life, and works through behavioral, educational and administrative diagnoses in order to identify the desired content of a program and how it should be delivered. To influence health behaviors, focus should be aimed at predisposing, enabling and reinforcing variables (see Figure 2).

Very similar are Sullivan's *Comprehensive Health Education Model* and Ross and Mico's *Model for Health Education Planning* (Bates & Winder, 1984), which identify six steps and phases, respectively, in the planning process.

Dignan and Carr (1987) base their *Health Education/Promotion Planning Model* on the theoretical foundations of the health belief model, the communication/ persuasion matrix, the communication/behavior change (CBC) framework and the social marketing framework. Their seven-step process can be targeted towards individuals, groups or communities.

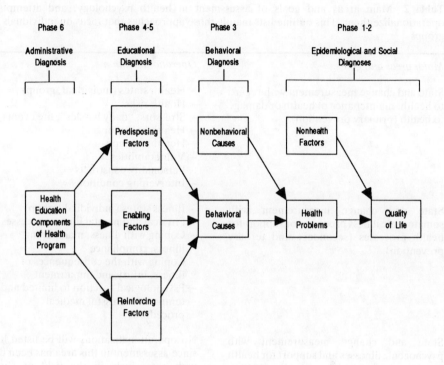

Phase 6	Phase 4-5	Phase 3	Phase 1-2
Administrative Diagnosis	Educational Diagnosis	Behavioral Diagnosis	Epidemiological and Social Diagnoses

Figure 2. The PRECEDE framework (Green et al., 1980).

In their *Conceptual Model for the Analysis of Health Education Planning and Resource Development*, Bates and Winder (1984) propose a cycle of developing, implementing and evaluating a health education plan that should provide increasingly better and more effective education services.

Assessment and Applications

Assessment

Many different aspects, primarily methodological and strategic, of assessment in health psychology have been presented but remained largely in the background. Several are included in the two handbooks edited by Karoly (1985, 1988). However, even a broad methodological approach does not provide an exemption from the need to formulate concrete psychodiagnostic goals and to operationalize them. In so far as possible, assessment should be based on psychological theories of health and disease and on testable models (see above), and should take into account findings from social psychology, developmental psychology and differential psychology.

Table 2 Main areas and goals of assessment in health psychology, and attempts to operationalize them. This outline lists mainly those approaches that focus on individuals and groups

Major areas and goals	*Operationalization*
State and change measurement with regard to health, maintenance of health or damage to health (primary prevention)	– Health states (individual, group) – Health risks – Stressors, "daily hassles", life events – Health behavior – Health concepts – Vulnerabilities – Personality constructs – Intervening conditions
State and change measurement with somatogenic illness processes or support for health processes (secondary and tertiary prevention)	– Illness states (individual, group) – Physical and mental illness processes – Coping with illness, maintaining illness, compliance – Coping with the consequences of illness, injury and impairment – Psychological reaction to limited and temporary stressful medical procedures
State and change measurement with psychogenic illnesses and support for health processes (secondary and tertiary prevention)	No operationalizations will be listed here, since assessment in this area has been dealt with extensively in the field of clinical psychology

Table 2 shows some of the more important diagnostic goals and areas that are aimed primarily at the individual or group. These aspects must not be considered in isolation, but rather should their complex dynamic interplay be weighed. For purposes of this discussion, we shall concentrate on the first area in Table 2.

Other important subgoals of health psychology assessment include the *ecological perspective* (cf., Kaminski, 1988; Winett, 1985; Winett, King & Altman, 1989), the *epidemiology* and the *evaluation* of health programs (cf., Dignan & Carr, 1987; Green & Lewis, 1986). In these areas, where there is a great deal of research activity, different aspects than in the more case-oriented assessment are emphasized.

With regard to assessment in health psychology, the framework needs to be defined (cf., Schmidt, 1990). The different definitions and theories of health psychology present, of course, very different diagnostic requirements. Some of the more important constructs of psychodiagnostics in this field are implied in Becker's (1982) equation-like representation of the conditions hazardous and conductive to health (described above). What makes the assessment of such constructs so difficult, in addition to their complexity and their often unkown interaction, is the subjective evaluation of situations and resources and the many intervening personality characteristics and states (cf., Beutel, 1988; Becker, 1986). Health psychology diagnostics is mostly based on (semistructured) interviews and short questionnaires. Some of these questionnaires are relatively nonspecific measures, commonly used in clinical psychology and personality psychology (cf., Dana & Hoffmann, 1987), and some are very specific measures that assess certain constructs or behaviors in particular areas (e.g., eating habits, exercising).

There are only a few comprehensive instruments for diagnosing health. One approach is the Trierer Persönlichkeitsfragebogen (TPF; Trier Personality Questionnaire) developed by Becker (1989). Dana & Hoffman (1987) reviewed questionnaires and rating scales for the following areas: health state (physical, social and mental), "wellness" and health risks or hazards. In a book edited by Karoly (1985), several chapters contain examples of questionnaires on health psychology and fields of application.

Systematic observations and standardized behavior ratings are extremely rare in health psychology, although there have been some interesting developments in computer-supported techniques (cf., Perrez, 1988). Psychophysiological methods and biochemical approaches are, in principle, very interesting for health psychology, but many methodological problems are associated. Furthermore, family diagnostics and the assessment of social support systems (cf., Baumann, 1987; Laireiter & Baumann, 1988; Leppin & Schwarzer, 1990) play a significant role.

Despite the overemphasis on self-description in the modalities of assessment in health psychology and the often arbitrary formulation of psychodiagnostic goals and constructs, it is still encouraging that the need for measurement has lately been emphasized more. These developments (e.g., Karoly 1985; 1988) could represent the beginning of real improvements in health psychology psychodiagnostics.

Applications

The common goal of health psychology interventions is best exemplified by the WHO-statement "Health for all by the year 2000" and by the effort to provide "healthy environments for healthy people"; however, strategies for attaining this goal are manifold and are dependent upon a particular theoretical background for the diagnosis of intervention, the target groups and problems considered, the setting and the time frame, and the individual or organization conducting the intervention.

The most widely used approach is that of *health education*, which focuses on influencing health-related behaviors positively, and the broader concept of *health promotion*, which has been defined as "any combination of health education and related organizational, economic, and environmental supports for behavior conducive to health" (Green, 1984).

For the most part, *health education* efforts are aimed at *individuals* or *groups* of people who are "at risk" for developing a disease or damaging their health, either by engaging in certain risk behaviors (see below) or by simply belonging to a particular "risk group" (e.g. older people, adolescents, people from a lower social class, overweight people, self-help groups). More emphasis has recently been put on maintaining health in "healthy people".

Health promotion is concerned primarily with larger populations. Interventions on the *organizational/environmental* level have resulted in a number of community health promotion programs, revealing links between reductions in morbidity and mortality and changing health practices (e.g. the Stanford Five City Project, the Framingham Heart Study, or the North Karelia, Finland, community studies, to mention only a few of the more prominent examples; Ward, 1986). Discussion about legal or policy changes on the *institutional/societal level*, on the other hand, are still quite controversial and have not yet reached a state of acceptable compromise.

As *target problems*, "unhealthy environments" and policies have been less effectively dealt with than "unhealthy behaviors". However, in order to plan theoretically sound and efficient interventions, more conceptual and methodological work needs to be done on the distinction between initiating and maintaining health-promoting behavior versus stopping risky behavior, possible motivations for engaging in health-related behaviors, the relationship between different health behaviors, their organization into a specific "life style", and the connection between life styles and health status.

Health education and health promotion can take place in a variety of *settings*. Outside the family, *communities, work-sites* and especially *schools* have played a major role in providing health-related information and activities. Compared to the United States, curriculum development and program planning in Europe need more conceptual and methodological refinement. However, medical and health centers, community agencies, work-sites and educational institutions are making progress in initiating health-promoting changes here, too.

Obviously, the question of who should *provide* health education or promotion (or who is able to do so) is a lot easier to be answered if thorough professional training is available (as, for example, in American Schools of Public Health; Dorsel & Baum, 1989; Stone, 1983). The situation in Europe is a lot more heterogeneous in this regard – a diversity of individuals with different professional backgrounds and from different private or public institutions and organizations offer their services in this field. Major improvements in the area of education and training of health promotion professionals are necessary.

Depending on the specific goals and intentions, one can choose from the following *health education methods and strategies* listed by Dignan and Carr (1987): audiovisual aids, behavior modification, community development, educational television, individual instruction, inquiry learning, lecture-discussion, mass-media presentations, organizational development, peer group discussion, programmed learning, simulations and games, skill development, social action and social planning. Table 3 shows a modification of the two-dimensional taxonomy of health education methods developed by Tones (1986). Each method has its own characteristics and potentials for achieving certain health education outcomes.

More studies need to focus on the many different possible combinations of materials, settings, methods and personnel in order to find out which intervention design will uniquely fit a specific target population. In the United States, four comprehensive *health behavior indicator systems* (Objectives for the Nation, Cancer Control Objectives, Behavioral Risk Factor Surveillance System, Model Standards for Community Preventive Health Services; cf., Kolbe, 1988) have been implemented in order to plan, monitor and manage health promotion programs by measuring the prevalence, determinants and consequences of health behaviors as well as the effectiveness of interventions.

Table 3 Health education methods (adapted from Tones, 1986)

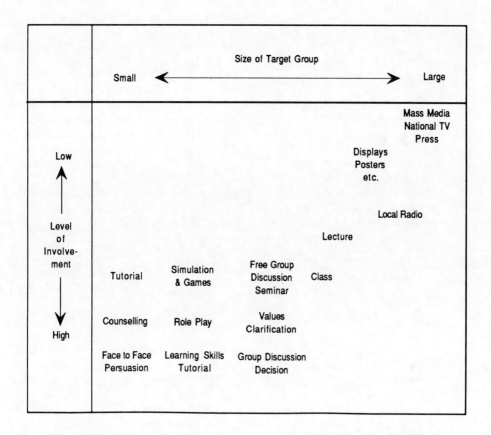

In planning health promotion programes, major consideration should be directed to measuring and evaluating the outcome (cf., Green & Lewis, 1986), the cost effectiveness and the limitations of health promotion, the influence of social relationships and environments, ecological conditions (cf., Brown & Margo, 1978) and ethical aspects of inducing behavior changes (cf., Burdine, McLeroy & Gottlieb, 1987), as well as to questions regarding the "responsibility" for maintaining or regaining health versus functions or perceived benefits of risk behavior (see Wenzel, 1986).

References

Ajzen, I., and Fishbein, M. (1980). *Understanding attitudes and predicting social behavior.* Englewood Cliffs, N.J.: Prentice-Hall

Ajzen, I., and Timko, C. (1986). Correspondence between health attitudes and behavior. *Basic and Applied Social Psychology, 7,* 259–276.

Albee, G. W. (1983). Von der Prävention psychopathologischer Erscheinungen zur Förderung menschlicher Handlungsfähigkeit [From the prevention of psychopathological disorders to the promotion of human action skills]. In S. Fliegel, B. Röhrle, and W. Stark (Eds.), *Gemeindepsychologische Perspektiven. Bd. 2: Interventionsprinzipien* (pp. 17–31). Tübingen: Deutsche Gesellschaft für Verhaltenstherapie.

Antonovsky, A. (1979). *Health, stress, and coping.* San Francisco: Jossey-Bass.

Bates, I. J., and Winder, A. E. (1984). *Introduction to health education.* Palo Alto: Mayfield Publishing Company.

Baumann, U. (Ed.). (1987). Soziales Netzwerk – Soziale Unterstützung. Themenheft [Social network – social support. Special issue]. *Zeitschrift für Klinische Psychologie, 16,* 305–443.

Bausell, R. B. (1985). The Prevention Index – A method of assessing the effects of a preventive lifestyle. *Evaluation and the Health Professions, 8,* 3–6.

Bausell, R. B. (1986). Health-seeking behaviors: Public versus public health perspectives. *Psychological Reports, 58,* 187–190.

Becker, P. (1982). *Psychologie der seelischen Gesundheit Band 1: Theorien, Modelle, Diagnostik* [Psychology of mental health Vol. 1: Theories, models, assessment]. Göttingen: Hogrefe.

Becker, P. (1986). Theoretischer Rahmen [Theoretical framework]. In P. Becker and B. Minsel, *Psychologie der seelischen Gesundheit Band 2: Persönlichkeitspsychologische Grundlagen, Bedingungsanalysen und Förderungsmöglichkeiten* (pp. 1–90). Göttingen: Hogrefe.

Becker, P. (1989). *Der Trierer Persönlichkeitsfragebogen (TPF). Testmappe mit Handanweisung* [Trierer Personality Inventory. Testkit and manual.]. Göttingen: Hogrefe.

Bedworth, D. A., and Bedworth, A.E. (1978). *Health education – A process for human effectiveness.* New York: Harper and Row.

Bengel, J. (1989). Ärztliche Gesundheitsberatung aus Sicht der Evaluation [Health education by physicians from an evaluation point of view]. In W. Schönpflug (Ed.), *Bericht über den 36. Kongreß der Deutschen Gesellschaft für Psychologie in Berlin 1988* (Vol. 2, pp. 121–130). Göttingen: Hogrefe.

Beutel, M. (1988). *Bewältigungsprozesse bei chronischen Erkrankungen* [Coping processes in chronic diseases]. Weinheim: Edition Medizin, VHC.

Bloom, B. L. (1988). *Health Psychology. A psychosocial perspective.* Englewood Cliffs, N.J.: Prentice Hall.

Boesch, E. E. (1976). *Psychopathologie des Alltags* [Psychopathology of everyday life]. Bern: Huber.

Boyd, J. S., and Moscicki, E. K. (1986). Fire arms and youth suicide. *American Journal of Public Health, 76,* 1240–1242.

Braun, H., Martini, H., and Minger, H. (1989). *Kommunale Sozialpolitik in den neunziger Jahren* [Communal social politics in the nineties]. Köln: Deutscher Gemeindeverlag.

Brown, E. R., and Margo, G. E. (1978). Health education: Can the reformers be reformed? *International Journal of Health Services, 8,* 3–26.

Buchmann, M., Karrer, D., and Meier, R. (1985). *Der Umgang mit Gesundheit und Krankheit im Alltag* [Coping with health and illness in everyday life]. Bern: Haupt.

Burdine, J. N., McLeroy, K. B., and Gottlieb, N. H. (1987). Ethical dilemmas in health promotion: An introduction. *Health Education Quarterly, 14,* 7–9.

Carlton, B. (1985). Preventive health's emerging problem: Individual behaviour change or social and economic change? *Hygie, 4,* 46–50.

Clearing-Sky, M. (1988). Exercise: Issues for prescribing psychologists. *Psychology & Health, 2,* 189–207

Cube, F. von, and Storch, V. (Eds.).(1988). *Umweltpädagogik. Ansätze, Analysen, Ausblicke [Environmental pedagogics. Approaches, analyses, outlook].* Heidelberg: Schindele.

Cummings, K. M., Becker, M. H., and Maile, M. C. (1980). Bringing the models together: An empirical approach to combining variables used to explain health action. *Journal of Behavioral Medicine, 3*, 123–145.

Dana, R. H., and Hoffmann, T. A. (1987). Health assessment domains: Credibility and legitimization. *Clinical Psychology Review, 7*, 539–555.

Diaz-Guerrero, R. (1984). Behavioral health across cultures. In J. D. Matarazzo, Sh. M. Weiss, J. A. Herd, N. E. Miller, and St. M. Weiss (Eds.), *Behavioral health: A handbook of health enhancement and disease prevention* (pp. 164–178). New York: Wiley.

Diekstra, R. F., and Jansen, M.A. (1988). Psychology's role in the new health care systems: The importance of psychological interventions in primary health care. *Psychotherapy, 25*, 344–351.

Dignan, M. B., and Carr, P.A. (1987). *Program planning for health education and health promotion*. Philadelphia: Lea and Febiger.

Dorsel, T. N., and Baum, A. (1989). Undergraduate health psychology: Another challenge for an ambitious field. *Psychology and Health, 3*, 87–92.

Elias, M. J. (1987). Establishing enduring prevention programs: advancing the legacy of Swampscott. *American Journal of Community Psychology, 15*, 539–553.

Endler, N. S. (1988). Hassles, health, and happiness. In M. P. Janisse (Ed.), *Individual differences, stress, and health psychology* (pp. 24–56). New York: Springer.

Erben, R. (1983). *Auf dem Wege zur konkreten Utopie – Entwicklungen und Perspektiven der Gesundheitserziehung in Europa* [On the way towards concrete utopia – Developments and perspectives of health education in Europe]. Unpublished doctoral dissertation. Freie Universität, Berlin.

Evans, G. W., and Cohen, S. (1987). Environmental stress. In W. Stokols and J. Altman (Eds.), *Handbook of environmental psychology* (Vol. 1, pp. 571–610). New York: Wiley.

Franzkowiak, P. (1986). Kleine Freuden, Kleine Fluchten. Alltägliches Risikoverhalten und medizinische Gefährdungsideologie [Small pleasures – small flights. Everyday life risk behavior and medical risk ideology]. In E. Wenzel (Ed.), *Die Ökologie des Körpers* (pp. 121–174). Frankfurt/M.: Suhrkamp Verlag.

Fuchs, R., Hahn, A., Jerusalem, M., Leppin, A., Mittag, W., and Schwarzer, R. (1989). *Auf dem Weg zu einer sozialkognitiven Theorie des Gesundheitsverhaltens* [On the way towards a social-cognitive theory of health behavior]. Arbeitsberichte des Instituts für Psychologie Nr. 11. Berlin: Freie Universität, Institut für Psychologie.

Gochman, D. S. (Ed.). (1988). *Health behavior – emerging research perspectives*. New York: Plenum.

Goldsmith, M. F. (1986). Worksite wellness programs: Latest wrinkle to smooth health care costs. *Journal of the American Medical Association, 256*, 1089–1091, 1095.

Green, L. W. (1984). Health education models. In J.D. Matarazzo, Sh. M. Weiss, J. A. Herd, N. E. Miller, and St. M. Weiss (Eds.), *Behavioral health. A handbook of health enhancement and disease prevention* (pp. 181–198). New York: Wiley.

Green, L. W. (1974). Editorial. In M.H. Becker (Ed.), The health belief model and personal health behavior (special issue). *Health Education Monographs, 2*, 324–325.

Green, L. W., Kreuter, M. W., Deeds, S. G., and Partridge, K. B. (1980). *Health education planning – a diagnostic approach*. Palo Alto: Mayfield Publishing Company.

Green, L. W., and Lewis, F. M. (1986). *Measurement and evaluation in health education and health promotion*. Palo Alto: Mayfield Publishing Company.

Harris, P. R. (1980). *Promoting health – preventing disease: Objectives for the nation*. Washington, D. C.: US Government Printing Office.

Herzlich, C. (1973). *Health and illness: A social psychological analysis*. London: Academic Press.

Horn, D. (1976). A model for the study of personal choice health behavior. *International Journal of Health Education, 19*, 89–100.

Hoyman, H. S. (1975). Rethinking an ecologic-system model of man's health , disease, aging, death. *The Journal of School Health, 55*, 509–518.

Jemmott, J. B. III. (1987). Social motives and susceptibility to disease: Stalking individual differences in health risks. *Journal of Personality, 55*, 267–298.

Junge, B. (1986). Rückgang der Sterblichkeit in Japan, den USA und der Bundesrepublik Deutschland – der Beitrag der einzelnen Todesursachen [Reduction of mortality rates in Japan, USA, and the Federal Republic of Germany – contributions of the single causes of death]. *Öffentliches Gesundheitswesen, 48*, 185–192.

Kaminski, G. (1988). Ökologische Perspektiven in psychologischer Diagnostik? [Ecological perspectives in psychological assessment]. *Zeitschrift für Differentielle und Diagnostische Psychologie, 9*, 155–168.

Kar, S. B. (1986). Communication for health promotion: A model for research and action. *Advances in Health Education and Promotion, 1*, 267–307.

Karoly, P. (1985). *Measurement strategies in health psychology*. New York: Wiley.

Karoly, P. (Ed.). (1988). *Handbook of child health assessment*. New York: Wiley.

Keller, E. S., Winett, R. A., and Everett, P. E. (1982). *Preserving the environment. New strategies for behavior change*. New York: Pergamon.

Kiesler, C.A., and Morton, T. L. (1988). Psychology and public policy in the "health care revolution". *American Psychologist, 43*, 993–1003.

Kirscht, J. P. (1988). The Health Belief Model and predictions of health actions. In D. S. Gochman (Ed.), *Health behavior – emerging research perspectives* (pp. 27–41). New York: Plenum.

Kobasa, S. C. (1982). The hardy personality: Toward a social psychology of stress and health. In G. S. Sanders and J. Suls (Eds.), *Social psychology of health and illness* (pp. 3–32). Hillsdale, N. J.: Erlbaum.

Kolbe, J. L. (1988). The application of health behavior research – Health education and health promotion. In D. S. Gochman (Ed.), *Health behavior – Emerging research perspectives* (pp. 381–396). New York: Plenum.

Kosa, J., and Robertson, L. S. (1969). The social aspects of health and illness. In J. Kosa and I. K. Zola (Eds.), *Poverty and health: a sociological analysis* (pp. 35–68). Cambridge: Harvard University Press.

Krantz, D. S., Grunberg, N. E., and Baum, A. (1985). Health psychology. *Annual Review of Psychology, 36*, 349–383.

Kressin, U. (1987). *Primäre Gesundheitserziehung in der Bundesrepublik Deutschland* (2nd ed.) [Primary health education in West Germany]. Konstanz: Hartung-Gorre Verlag.

Kristiansen, C. M. (1985). Value correlates of preventive health behavior. *Journal of Personality and Social Psychology, 49*, 748–758.

Laireiter, A., and Baumann, U. (1988). Klinisch-psychologische Soziodiagnostik: Protektive Variablen und soziale Anpassung [Clinical psychological socio-diagnosis: Protective variables and social adjustment]. *Diagnostica, 34*, 190–226.

Langlie, J. K. (1977). Social networks, health beliefs, and preventive health behavior. *Journal of Health and Social Behavior, 18*, 244–260.

Lau, R. R. (1988). Beliefs about control and health behavior. In D. S. Gochman (Ed.), *Health behavior – emerging research perspectives* (pp. 43–63). New York: Plenum.

Lau, R. R., Hartman, K. A., and Ware, J. E. jr. (1986). Health as a value: Methodological and theoretical considerations. *Health Psychology, 5*, 25–43.

Lau, R. R., and Ware, J. E. jr. (1981). Refinements in the measurement of health specific locus of control beliefs. *Medical Care, 19*, 1147–1158.

Lazes, P. M., Kaplan, L. H., and Gordon, K. A. (1987). *The handbook of health education* (2nd ed.). Rockville: Aspen Publishers, Inc.

Leppin, A., and Schwarzer, R (1990). Social support and physical health. An updated meta-analysis. In L. R. Schmidt, P. Schwenkmezger, J. Weinman, and S. Maes (Eds.), *Theoretical and applied aspects of health psychology*. London: Harwood.

Lohaus, A., and Schmitt, G. M. (1989). Kontrollüberzeugungen zu Krankheit und Gesundheit (KKG): Bericht über die Entwicklung eines Testverfahrens [Control beliefs concerning illness and health: Report about the development of a testing procedure]. *Diagnostica, 35*, 59–72.

Lütjen, R., and Frey, D. (1987). Gesundheitspsychologie – sozialpsychologische Aspekte von Gesundheit und Krankheit [Health psychology – social-psychological aspects of health and illness]. In J. Schultz-Gambard (Ed.), *Angewandte Sozialpsychologie. Konzepte, Ergebnisse, Perspektiven* (pp. 293–306). München: Psychologie Verlags Union.

Matarazzo, J. D. (1980). Behavioral health and behavioral medicine. Frontiers for a new health psychology. *American Psychologist, 35*, 807–817.

Matarazzo, J. D. (1984a). Behavioral immunogens and pathogens in health and illness. In B. L. Hammonds and C. J. Scheier (Eds.), Psychology and health (pp. 9–43). Washington, D.C.: APA.

Matarazzo, J. D. (1984b). Behavioral health: A 1990 challenge for the health services professions. In J. D. Matarazzo, Sh. M. Weiss, J. A. Herd, N. E. Miller, and St. M. Weiss (Eds.), *Behavioral health: A handbook of health enhancement and disease prevention* (pp. 3–40). New York: Wiley.

Matarazzo, J. D., Weiss, Sh. M., Herd, J. A., Miller, N. E., and Weiss, St. M. (Eds.). (1984). *Behavioral health: A handbook of health enhancement and disease prevention*. New York: Wiley.

McClelland, D. C. (1989). Motivational factors in health and disease. *American Psychologist, 44*, 675–683.

Milio, N. (1976). A framework for prevention: Changing health-damaging to health-generating life patterns. *American Journal of Public Health, 66*, 435–439.

Miller, N. E. (1984). Learning: Some facts and research relevant to maintaining health. In J. D. Matarazzo, Sh. M. Weiss, J. A. Herd, N. E. Miller, and St. M. Weiss (Eds.), *Behavioral health: A handbook of health enhancement and disease prevention* (pp. 199–208). New York: Wiley.

Millstein, S. G. (1989). Adolescent health. *American Psychologist, 44*, 837–842.

Mischel, W. (1974). Processes in delay of gratification. In L. Berkowitz (Ed.), *Advances in experimental social psychology* (Vol. 7, pp. 249–292). New York: Academic Press.

Moos, R. H. (1979). Social-ecological perspectives on health. In G. Stone, F. Cohen, N. E. Adler, and Associates (Eds.), *Health psychology – A handbook* (pp.523–547). San Francisco: Jossey-Bass Publishers.

Oliver, V. (1974). Some limitations of rational-choice models. *International Journal of Health Education, 18*, 7–13.

Perrez, M. (1988). Bewältigung von Alltagsbelastungen und seelische Gesundheit [Coping with daily hassles and mental health]. *Zeitschrift für Klinische Psychologie, 17*, 292–306.

Presse- und Informationsamt der Bundesregierung (Ed.). (1989). *Sozialpolitische Umschau* Nr. 210 [Review in social politics]. Bonn: Hektographie.

Ridder, P. (1987). Kritische Übersicht über das Begriffsfeld [Critical overview about definitions in preventive medicine]. In H. Schaefer, H. Schipperges, and G. Wagner (Eds.), *Präventive Medizin* (pp. 39–64). Berlin: Springer.

Rodin, J., and Salovey, P. (1989). Health psychology. *Annual Review of Psychology, 40*, 533–579.

Rosenstock, I. M. (1966). Why people use health services. *Milbank Memorial Fund Quarterly, 44*, 94–127.

Sartorius, N. (in press). Psychology and health care: A WHO perspective. In M. Johnston (Ed.), *Health psychology in Europe*.

Schipperges, H. (1982). *Der Arzt von morgen* [The physician of the future]. Berlin: Severin and Siedler.

Schmidt, L. R. (in press). Psychodiagnostik in der Gesundheitspsycholgie [Assessment in health psychology]. In R. Schwarzer (Ed.), *Gesundheitspsychologie*. Göttingen: Hogrefe.

Schwenkmezger, P. (1977). *Risikoverhalten und Risikobereitschaft* [Risk taking behavior and risk taking attitude]. Weinheim: Beltz.

Schwenkmezger, P. (in press). Ärger, Ärgerausdruck und Gesundheit [Anger, anger expression, and health]. In R. Schwarzer (Ed.), *Gesundheitspsychologie*. Göttingen: Hogrefe.

Seeman, M., and Seeman, T. E. (1983). Health behavior and personal autonomy: A longitudinal study of the sense of control in illness. *Journal of Health and Social Behavior, 24*, 144–160.

Sek, H. (1987). Psychological concepts of health, modes of prevention and counseling for health promotion. *Polish Psychological Bulletin, 18*, 77–88.

Stark, W. (Ed.). (1989a). *Lebensweltbezogene Prävention und Gesundheitsförderung – Konzepte und Strategien für die psychosoziale Praxis* [Environment-related prevention and health promotion – Concepts and strategies for the psychosocial practice]. Freiburg: Lambertus.

Stark, W. (1989b). Prävention als Gestaltung von Lebensräumen [Prevention as the designing of living spaces]. In W. Stark (Ed.). *Lebensweltbezogene Prävention und Gesundheitsförderung* (pp. 11–37). Freiburg: Lambertus.

Stone, G. C. (1979). Health and the health system: A historical overview and conceptual framework. In G. C. Stone, F. Cohen, N. E. Adler, and Associates (Eds.), *Health psychology – A handbook. Theories, applications, and challenges of a psychological approach to the health care system* (pp. 1–17). San Francisco: Jossey-Bass.

Stone, G. C. (1983). National working conference on education and training in health psychology. *Health Psychology, 2*, 1–153.

Stone, G. C., Cohen, F., Adler, N. E., and Associates. (1979). *Health psychology – A handbook. Theories, applications, and challenges of a psychosocial approach to the health care system.* San Francisco: Jossey-Bass Publishers.

Tones, K. (1986). The methodology of health education. *Journal of the Royal Society of Medicine, 79*, 5–7.

Triandis, H. C. (1977). *Interpersonal behavior.* Monterey, Calif.: Brooks/Cole.

Ullman, D. (1988). *Getting beyond wellness macho: The promise and pitfalls of holistic health. Utne Reader (Jan./Feb.), 68–72.*

Utz, H. E. (1979). *Empirische Untersuchungen zum Belohnungsaufschub* [Research on delay of gratification]. München: Minerva.

Voigt, D. (1978). *Gesundheitsverhalten: Zur Soziologie gesundheitsbezogenen Verhaltens. Hypothesen – Theorien – empirische Untersuchungen* [Health behavior: The sociology of health related behavior. Hypotheses – theories – empirical studies]. Stuttgart: Kohlhammer.

Wallston, B. S., and Wallston, K. A. (1978). Locus of control and health: A review of the literature. *Health Education Monographs, 6*, 107–117.

Wallston, B. S., and Wallston, K. A. (1984). Social psychological models of health behavior: An examination and integration. In A. Baum, S. Taylor, and J. E. Singer (Eds.), *Handbook of psychology and health, Vol. IV: Social aspects of health* (pp. 25–53). Hillsdale, N. J.: Erlbaum.

Wallston, K. A., and Wallston, B. S. (1982). Who is responsible for your health? The construct of Health Locus of Control. In G. Sanders and J. Suls (Eds.), *Social psychology of health and illness* (pp. 65–95). Hillsdale, N. J.: Erlbaum.

Wallston, K. A., Wallston, B. S., and DeVellis, R. (1978). Development of the Multidimensional Health Locus of Control (MHLC) Scales. *Health Education Monographs, 6*, 161–170.

Ward, W. B. (Ed.). (1986). *Advantage in health education and promotion Vol. 1.* Greenwich: Jai Press Inc.

Wenzel, E. (Ed.). (1986). *Die Ökologie des Körpers* [The ecology of the body]. Frankfurt/M.: Edition Suhrkamp.

Winett, R. A. (1985). Egobehavioral assessment in health life-styles: Concepts and methods.

World Health Organization (1981). *Global strategy for health for all by the year 2000*. Geneva: World Health Organization.

Wurtele, S. K., and Maddux, J. E. (1987). Relative contributions of protection motivation theory components in predicting exercise intentions and behavior. *Health Psychology, 6,* 453–466.

Yankelovitch, Skelly, and White (1979). *The General Mills American Family Report, 1978–79: Family health in an era of stress*. Minneapolis: General Mills, Inc.

Yates, B. T. (1984). How psychology can improve effectiveness and reduce costs of health services. *Psychotherapy, 21,* 439–451.

Zuckerman, M. (1988). Sensation seeking, risk taking, and health. In M. P. Janisse (Ed.), *Individual differences, stress, and health psychology* (pp. 72–88). New York: Springer.

Types of Models in Understanding and Describing Diseases

Petra Netter

The present contribution examines the procedure of model making in disease research, discussing the significance of the following points when applying models for gaining insight into structures and functions of mind-body relationships and procedures for their analysis: aims and goals, approaches and procedures, areas of content, types of relationships encountered in different models of disease, and various pitfalls and fallacies.

In this analysis our considerations will be mainly based on psychosomatic complaints, which are closely related to neurotic and somatic anxiety, but some aspects and principles of models may more readily be demonstrated by those developed for other psychosomatic diseases like myocardial infarction and disturbances related to pregnancy.

When trying to classify models involved in research on mind and body and on behavior, environment, and disease all the aspects listed above may serve as classes according to which models may be grouped.

One has to be aware, however, that the final model is the result of a process from the design of a study to the interpretation of converging results from different sources of information. Each step from raising a scientific question across selection of subjects, methods of assessment and statistical procedures of evaluation to conceptual arrangement and interpretation of results is governed by a specific model guiding the researcher's concepts for selecting the steps and ideas from the pool of possible elements and relationships. Therefore the phase of investigation is included in the categories according to which models may be classified (Table 1) each of which will be discussed in the following sections and illustrated by models encountered in the literature on psychosomatic diseases.

It must be emphasized, however, that each model could be located in a pluridimensional space of categories and in addition would sometimes even meet two or three subcategories of goals, relationships, and content. We will refrain from classifying each model according to all categories at the same time but will select them according to their most salient qualities.

Models According to Phase of Investigation

The phases of an investigation themselves may be depicted by a model which may elucideate at which steps models may determine the researcher's strategies (Fig. 1).

The first step in this figure – that is, the model of disease generating the leading questions of an investigation is also the final outcome of the study, as indicated by the arrow pointing backwards from interpretation to the start. Since this part is related to the goals, relationships and]contents of disease models which will be dealt with in later sections, we shall begin with models related to sample selection. An example, depicted in Fig. 2, is adopted when using healthy subjects in psychosomatic or psychiatric research.

Dedicated to G.A.Lienert for his 70th birthday

Table 1 Categories of classification of models

---

1. Phase of Investigation
   (Models of sample selection or models of design, vs. models of disease)
2. Approaches and Evaluation
   Theory or logical considerations
   Experiments
   Epidemiology   Statistical Models

3. Goals
   Structure – Function
             – Prediction
             – Diagnosis
             – Causes
4. Relationships
   Correlational – Cause-Effect
   Uni-, Bi-, Pluridirectional
   Linear – Nonlinear
5. Content
   Symptoms

   Behavior   Cognitive
                         Motivational
                         Motor

   Biochemistry   Brain
                         periphery

   Morphology (Brain Structures)
   Input Variables (Stressors)

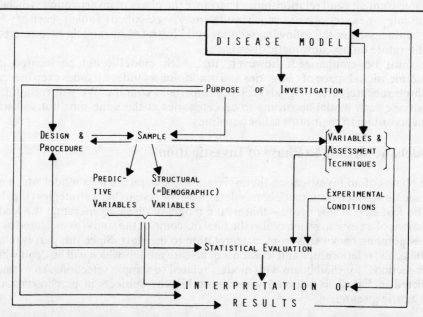

Figure 1. Steps involved in planning, performing, and evaluating an investigation in disease research.

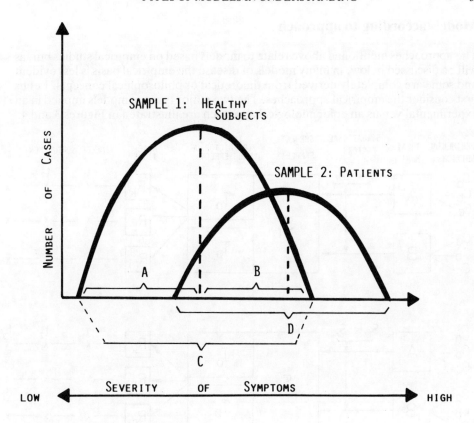

Figure 2. Model for sample selection

Here pathological conditions are conceived as one pole of a linear continuum, from health to pathology, assuming that subjects without or with few symptoms relate to those with more or more severe symptoms in the same way as the total healthy population relates to the clinical group.

The selection of variables and experimental conditions to be investigated is similarly determined by the disease concept and guided by models about organizational structure of mind-body relationships and about classes of stressors. A further step concerned with models is statistical evaluation, which is closely linked to the choice of design and procedure. This again depends on the questions investigated and decides whether the sample is randomly assigned to experimental conditions or has to be analyzed with respect to structural variables as in surveys applied in the epidemiological approach on large unselected samples. The latter aspect is of particular relevance to interpretations of results and thus to concepts about the disease model. It forms part of the second category in Table 1 according to which models may be classified, and will therefore be considered in the next section.

Models according to approach

The approaches mentioned above relate to models based on empirical studies but, as will be discussed below, in many models of disease the empirical basis is less evident and some are completely derived from theoretical or philosophical concepts. Let us first consider the empirical approaches. The two major types of models implied in an experimental versus an epidemiological approach are illustrated in Figures 3 and 4.

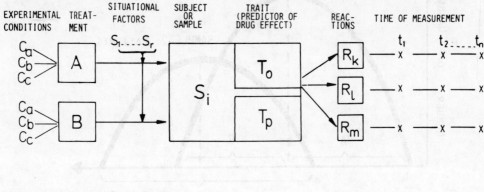

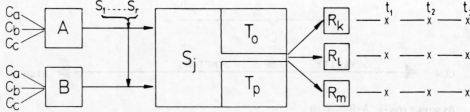

Figure 3. Model relating treatment, subjects, and responses in experimental studies.

Whereas experimental studies are based on unidirectional cause-effect concepts in which indepedent and dependent variables may be clearly separated and tested independently (Fig. 3), relationships in epidemiological investigations may be concealed or produced by intervening variables and confounding factors as indicated in Fig. 4.

This may occur,

a) because the consequence determines the preceding factors (for instance: type of therapy is chosen for avoiding risks as in an oral contraceptive study where subjects at risk of thrombosis were found to be more frequent in the nontreated group; or an unspecific treatment of symptoms chosen is inefficient and seemingly causes the symptoms, as when diazepam is applied for preventing abortions and, being ineffective, seems to be responsible for prematurely terminated pregnancies;

b) because the subject him- or herself chooses environmental conditions via behavior, causing diseases which may be genetically linked to the behavior which determined the choice of environment (for instance: the concept that smoking behavior and development of cancer may be determined by the same underlying personality dimension of extraversion (Eysenck, 1985);

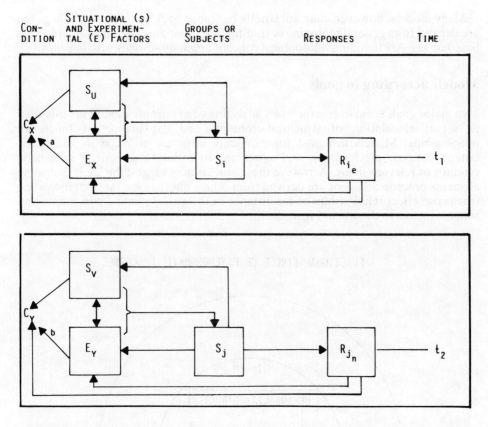

Figure 4. Model relating treatment, subjects, and responses in epidemiological studies.

Si, Sj = Subjects; Ex, Ey = Treatments; Su, Sv = Situational Factors;
R_{ie}. R_{jn} = Responses; t_1, t_2 = times of observation; (Demonstration of incomparability and confounding)

c) because the interval between exposure to the risk factor and onset of the event is too short to be effective particularly in longitudinal studies where duration of exposure is confounded with slowly growing noxious events with an exact termination, as for instance death or abortion.

The statistical models required for analyzing causal and pseudo-relationships in experimental and epidemiological designs will of course be relevant to aspects of relationships as outlined in section 4 but have to be mentioned in this context as well,

a) as consequences of design and

b) as tools controlling for confounding factors by stratification of the sample, or by path analytic techniques and log linear models of data analysis.

Many models, however, may not strictly be traced back to empirical findings but are derived from general reasoning or traditions of theorizing as expressed in models based on the Aristotelain philosophical concept about mind-body relationships.

Models according to goals

Two major goals seem to emerge when analyzing what purpose models are intended to serve: elucidation of structural contents and explanation of functional relationships. Models designed for providing structure will classify diagnostic criteria, causes, mechanisms, and symptoms in order to provide a systematic synopsis of relevant items. Arrows in these models may suggest the ideas that some elements precede others or are derived from others but they are far from indicating true cause-effect relationships as for instance in the model relating personality and somatic factors to disease in Figure 5.

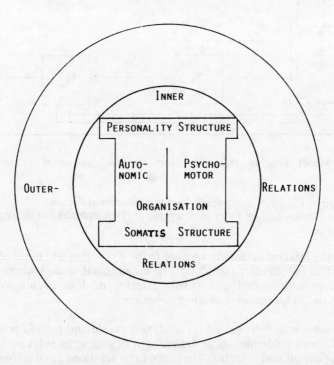

FUNCTIONAL CIRCLE OF PSYCHOSOMATIC PROCESSES

Figure 5.   Model relating personality and somatic factors to disease (Delius, 1966) Type of model: Structure + "Pseudo-cause-effect", unidirectional, natural history.

There is a sort of continuum between the goals of identifying structures and explaining functions as demonstrated by models which try to arrange observations according to a latent continuum as proposed by the author in an attempt to relate increasing somatic symptomatology to decreasing psychological complaints and vice versa according to an underlying dimension of somatization or repression increasing from manifestation of purely psychological to purely somatic symptoms (Netter, 1981, Netter & Neuhäuser, 1982).

A similar concept has also been established by Temoshok in a model taken from Bahnson (1979) for different types of diseases located on the axes of two defense mechanisms (repression and projection, Figure 6).

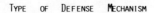

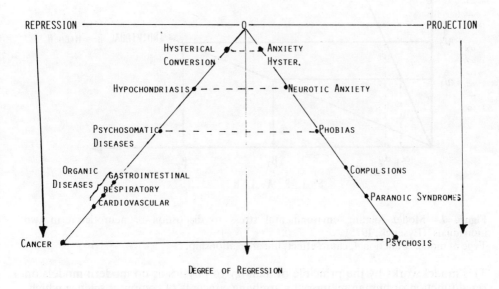

Figure 6. Defense mechanisms in different diseases (Temoshok, mod. by Bahnson, 1979). Type of model: Structural + functional: predictive

In these types of models the purpose is not only creation of order but also comprehension of the principles according to which phenomena are functionally organized.

Proceeding to the more functional goals of models we come to models predominantly interested in either prediction or diagnostic conclusions or simply cause-effect relationships.

An example of a predictive model is Eysenck's attempt to explain why individuals with high emotional lability tend to experience more stress than stable subjects to identical stressors (Eysenck, 1975, Figure 7).

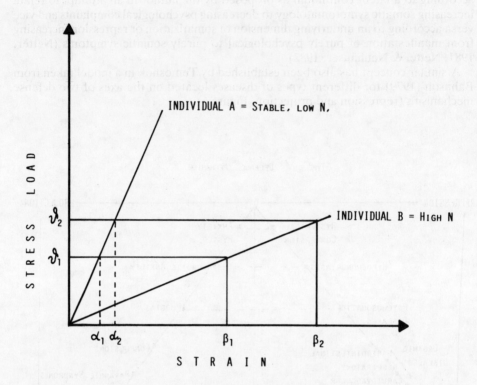

Figure 7. Model relating environmental stress to dispostion of neuroticism in two individuals. (Eysenck, 1975).
Type of model: Functional, cause-effect, linear relationship.

This model works by the principle of analogy to physics as do modern models on renal function or human memory by applying concepts of computer science which, like the Eysenck model, wish to achieve mathematical prediction of symptoms.

Most models of course, take into consideration that development of diseases cannot be predicted on the simple basis of input and dispositional variables but have to incorporate cognitive processes as intervening variables. An example is presented in Figure 8, a modified Lazarus model of stress response in which appraisal and coping processes, determined by the environmental stressor and the subject's set of dispositions and experiences, will modify the response. This model also shows that relationships are not just unidirectional but may contain multiple feed-back loops. A model like this may also be conceived as aiming at prediction of behavior although the intervening processes are merely hypothesized and not easily quantified.

The second category of functional models is concerned with diagnosis. This may be achieved by starting from an unspecific symptom which may be traced back to the underlying disease by several diagnostic steps along a "decision tree" as represented in Figure 9 for the symptom of exhaustion and fatigue. The diagnosing physician has to find his way in the opposite direction to the arrows indicating chronological or causal chains of events.

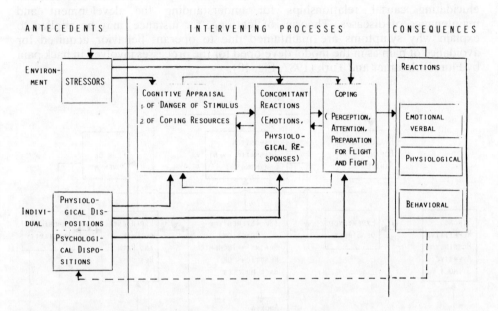

Figure 8. Typical stress model (Elements as in the one by Lazarus, mod. after Hodapp & Weyer, 1982)
Type of model: structural + functional, bidirectional

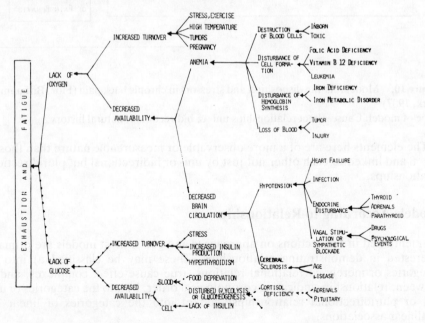

Figure 9. Diagnostic "tree" from psychosomatic symptom to underlying disease (Netter, 1982). Type of model: Functional: diagnostic

Finally, the third category of functional models is predominantly interested in elucidating causal relationships for understanding the development and maintenance of diseases. Theories of learning, for instance, may be applied to explain why symptoms are maintained due to operant behavior acquired for avoidance of pain as in the model developed for the processes involved in back pain by Flor, Birbaumer and Turk (1987, Fig. 10).

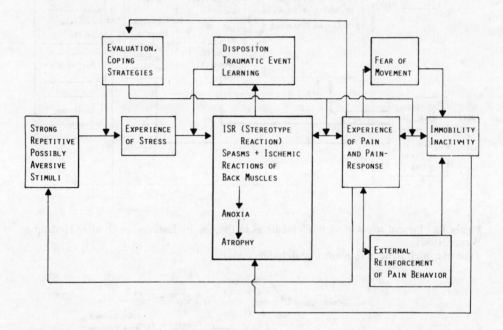

Figure 10.   Model relating disposition and stressors in chronic back pain (Flor, Birbaumer & Turk, 1987)
Type of model: Cause-effect relationships uni- & bidirectional, natural history.

The elements here are of a more observable or measureable nature than those in Fig. 8 and linked to each other not just by uni- or bidirectional but pluridirectional relationships.

Models According to Relationships

As mentioned in the sections on approaches and goals, most models are primarily interested in demonstrating relationships. These may be classified a) into the categories of merely correlational relations, true cause-effect complexes, and, in between, relationships indicating chronological order; b) into the categories of uni-, bi-, or pluridirectional relationships; and c) into the categories of linear and nonlinear associations.

As to a): As mentioned in the section on approaches, true cause-effect relations may much more readily be derived from experiments than from data based on surveys. This holds for relations between symptoms as well as for those between risk factors or behavior and resulting disease. In epidemiological studies concurrent associations have to be disentangled into their chronological order and liberated from confounding bias by procedures of stratification or path analysis. A model demonstrating how associations perceived as cause-effect relationships may turn out to be based on intervening bias is demonstrated by an example taken from a study on pregnancy and child development in Figure 11. The model relates participation in antenatal training of the mother to perinatal mortality by incorporating all available factors correlated directly or via intervening variables to the input variable of health behavior and to the output: fate of the infant.Φ-coefficients of associations computed for relationships, though seemingly negligible, in this large sample are all significant and taken together can explain the pseudocorrelation between beneficial effect of antenatal training and low infant mortality.

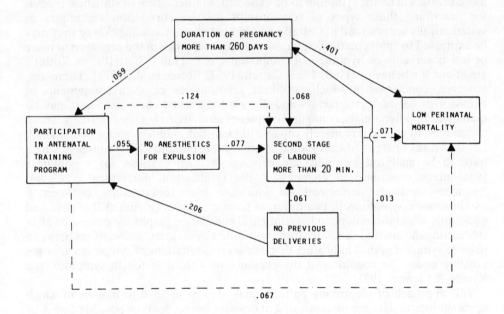

Figure 11. A Model explaining pseudo-cause-effect-relationships (---) by true causal relationships (——); figures indicate correlation coefficients (Φ) in a sample of 5126 cases, (Netter & Mau, 1976)
Type of model: correlational + cause-effect.

This example demonstrates that statistical analysis of epidemiological data has to take into account intervening variables just like the models in Fig. 8 and 10 assume psychological processes as hidden links between input and output.

As to b): The concept of uni-, bi- or pluridirectional relationships has been touched on in several of the models presented so far. This aspect is mentioned briefly to draw attention to the fact that many disease models – in particular those incorporating environmental factors – regard diseases as the consequence of external stimuli, ignoring mutual influences between disease and behavioral factors determining exposure (Fig. 4), or bidirectional relationships like that between pain response and reinforcement of pain behavior in Fig. 10. In this figure, experience of pain is related to four further elements of the model – a phenomenon also encountered in experimentally induced somatic symptoms. These pluridimensional relations demonstrate the difficulty of diagnostic processes in these types of models, in which intuition frequently replaces reasoning since solid probabilities are lacking for grouping the pluridimensional relationships according to frequencies and salience.

As to c): The models presented so far were all based on linear concepts: that is, the longer the duration of the risk factor or the higher its intensity, the more likely or the more severe will be the symptom to be expected. Mathematical or statistical models for describing these types of relationships will be correlation techniques as systematically represented in Cattell's covariation chart (Cattell, 1952) or they may be expressed by mathematical equations relating responses of the organism to more or less observable or hypothetical components as in Hull's, Cattell's, or Rotter's equations for behavior (Hull, 1952; Cattell, 1957; Rotter et al., 1972). There are, however, conditions in which nonlinear relationships between components of behavior or between risk factors and disease have to be considered and may be quantified by polynomials, configural frequency analysis, or log linear models. These techniques, of course, are merely capable of identifying configurations of elements, i.e. structures or types of conditional relationships, the underlying causes of which have to be analyzed by additional experiments. An example for a nonlinear syndromatic coherence of elements is the result of a hierarchical configural frequency analysis performed to elucidate the relationships between 5 psychosomatic symptoms in two different female samples (Figure. 12). Triple and quadruple associations depicted as configural association graphs are computed after subtracting the amount of covariation contributed by bivariate associations between pairs of symptoms, thus indicating that certain constellations of symptoms are only possible under the condition of the presence of a third or fourth symptom (see Krauth & Lienert, 1973).

This approach of identifying patterns may also be applied to models in which epidemiological data are incorporated to describe antecedents or possible causes of health behavior or disease. Besides configural frequency analysis presented in Figure 12, log linear models have been applied to sets of qualitative data of this type classified according to several variables at a time (for instance the relationship between psychosomatic complaints of mothers and perinatal mortality of infant taking into account social class, number of previous abortions and previous deliveries). Data are tested for goodness of fit by chi^2-tests which can provide us with one of the following results: 1) The kind of association between variable 1 and 2 differs within subgroups stratified according to variables 3-n, 2) the association in the total group is feigned by heterogeneities in the data and there is no association within each subgroup or 3) the association in the total group is roughly the same as in subgroups (Netter & Wermuth, 1975).

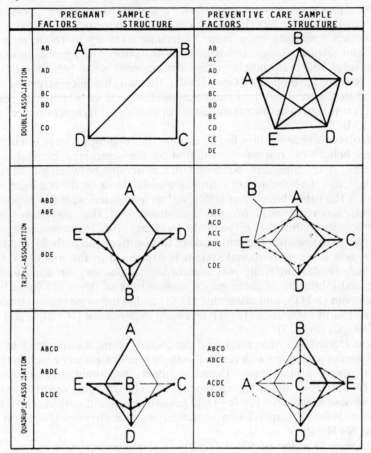

Figure 12. Configural frequency association graphs of 5 psychosomatic complaints. (Netter, 1981).

p≤ 0.01 = Bold lines   A=Loss of Appetite
p≤ 0.05 = Thin lines   B=Fatigue
   = Double associations C=Headaches
   =Triple associations   D=Circulatory Dysregulation
   = Quadruple associations E=Constipation
Type of model: Correlational, nonlinear

Models According to Content

As became evident from presenting models designed for different purposes and diseases, the content of a model may vary according to symptoms, to a bahavior involved, to morphological structures and biochemical processes and according to whether risk factors are incorporated.

Symptoms may be of a more clinical nature, as in models presented in Figure 10 or

12, or may comprise laboratory symptomatology (Fig. 9), or be viewed as nosological entities as in Figure 6.

Behavioral processes may comprise those related to risk exposure, preventive care (Fig. 11), cognitive processes (Fig. 8) or symptom management (Fig. 10).
Several models operating on a more molecular level try to relate motivational processes and resulting motor behavior such as anxiety and aggression to specifiic brain structures and brain biochemistry. An example is the behavioral inhibition system, a concept developed by Gray (1982), the morphological structure of which is depicted in Figure 13 A and the functional aspects of which with respect to transmitters involved in neurotransmission responsible for its functions are indicated in Figure 13 B.

These molecular relationships finally explain the relation between environmental stimuli and behavioral responses mediated by the septo-hippocampal inhibition system (Gray, 1982). Similarly, but based on a closer link between biochemical and behavior systems, the behaviors of submission and defense on the one hand and fight and flight on the other have been conceived as associated with the hypothalamo-pituitary-adrenocortical axis on the one hand and the amygdala-sympatho-medullary activity on the other in the model by Henry (1982) as shown in Figure 14.

The intention to organize the multitude of transmitters and pathological behavior into a common three-dimensional system is expressed in the model by Cloniger (1987) which relates different psychopathological diseases or abnormalities to activation and inhibition of three major transmitters of the brain (noradrenaline (NA), serotonin (5-HT), and dopamine (DA)) and at the same time to three major motivations (harm avoidance (H+/H-), reward dependence (R+/R-), and novelty seeking (N+/N-) (Fig. 15).

The model combines structural and functional elements resulting in $2^3 = 8$ different types of pathology with respect to three types of anxiety which they exhibit to different degrees of intensity (somatic anxiety predominantly present in the histrionic (N+H−R+) and antisocial type (N+H−R−), cognitive anxiety exhibited primarily by obsessional (N−H+R−) and passive dependent subjects (N−H+R+), and reactive dyshoria displayed in particular by cyclothymics (N−H−R+) and histrionics (N+H−R+).

As we have seen in the previous sections, one major aspect of content, besides behavior, biochemistry, and symptomatology, is the environment which is often incorporated into disease models which try to attract public attention of health care problems and preventive medicine. Such models are for instance very popular for elucidating structure of risk factors for the development of myocardial infarction. These may vary with respect to complexity and explanatory benefit. In the model by Cooper (1983) for instance, the arrows just represent the endeavor for order without indicating mutual interrelationships between risk factors or results (Fig. 16).

Whereas in more sophisticated models, like that by Schaefer and Blohmke (1977, Fig. 17) a hierarchy of risk factors is presented for the sociopsychological variables as well as for the somatic ones. But there is probably little empirical evidence for the decision to relate, for instance, social change to anxiety and aggression but not to discontent or worries in Figure 17 or to locate personality two levels above anxiety. These complex models present the danger of believing too readily in the relationships represented, interpreting arrows as indicating chronologically arranged cause-effect relationsips and thus ignoring pluridimensionality, nonlinearity, and possible confounding factors.

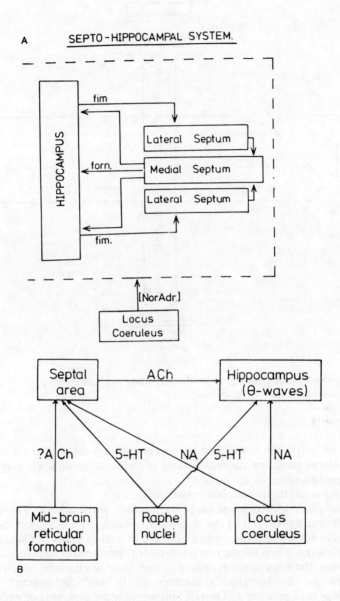

Figure 13. The interrelations between structures that may mediate responses to signals of punishment and nonreward, A. Interconnections between septal area and hippocampus. B. Ascending serotonergic (5-HT), noradrenergic (NA), and cholinergic (ACh) projections to the septal area and hippocampus, (NA= noradrenaline, 5HT=serotonin, ACH=acetylcholin) Type of model: Structural + functional, bi- and pluridirectional

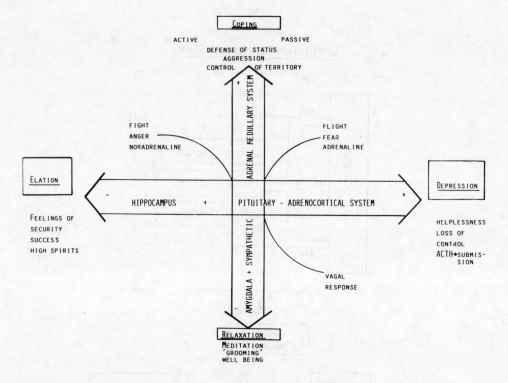

Figure 14.   Neuroendocrinological model according to Henry (1982).
Type of model: Structural + functional

Conclusions

If we try to justify the use of models in research on diseases from what has been
outlined about goals, relationships, and contents of models we may come to the
following conclusions:

Models may assist the researcher in two major ways:

1) They may help him to define his goals, samples, and methods of investigation just
like the structure provided by the chapters in a book. In this respect models provide
a synopsis or review and the feeling of order as well as a sort of checklist of aspects
to be considered when listing one's intentions, procedures and research outcome.
Furthermore, the simultaneous optical presentation of elements which in reality may
be hidden in chronological sequences or in multidimensional casuse-effect
relationships may provide a "Gestalt"-impression the elements of which in a verbal
report could only be dissected into a linear temporal order of presentation in which
necessarily connections and links would have to be cut into parts. Most recipients of
messages are more capable of memorizing figures and pictures than abstract verbal
thoughts and therefore reinforce scientists for producing models by citing and
teaching them.

2) A second major intention of a scientist for presenting models, however, is the
more scientific purpose to provide general principles according to which scattered

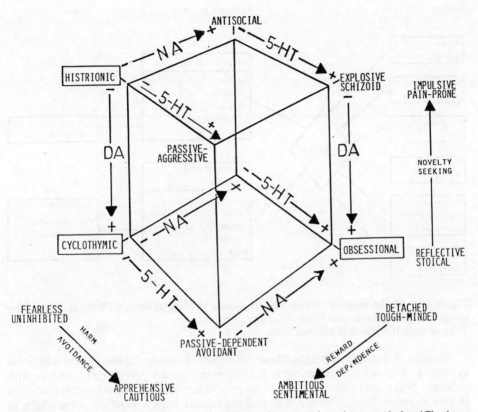

Figure 15. Three-way interaction of personality and monoaminergic transmission (Cloniger, 1987). (DA = dopamine, NA = notadrenaline, 5HT = serotonin) Type of model: Predominantly structural.

elements of information and experimental findings can be explained. The idea to find rules and laws has guided scientists throughout centuries and many of them have not resisted the temptation to base their theories on a single principle or cause like libido, repression, stress, or lack of parental affection as an explanation for any type of deviant development. There is a narrow road between the ingenious idea of the intuitive researcher who all of a sudden can explain the puzzling structure of protein molecules by the double helix as the basic principle of genetic transfer of information and the phantasies of a monomanic schizoid mind who believes he has found the word formula. The reason is the controversy that on the one hand models are perceived as the more elegant and convincing the less corollaries, exceptions, and conditional principles they involve, but that reality on the other is frequently more complicated and controversial than authors and editors may desire. If however, the introduction of a third dimension, a nonlinear relationship, a mathematical function underlying a temporal sequence or pattern of symptoms may suddenly serve as an eye-opener suitable to organize controversial elements into one common theory it is eagerly accepted – until new researchers produce experimental findings that do not match the model and force the scientific world to revise it.

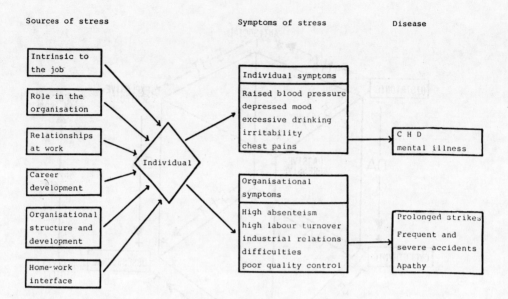

Figure 16.   Model relating coronary heart disease (CHD) or mental illness and respective symptoms to environmental factors (Cooper, 1983)
Type of model: Structural: classification.

A model of this type is perhaps Gray's attempt to define the behavioral inhibition systems as a common denominator for the many results produced by studies with different drugs, and with electrical or surgical interventions. Most models discussed in this chapter, however, are less ambitious and take a position somewhere in between the purpose of order or structure and the intention of detecting general principles. Most models – no matter whether they are mainly composed of physiological networks of responses, or interrelated social factors troubling epidemiologists as confounding factors or of sequences of motives or learning processes – are merely designed to draw the researcher's attention to the facts of pluridimensionality or multicausality without aiming at the goals of providing a new theory.

In summary, most of us would probably feel lost without models of diseases and their development as guidelines along which to organize research, but all of us should be aware that they are just "pictures in our heads" that we construct as substitutes of the real world in order to comprehend its complexity but which have to remain subject to change.

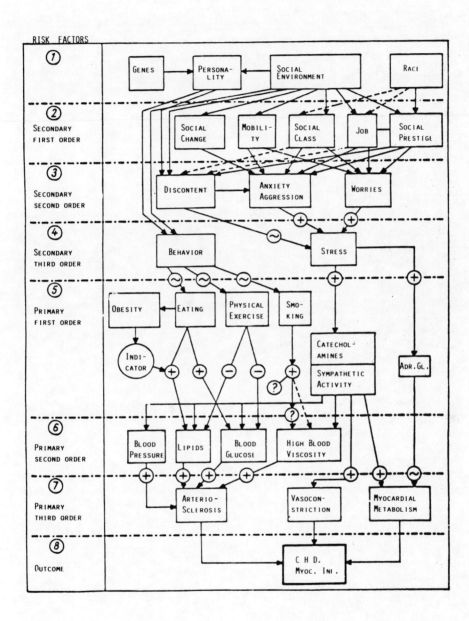

Figure 17. Hierarchy of risk factors (Schäfer & Blohmke, 1977)
Type of model: Cause-effect relationships, natural history, unidirectional.

References

Bahnson, C.B. (1979). Das Krebsproblem in psychosomatischer Dimension [The psychosomatic dimension of cancer]. In T. Uexküll (Ed.), *Lehrbuch der psychosomatischen Medizin* (pp. 685–659). München: Urban & Schwarzenberg.

Cattell, R. B. (1952). The three basic factor-analytic research designs – their interrelations and derivation. *Psychological Bulletin, 49*, 499–520.

Cattell, R. B. (1957). *Personality and motivation strucure and measurement*. Yonkers: New World.

Cloninger, C. R. (1987). Recent advances in the genetics of anxiety and somatoform disorders. In H. Y. Meltzer (Ed.), *Psychopharmacology: The third generation of progress* (pp. 955–965). New York: Raven Press.

Cooper, C. L. (1983). Identifying stressors at work: Recent research development. *Journal of Psychosomatic Research, 27*, 369–376.

Delius, L. (1966). *Psychovegetative Syndrome* [Psychovegetative syndroms]. Stuttgart: Thieme.

Eysenck, H. J. (1975). The measurement of emotion: Psychological parameters and methods. In L. Levi (Ed.), *Emotions – their parameters and measurement* (pp. 439–467). New York: Raven Press.

Eysenck, H. J. (1985). Personality, cancer and cardiovascular disease: A causal analysis. *Personality and Individual Differences, 6*, 535–556.

Flor, H., Birbaumer, N., and Turk, D. C. (1987). Ein Diathese-Stress-Modell chronischer Rückenschmerzen: Empirische Überprüfung and therapeutische Implikationen [A diathese-stress-model of chronic back pain: Results and therapeutic implications]. In W. D. Gerber, W. Miltner, and K. Mayer (Eds.), *Verhaltensmedizin: Ergebnisse und Perspektiven interdisziplinärer Forschung* (pp. 37–54). Weinheim: VCH-Verlagsgesellschaft.

Gray, J. A. (1982). *The neuropsychology of anxiety*. Oxford: University Press.

Henry, J. P. (1982). The relationship of social to biological processes in disease. *Social Science and Medicine, 16*, 369–380.

Hodapp, V., and Weyer, G. (1982). Zur Streβ-Hypothese der essentiellen Hypertonie [The stress hypothesis of essential hypertension]. In D. Vaitl (Ed.), *Essentielle Hypertonie. Psychologisch-medizinische Aspekte* (pp. 112–139). Berlin: Springer.

Hull, C. L. (1952). *A behavior system*. New Haven: Yale University Press.

Krauth, J., and Lienert, G. A. (1973). *Die Konfigurationsfrequenzanalyse und ihre Anwendung in Medizin und Psychologie* [The configuration-frequency analysis and its application in medicine and psychology]. Freiburg: Alber.

Netter, P. (1981). Konfigurationsfrequenzanalyse von funktionellen Beschwerden bei Spontanangabe und standardisierter Befragung [Configuration-frequency analysis of psychosomatic complaints in spontaneous reports and standardized questionnaires]. In W. Janke (Ed.), *Beiträge zur Methodik der differentiellen, diagnostischen und klinischen Psychologie* (pp. 391–420). Königstein i. Ts.: Hain.

Netter, P (1982). Medizinische Grundlagen für die Schwerpunktausbildung "Klinische Psychologie" [Medical bases in the curriculum of clinical psychology]. In W. R. Minsel and R. Scheller (Eds.), *Psychologie und Medizin, Band III: Brennpunkte der Klinischen Psychologie* (pp. 54–87). München: Kösel.

Netter, P., and Mau, G. (1976). Erfassung der Wirkung therapeutischer Maßnahmen und anderer Einflußfaktoren auf Schwangerschaftsverlauf und Kindesentwicklung [Measuring the effects of different interventions on pregnancy and early child development]. In S. Koller and J. Berger (Eds.), *Klinisch-statistische Forschung* (pp. 83–199). Stuttgart: Schattauer.

Netter, P., and Neuhäuser, S. (1982). Überlegungen, Wege und Beispiele zur Identifikation von Untertypen der essentiellen Hypertonie [Considerations, ways and examples to identify subtypes of essential hypertension]. In Vaitl, D. (Ed.), *Essentielle Hypertonie. Psychologisch-medizinische Aspekte* (pp. 140–161). Berlin: Springer.

Netter, P., and Wermuth, N. (1975). Psychosomatic complaints as related to contraceptive practice and frequency of intercourse. In H. Hirch (Ed.). *Proceeding of the IVth International Congress of Psychosomatic Obstetrics and Gynecology in Tel Aviv 1974* (pp. 189–196). Basel: Karger.

Rotter, J. B., Chance, J. E., and Phares, E. J. (1972). *Applications of a social learning theory of personality*. New York: Holt, Rinehart and Winston.

Schäfer, H., and Blohmke, M. (1977). *Herzkrank durch psychosozialen Streß* [Heart diseases and psychosocial stress]. Heidelberg: Springer.

Diet and Health: An Overview of Behavioral and Autonomic Effects of Food Constituents

Ursula Diebschlag, Dirk Hellhammer, Hendrik Lehnert and
Robert Murison

Introduction

Brain cells and brain function are dependent upon an adequate supply of nutrients. Food deprivation or deficiencies of certain nutrients such as vitamins or minerals affect neuronal development and metabolism, thus disturbing mental and bodily health (Leprohon-Green & Anderson, 1986; Nowak & Munro, 1977; Yogman, 1986). Even under normal conditions, the brain requires a substantial amount of energy for metabolic activities, and seems to respond sensitively to slight alterations in the nutrient state of the body (Sokoloff, Fitz Gerald, & Kaufman, 1977). In particular, the brain demands a continuous supply of glucose and oxygen, which are constantly available, since they can easily cross the blood – brain barrier. Lipids, however, enter the brain by slow diffusion, and provide sufficient resources of essential fatty acids and lipoids (e.g. cholestrol), which seem to influence the composition of microsomal and synaptosomal membranes in the brain (Foot, Cruz & Clandini, 1982; Tahin, Blum & Carafoli, 1981).

Besides such general and non-specific effects of nutrients on brain function, there are certain amino acids which discretely modulate neuronal activities, and, consequently, regulate behavioral and autonomic responses. These amino acids can act as substrates for protein synthesis, precursors for neurotransmitters and may provide energy by oxidation (Sokoloff et al., 1977). The following overview will focus on two amino acids, tryptophan and tyrosine, respectively. Tryptophan is necessary for the synthesis of serotonin (5-hydroxytryptamine; 5-HT), histamine and glycine (Fernstrom, Larin & Wurtman, 1973). Tyrosine, on the other hand, is the precusor amino acid for the catecholamines dopamine (DA), norepinephrine (NE) and epinephrine (E) (Gibson & Wurtman, 1977). All these subtrates play a key role as neurotransmitters in the central and autonomic nervous system. Thus, it is intriguing to speculate that neuronal and behavioral functions are dependent on the availability of their precursor amino acids, or even that we may self-regulate our own psychobiological status by a selective intake of food constituents. This overview will summarize some preliminary data providing some evidence for such relationships.

51

Tryptophan and Health

Tryptophan and Brain Serotonin

Tryptophan and the other large neutral amino acids (LNAA), such as phenylalanin, leucine, isoleucine, valine and tyrosine are present in all protein-rich food. After digestion all LNAA are distributed to the body via the blood stream. Before they can reach the brain, however, they have to pass the blood-brain barrier. Here, an active transport mechanism is necessary for their uptake into the brain (Wurtman & Pardridge, 1979). Since all LNAA compete for attachment to the same type of carrier molecule, the uptake of tryptophan is largely dependent on the presence of the other competing amino acids in plasma. Thus, tryptophan transport into the brain can be enhanced by either increasing its plasma levels, or, on the other hand, by lowering blood levels of the competing LNAA. The essential feature is the serum tryptophan/LNAA ratio. This ratio predicts how much tryptophan will actually enter the brain (Fernstrom, 1987).

A normal protein-rich meal contains 1–1,5% of tryptophan, but about 25% other large neutral amino acids. Consequently such a diet will not increase, but rather decrease the tryptophan influx into the brain (Fernstrom, 1983; Fernstrom & Wurtman, 1972). On the other hand, a meal rich in carbohydrates but poor in proteins increases brain tryptophan levels. How is this possible? The intake of carbohydrates enhances blood glucose levels, thereby raising insulin levels. Insulin causes all the other competing LNAA to be incorporated into muscle tissue. However, tryptophan remains almost unaffected, since about 80% of this amino acid is bound to albumin molecules. Moreover, insulin dissociates the free fatty acids from albumine, thus increasing the binding capacity for free tryptophan molecules in plasma. Both mechanisms cause a positive ratio of tryptophan to the other competing LNAA, and, therefore, an increasing tryptophan transport through the blood-brain barrier (Lieberman, Spring & Garfield, 1986; Spring, Chiodo & Bowen, 1987).

After reaching serotonergic neurons in the brain, tryptophan is hydroxylated to 5–hydroxytryptophan (5–HTP), and then decarboxylated to 5–HT (see Figure 1). The enzyme that catalyzes the initial and rate-limiting reaction is normally only partly saturated so that treatments which raise brain tryptophan levels rapidly increase serotonin production (Fernstrom, 1987). In particular, carbohydrate-rich meals result in an increase of serotonergic activity in the brain, and subsequently, in variations of those neuronal functions modulated by serotonin.

There is very broad literature on the relationship between serotonin and behavior, disease, as well as endocrine and autonomic function. The following discussion is a simplified summary, as seen in Figure 2 (for further reviews see Hellhammer, 1983; Soubrie, 1986; Wurtman, Hefti & Melamed, 1981).

Serotonergic cell bodies from the midbrain ascend to many cortical and subcortical regions, and descend to the lower brainstem and the spinal cord, for example to preganglionic neurons of the autonomic nervous system. The anatomical distribution of serotonergic fiber systems suggests a rather unspecific effect on brain areas and function. Stimulation of these fiber systems alters cognitive, emotional and motivational responses, activity and arousal, as well as autonomic function. Apart from this heterogeneity of effects there is also some homogeneity: It seems

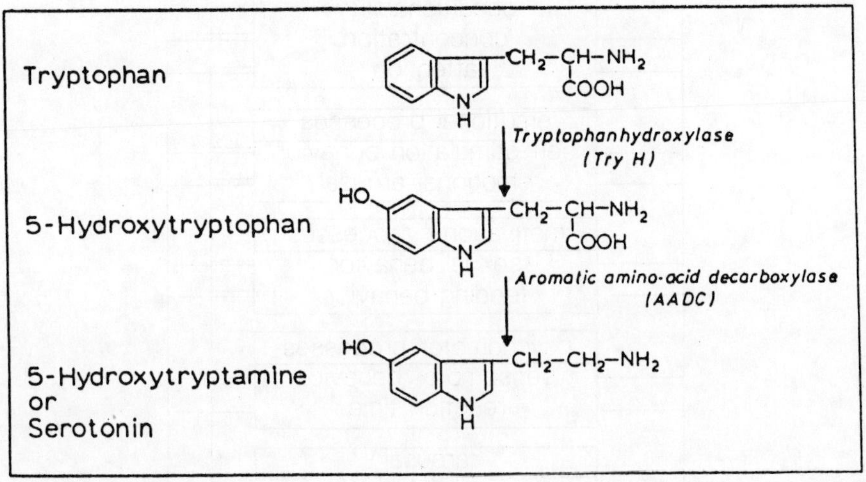

Figure 1. Biosynthesis of serotonin. From "Chemoarchitecture of the brain" (p.13) by R. Nieuwenhuys, 1985, Berlin: Springer.

that serotonergic activity dampens cognitive, emotional, motor and autonomic arousal, as well as pain sensitivity. Thus the serotonergic system has been considered to promote a trophotropic or parasympathetic-like state in the organism. Such a state seems to be experienced as relaxation, lack of initiative and motivation, enhanced threshold for positive and negative affects and impaired psychomotor performance. Just the opposite spectrum of effects seems to be regulated by some of the catecholaminergic fiber systems in the central nervous system. Noradrenergic and dopaminergic pathways descend and ascend to almost the same areas as the serotonergic system. It has been suggested that the catecholaminergic systems promote an ergotropic or sympathetic-like status of the brain. Moreover it has been proposed that both the serotonergic and the catecholaminergic systems closely interact with each other. In particular, there is a strong interaction between the cell bodies of the dorsal noradrenergic and the serotonergic system.

Taken together an increased uptake of tryptophan may enhance serotonergic function, and indirectly decrease catecholaminergic activity. Thus, one would expect concomittant psychobiological alterations, such as a dampening of arousal, of activity and autonomic activation, a reduced sensitivity to pain, as well as a decrease in emotional and motivational responsiveness and performance. Indeed, many studies have shown that such effects can be observed after tryptophan administration, and, to a small extent, after dietary manipulations (Spring, 1986). One may consequently suggest that some individuals may regulate their own mental and autonomic arousal by selective food intake. Insight into these psychobiological mechanisms may particulary help to clarify the nature of health disturbances associated with carbohydrate craving.

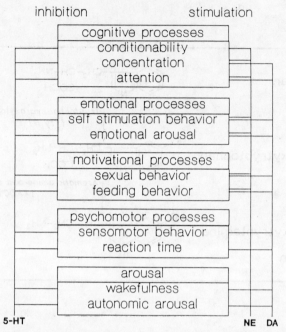

Figure 2. Simplified diagram of biogenic amine effects on behavior.

Tryptophan and Disease

Carbohydrate craving is normally associated with a high intake of calories, and consequently is associated with overweight. Overweight is considered a major risk factor for several health disturbances. Given the possibility that an individual might experience that the intake of carbohydrates reduces stress and autonomic arousal, he or she may well establish carbohydrate craving as a suitable strategy to cope with stress. Indeed, about two-thirds of all obese people are carbohydrate cravers, and in these patients carbohydrate-craving can be reduced by serotonin releasing drugs (Wurtman, 1984). These observations suggest a direct relationship between a carbohydrate-regulated tryptophan uptake into the brain and the behavioral relevance of subsequent serotonergic activity.

Moreover, one may expect a progressive increase of body weight following carbohydrate craving, accompanied by an increase in blood pressure, which again may promote such altered eating habits. Possibly, some hypertensive subjects have learned to regulate their own mental and autonomic activity by intake of carbohydrates. First evidence supporting such a hypothesis came from animal experiments. It was shown that oral administration of tryptophan is capable of reducing blood pressure in hypertensive rats (Sved, Van Itallie & Fernstrom, 1982). This effect was potentiated by fluoxetine, a serotonin agonist, and attenuated by valine, a competing amino acid. In cats, administration of tryptophan lowered blood pressure, inhibited preganglionic sympathetic discharging and even overrode an experimentally ischemia-induced surge in sympathetic traffic to the heart (Lehnert et al., 1987). These and other data suggest a significant control of serotonin precursors over sympathetic output. Furthermore, it was shown that a subgroup of obese patients who selectively preferred carbohydrates reduced carbohydrate consumption after administration of tryptophan or fenfluramine, a serotonin-releasing drug. In a subsequent study these carbohydrate cravers reported a positive mood after a carbohydrate-rich snack (Wurtman, 1984; J. J. Wurtman, J. R. Wurtman, Mark, Tsay, Gilbert & Growdon, 1985).

Putting this together, it seems reasonable to propose that some overweight and hypertensive subjects may profit from the positive mood state induced by carbohydrates. Such a proposed serotonergic mechanism may not be restricted to hypertension or obesity alone, since carbohydrate craving associated with serotonergic dysfunction has also been discussed for women with premenstrual distress and nicotine withdrawal (Benwell & Balfour, 1979; Benwell & Balfour, 1982; Rapkin, Edelmuth, Chang, Reading, McGuire & Su, 1987).

Recently, it has been shown that 67% of a subgroup of depressed patients with so-called "seasonal affective disorders" show carbohydrate craving. These patients have low cerebrospinal fluid levels of the serotonin metabolite 5- HIAA during their illness in the winter time, and it has been discussed that they try to compensate for their serotonin deficit by increased craving for carbohydrates, as a sort of self-medication (Coppen, Herzberg & Magga, 1967; Van Praag & Korf, 1974). Again, the serotonin agonist fenfluramine selectively suppressed carbohydrate craving in these patients.

With respect to arousal there is clear evidence for tryptophan to induce sleep onset. Although there are about 40 studies demonstrating this, there has not been any experiment investigating a possible potentiating effect of carbohydrates. However, it has been shown that carbohydrates potentiate the sleep-inducing effects of tryptophan (Adam & Oswald, 1979).

An increased sensitivity to pain may, in part, also be modulated by serotonin. Preliminary data show that tryptophan can raise pain thresholds, and this effect can be potentiated by carbohydrates (King, 1980). However, these effects are rather weak, and it seems unlikely that this mechanism is of clinical relevance.

Taken together, there is broad evidence today that individuals can regulate their tryptophan uptake into the brain by carbohydrates, thus affecting those psychobiological functions which are modulated by serotonergic activity. It seems that women respond more sensitively to these changes than men (Spring, Maller, Wurtman, Digman & Cozolino, 1983), but we do not yet understand why these sex differences occur.

Tyrosine and Health

The proposed functional (behavioral) balance between serotonergic and catecholaminergic system suggests that tyrosine, the precursor amino acid for norepinephrine and dopamine, may just exert effects on mental and autonomic functions opposite to those of tryptophan. However, the physiological consequences of enhanced tyrosine availability are very puzzling and not yet fully understood. On the other hand, there are numerous studies demonstrating that the noradrenergic system responds very sensitively to all kinds of stress. Prolonged stress, in particular, seems to result in an increased utilization of norepinephrine, thus causing a progressive depletion of norepinephrine stores (Reinstein, Lehnert, Scott & Wurtman, 1984; Weiss, P. G. Simson & P. E. Simson, 1989). From this viewpoint, it is interesting to investigate effects of tyrosine on brain catecholaminergic systems under stress, and, consequently, on health disturbances associated with stress.

Tyrosine and Brain Catecholamines

Subjects given tyrosine in a single oral dose exhibit high increases in plasma tyrosine levels, which last up to 8 hours and are accompanied by changes in the plasma tyrosine/LNAA ratio (Glaeser, Melamed, Growdon & Wurtman, 1979). Furthermore tyrosine administration causes elevations in the levels of tyrosine and the dopamine metabolite homovanillic acid (HVA) in the cerebrospinal fluid (Growdon & Melamed, 1980). This elevation suggests that the amino acid enters the brain and may affect the synthesis and release of dopamine. Additionally, it has been shown that the utilization of tyrosine is largely depended on the enzymatic activity of catecholaminergic neurons: If the neurons are active, more tyrosine is converted by the enzyme tyrosine-hydroxylase to dopamine and norepinephrine (see Figure 3). If the neurons are inactive, tyrosine-hydroxylase is inhibited by the end-product norepinephrine. Thus, additional tyrosine can not be utilized for further synthesis and release (Scally, Ulus & Wurtman, 1977).

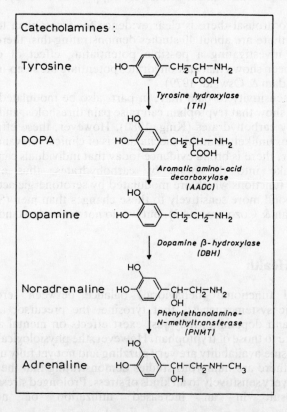

Figure 3. Biosynthetic pathway of the catecholamines dopamine, noradrenaline and adrenaline. From "Chemoarchitecture of the brain" (p.12) by R. Nieuwenhuys, 1985, Berlin: Springer.

Tyrosine and Disease

Patients with Parkinson's disease (Bernheimer, Birkmayer, Hornykiewicz, Jellinger & Seitelberger, 1973) and a subgroup of depressed patients (Schildkraut, 1965) suffer from a deficit of dopamine and norepinephrine. A similar depletion of brain catecholamines has also been discussed for attention deficit disorders (Lieberman, 1986). Attempts to treat these disorders with tyrosine or tyrosine-enriched diets have only been temporarily successful. Although a transient improvement has been observed, a relatively quick habituation seems to occur within several weeks. Thus, tyrosine does obviously not have the properties to act as a permanent therapeutic drug.

Under stress, a depletion of norepinephrine stores has been frequently observed (Milner & Wurtman, 1986), suggesting that, under these conditions, utilization exceeds synthesis of this amine. In animal experiments, tyrosine treatment results in an increase of norepinephrine-metabolites under stress (Lehnert, Reinstein, Stowbridge & Wurtman, 1984). Moreover, dietary tyrosine application prevents the depletion of norepinephrine, and, in addition, the behavioral depression which routinely occurs after stress exposure (Lehnert, Reinstein & Wurtman, 1984). These latter observations were of particular importance, suggesting that tyrosine may prevent poststress symptoms associated with norepinephrine depletion. Clinically, many health disturbances seem not to occur during but rather after a stress, such as asthma, migraine headaches, immune disorders, peptic ulceration, etc. Such disorders have been labelled in terms of "poststress", "parasympathetic rebound" or "exhaustion syndrome". Physiologically, such a status seems to be generally characterized by low sympathetic and high parasympathetic arousal (Meerson, 1984).

Recent observations confirmed such findings in man. They showed that tyrosine can minimize poststress symptoms such as impairment in vigilance and performance, sleepiness and subjective discomfort. Interestingly, it was found that the effect of tyrosine was greater when the stress was more intense, supporting the hypothesis of a relationship between stress, norepinephrine turnover and utilization of tyrosine (Lieberman, Corkin, Spring, Growdon & Wurtman, 1982; Lieberman et al., 1986).

On this basis we are presently interested in investigating whether tyrosine can prevent behavioral and autonomic consequences under poststress conditions. We are currently testing this hypothesis in a series of animal experiments, where rats are allowed to recover after immobilization stress. Under these conditions gastric ulcerations occur only within the poststress period and do not appear in vagotomized rats. Thus, the model seems to be suited to study such poststress disorders. Descending fibers from the dorsal noradrenergic bundle have frequently been shown to exert an inhibitory control over the preganglionic vagal nuclei in the brainstem (Loewy & Neil, 1981; Reis & Ledoux, 1987). Consequently, we predicted that a depletion of norepinephrine may result in a reduction of inhibitory noradrenergic control, thus facilitating poststress ulceration. Indeed, preliminary data from this animal model provides evidence for a strong beneficial effect of tyrosine in minimizing gastric ulceration (Murison, 1988). These data are very encouraging since they may help to better understand one (of many) participating mechanisms in the occurrence of poststress disorders.

Since brain catecholamines also participate in the regulation of blood pressure, effects of tyrosine have also been studied in both animal experiments and hypertensive patients. However, the data are very puzzling, suggesting both an inhibitory and an excitatory control of blood pressure. Data from animal experiments showed that tyrosine treatment results in an increase of norepinephrine metabolites in hypertensive rats, suggesting an increased utilization of tyrosine (Lehnert, Reinstein, Stowbridge & Wurtman, 1984). However, this amino acid has no consistent effect on blood pressure in normotensive animals, but it reduces blood pressure in hypertensive rats via a noradrenergic mechanism in the brain stem (Sved, Fernstrom & Wurtman, 1979). This effect is probably due to an activation of tyrosine hydroxylase in hypertensive rats, resulting in a rapid utilization of the amino acid. On the other hand, tyrosine elevates blood pressure in hypotensive animals (Conlay, Maher & Wurtman, 1981). Preliminary data from a study in borderline hypertensive patients under stress suggest that tyrosine exerts a significant attenuation of the stress-induced elevation of systolic blood pressure. Again, tyrosine appears to lower blood pressure selectively in the hypertensive state and reaction (Diebschlag, Lehnert, Reche, Warnecke, Hellhammer & Beyer, in press). Taken together, it seems that tyrosine can both up- and down- regulate blood pressure, thus allowing an optimal adaptation of sympathetic arousal to stress.

Conclusion

Brain neurotransmitter synthesis is influenced directly by the availability of precursors, which are nutrients in the diet and blood. Changes in nutrient availability such as those which may occur with variations in meal composition and quantity may have effects on normal brain function, behavior, and health. The growing knowledge in this field may help to develop new diagnostic approaches or even combined dietary and behavioral treatments of such disorders.

The present overview focused mainly of the precursors of the biogenic amines. Similar manipulations are well documented for acetylcholine, providing evidence for effects of dietary choline or lecithin on behavior and the treatment of several diseases, such as tardive dyskinesia, Huntington's and Alzheimer's disease, ataxia, Tourette's and myasthemic syndrome (Wurtman et al., 1981).

Presently, however, we do not fully understand the possible impact of relationships between nutrients and behavior for the occurrence and pathogenesis of diseases. Further research may at some time allow us to improve strategies in health psychology on the basis of our knowledge about the psychobiological mechanisms behind health-damaging eating habits.

This research was supported, in part, by the
Deutsche Forschungsgemeinschaft (He 1013/3 – 1)

References

Adam, K. and Oswald, I. (1979). One gram of 1–tryptophan fails to alter the time taken to fall asleep. *Neuropharmacology, 18*, 1025.

Benwell, M. E. and Balfour, D. J. (1979). Effects of nicotine administration and its withdrawal on plasma corticosterone and brain 5–hydroxyindoles. *Psychopharmacology, 63*, 7.

Benwell, M. E. and Balfour, D. J. (1982). The effects of nicotine administration on 5–HT uptake and biosynthesis in rat brain. *European Journal of Pharmacology, 84*, 71.

Bernheimer, H., Birkmayer, W., Hornykiewicz, O., Jellinger, K. and Seitelberger, F. (1973). Brain dopamine and the syndromes of Parkinson and Huntington. *Journal of Neurological Science, 20*, 415.

Conlay, L. A., Maher, T. J. and Wurtman, R. J. (1981). Tyrosine increases blood pressure in hypertensive rats. *Science, 212*, 559.

Coppen, A., Herzberg, B. and Magga, R. (1967). Tryptophan in the treatment of depression. *Lancet, 2*, 1178.

Diebschlag, U., Lehnert, H., Reche, A., Warnecke, W., Hellhammer, D. and Beyer, J. (in press). Effects of the precursor amino acids 1–tyrosine and 1–tryptophan on stress–induced blood pressure increases in borderline hypertensives. *Acta Endocrinologica*.

Fernstrom, J. D. (1983). Role of precursor availability in the control of monoamine biosynthesis in brain. *Physiological Reviews, 63,* 484.

Fernstrom, J. D. (1987). Food-induced changes in brain serotonin synthesis: Is there a relationship to appetite for specific macronutrients? *Appetite, 8*, 163.

Fernstrom, J. D., Larin, F. and Wurtman, R. J. (1973). Correlation between brain tryptophan and plasma neutral amino acid levels following food consumption in rats. *Life Sciences, 13*, 517.

Fernstrom, J. D. and Wurtman, R. J. (1972). Brain serotonin content: physiological regulation by plasma neutral amino acids. *Science, 178*, 414.

Foot, M., Cruz, T. F. and Clandini, M. T. (1982). Influence of dietary fat on the lipid composition of rat-brain synaptosomal and microsomal membranes. *Biochemical Journal, 208*, 631.

Gibson, C. J. and Wurtman, R. J. (1977). Physiological control of brain catecholamine synthesis by brain tyrosine concentrations. *Biochemistry and Pharmacology, 26*, 1137.

Glaeser, B. S., Melamed, E., Growdon, J. H. and Wurtman, R. J. (1979). Elevation of plasma tyrosine after a single oral dose of 1–tyrosine. *Life Sciences, 25*, 265.

Growdon, J. H. and Melamed, E. (1980). Effects of oral 1–tyrosine administration on CSF tyrosine and HVA levels in patients with Parkinson's disease. *Neurology, 30*, 396.

Hellhammer, D. (Ed.). (1983). *Gehirn und Verhalten (Brain and Behavior)*, Münster: Aschendorff.

King, R. B. (1980). Pain and tryptophan. *Journal of Neurosurgery, 53*, 44.

Leprohon-Greenwood, C. E. and Anderson, G. H. (1986). An overview of the mechanisms by which diet affects brain function. *Food Technology, 1*, 132.

Lehnert, H., Lombardi, F., Raeder, E. A., Lorenzo, A. V., Verrier, R. L., Lown, B. and Wurtman, R. J. (1987). Increased release of brain serotonin reduces vulnerability to ventricular fibrillation in the cat. *Journal of Cardiovascular Pharmacology, 10*, 389.

Lehnert, H., Reinstein, D. K., Strowbridge, B. W. and Wurtman, R. J. (1984). Neurochemical and behavioral consequences of acute, uncontrollable stress: effects of dietary tyrosine. *Brain Research, 303*, 215.

Lehnert, H., Reinstein, D. K. and Wurtman, R. J. (1984). Tyrosine reverses the depletion of brain norepinephrine and the behavioral deficits caused by tail-shock stress in rats. In E. Usdin, R. Kretnansky and I. Axelrod (Eds.), *Stress: The Role of Catecholamines and other Neurotransmitters*, (p.81). New York.

Lieberman, H. R. (1986). Behavioral changes caused by nutrients. *Bibliotheca Nutritia Dieta, 38*, 219.

Lieberman, H. R., Corkin, S., Spring, B. J., Growdon, J. H. and Wurtman, R. J. (1982). Mood and sensorimotor performance after neurotransmitter precursor administration. *Society for Neuroscience, 8*, 395.

Lieberman, H. R., Spring, B. J. and Garfield, G. S. (1986). The behavioral effects of food constituents: strategies used in studies of amino acids, protein, carbohydrates and caffeine. *Nutrition Reviews, 44*, 61.

Loewy, A. D. and Neil, J. J. (1981). The role of descending monoaminergic systems in central control of blood pressure. *Federal Proceedings, 40*, 2778.

Meerson, F. Z. (Ed.). (1984). *Adaptation, Stress and Prophylaxis*. Berlin: Springer.

Milner, J. D. and Wurtman, R. J. (1986). Catecholamine synthesis: physiological coupling to precursor supply. *Biochemical Pharmacology, 35*, 875.

Nowak, T. S. Jr and Munro, H. N. (1977). Effects of protein caloric malnutrition on biochemical aspects of brain development. In R. J. Wurtman and J. J. Wurtman (Eds.), *Nutrition and the Brain, 2*, (p.193). New York: Raven Press.

Rapkin, A. J., Edelmuth, E., Chang, L. C. Reading, A. E., McGuire, M. T. and Su, T. (1987). Whole-blood serotonin in premenstrual syndrome. *Obstetrics and Gynecology, 70*, 533.

Reinstein, D. K., Lehnert, H., Scott, N. A. and Wurtman, R. J. (1984). Tyrosine prevents behavioral and neurochemical correlates of acute stress in rats. *Life Sciences, 34*, 2225.

Reis, D. J. and Ledoux, J. E. (1987). Some central neural mechanisms governing resting and behaviorally coupled control of blood pressure. *Circulation, 76*, 2.

Scally, M. C., Ulus, I. H. and Wurtman, R. J. (1977). Brain tyrosine level controls striatal dopamine synthesis in haloperidol – treated rats. *Journal of Neural Transmission, 43*, 103.

Schildkraut, J. J. (1965). The catecholamine hypothesis of affective disorders: a review of supportive evidence. *American Journal of Psychiatry, 122*, 509.

Sokoloff, L., Fitz Gerald, G. G. and Kaufman, E. E. (1977). Cerebral nutrition and energy metabolism. In R. J. Wurtman and J. J. Wurtman (Eds.), *Nutrition and the Brain, 1* (p. 87). New York: Raven Press.

Soubrié, P. (1986). Reconciling the role of central serotonin neurons in human and animal behavior. *The Behavioral and Brain Sciences, 9*, 319.

Spring, B. J. (1986). Effects of food and nutrients on the behavior of normal individuals. In R. J. Wurtman and J. J. Wurtman (Eds.), *Nutrition and the Brain, 7*, (p.1). New York: Raven Press.

Spring, B. J., Chiodo, J. and Bowen, D. J. (1987). Carbohydrates, tryptophan and behavior: a methodological review. *Psychological Bulletin, 102*, 234.

Spring, B. J., Maller, O., Wurtman, J. J. Digman, L. and Cozolino, L. (1983). Effects of protein and carbohydrate meals on mood and performance: interactions with sex and age. *Journal of Psychiatric Research, 17*, 155.

Sved, A. F., Fernstrom, J. D. and Wurtman, R. J. (1979). Tyrosine administration reduces blood pressure and enhances brain norepinephrine release in spontaneously hypertensive rats. *Proceedings of the National Academy of Sciences USA, 76*, 3511.

Sved, A. F., Van Itallie, C. M. and Fernstrom, J. D. (1982). Studies on the antihypertensive action of 1–tryptophan. *Journal of Pharmacology and Experimental Therapeutics, 221*, 329.

Tahin, Q. S., Blum, M. and Carafoli, E. (1981). The fatty acid composition of subcellular membranes of rat liver, heart and brain: diet–induced modifications. *European Journal of Biochemistry, 121*, 5.

Van Praag, H. M. and Korf, J. (1974). Serotonin metabolism in depression; clinical application of the probenecid test. *Internationale Pharmakopsychiatrie, 9*, 35.

Weiss, J. M., Simson, P. G. and Simson, P. E. (1989). Neurochemical basis of stress–induced depression. In H. Weiner, I. Florin, R. Murison and D. Hellhammer (Eds.) *Frontiers of Stress Research*, (p.37). Toronto: Huber Publishers.

Wurtman, J. J. (1984). The involvement of brain serotonin in excessive carbohydrate snacking by obese carbohydrate cravers. *Journal of the American Dietetic Association, 84*, 1004.

Wurtman, R. J., Hefti, F, and Melamed, E. (1981). Precursor control of neurotransmitter synthesis. *Pharmacological Reviews, 32*, 315.

Wurtman, R. J. and Pardridge, W. M. (1979). Circulating trypophan, brain tryptophan and psychiatric disease. *Journal of Neural Transmission, 15*, 227.

Wurtman, J. J., Wurtman, R. J., Mark, S., Tsay, R., Gilbert, W. and Growdon, J. (1985). D-fenfluramine selectively suppresses carbohydrate snacking by obese subjects. *International Journal of Eating Disorders, 4*, 89.

Yogman, M. W. (1986). Nutrients and newborn behavior. *Nutrition Reviews: Diet and behavior. A multidisciplinary evaluation, 44*, 74.

Behavioral Aspects of the Modulation of Immunity

Novera Herbert Spector

It has been known since ancient times that the mental attitudes of an individual may affect his or her susceptibility to disease, as well as his or her ability to recover from disease. These ideas have been documented scientifically only in the twentieth century. Recently, we have witnessed a virtual explosion of new research in this fascinating area. Dozens of international workshops and symposia have been held recently on the subject of the interaction among the nervous, endocrine and immune systems, and these have included many reports on the immunological consequences of behavior. Both psychologic and sociologic aspects have been studied in much detail. Just a few of the recent volumes resulting from these workshop are listed in the references for this brief review. For example, papers arising from the first three International Workshops on Neuroimmunomodulation (NIM) cover research reported from hundreds of leading scientists from more than 40 countries (Spector et al., 1985; Janković *et al.*, 1986; Pierpaoli & Spector, 1987; Goetzl & Spector, 1989).

In this brief paper, I will not try to cover all aspects of behavior and NIM, but I will discuss three important and currently much debated aspects of these studies. First, it is important to understand what we mean by such terms as "stress," "distress," "eustress," "stressor" and so on. These terms appear more and more often, not only in popular literature, but in "scientific" papers as well... and they generate enormous confusion. Secondly, I will comment on the mechanisms involved in triggering changes in the host defence system. Finally, I will say a few words about a field which provides some of the best evidence for the effects of behavior on immunity: creating changes in immune responses by classical (Pavlovian) conditoning.

"Stress," "Distress," "Strain," and Total Confusion

In common parlance, as well as in much technical literature, the terms, *strain, stressor, stress and distress* are often used interchangeably. Furthermore, with very few exceptions, measurements of these entries are seldom done quantitively. This has led to enormous confusion, not only among hapless readers, but also among many writers who employ these terms. In my "Rambunctious remarks" (Spector, 1988), I made some comments on these problems which are relevant here.

In physics as it should be in physiology, stress has a precise meaning, When you apply *stress* (force) to a material, you can measure the *strain* in the material that has been stressed (pushed, distorted, bent, etc.). In psychology and sociology the word "stress" has been replaced (by some investigators) by "stressor" when they talk about the force that is applied from the outside. This is probably a good step in the right direction, but the word "stress" has been used also to substitute for what the physicists and what good physiologists have called "strain". Any stimulus, of any kind, from the *exterior*, or from the *interior* or the organism, is a *stress*.

Stimuli are constantly being received by the organism in the form of sensory input, in the form of antigenic input, and in other forms; and are constantly being received from the interior of the organism in the form of abstract thought, emotions, proprioceptors and autoimmune reactions (Figure 1). These stimuli (stressors) are constantly producing within the organism a series of responses which are continuous throught the lifetime of the individual.

Why Quibble?

One must make a very careful distinction between one stimulus and another because the number of such stimuli approaches infinity and the number of reactions is equally complex. This confusion of terms will lead to a confusion in our ideas, confusion in our data, and confusion in the design of future experiments. Further confusion is introduced by using the word "stress:" to mean either the stimulus (stressor) or the response (strain, etc.).

A step in the right direction would be simply to employ the word "distress." This could be any type of nociceptive stimulus and this would let us instantly take a leap equal to that which Hans Selye took after many years of talking about "stress responses."

A very brief look at history would be helpful here. The American physiologist, Walter Cannon, who invented the word "homeostasis," defined the "fear, fight, and flight reaction" in terms of catecholamines, in other words, the reaction of the adrenal medulla. Many years later Hans Selye redefined what he called "stress," or the reactions to a stressor, in terms of the adrenal cortex or corticosteroid response.

Today we know that at least a dozen hormones are involved in this type of response, including the catecholamines, the steroids, prolactin, growth hormone, and so on and so forth, as well as a host of neurally active peptides.

After Selye had for many years talked about the harmful effects of stress, Sam Corson from Ohio State University finally convinced him that "stress" in his sense could have beneficial as well as harmful effects, and Selye then began to write books about how to use stress to one's advantage (Selye, 1956, 1975a).

Selye then made distinctions among the words, *stress, eustress* eu, (from Greek, meaning, amoung other things, good), and *distress* (dys from Greek, sometimes opposed to eu, and meaning, among other things, poorly or poor, stretched here to mean bad) (Selye, 1975b; Milsum, 1985). Despite the use of this word by Selye and others, "eustress" has yet to appear in at least one major unabridged dictionary of the English language, and has not been used widely by most "stress" researchers.

Many people are still using the word *stress* when they mean distress. Indeed, dictionaries of the English language now include "*distress*" as one of the meanings of "*stress!*" At a recent gathering of immunologists and behavioral specialists in Arizona I raised this question. After listening for two days to people talking about stress and each one talking about something else, I said, "Hey, fellows, let's define our terms. I don't know what you mean by stress." Whereupon one psychologist jumped up, looking at me with disdain, and said, "Obviously you're unsophisticated. Every good psychologist knows exactly what we mean by stress," and then he gave a definition. Whereupon a psychiatrist at the other end of the table jumped up and said, "Oh no, that's not at all what we mean by stress." Within a few minutes there were five different definitions thrown on the table. I had no need to say anything more. I think that my point was validated, but I'm not sure that many people understood this.

The organism is constantly bombarded by stimuli. Often a stimulus produces only an imperceptible strain. When these strains are additive, they may reach a point (threshold) where a large and easily measurable response is evident. At this point, the accumulation of small quantitative changes may trigger a dramatic qualitative reaction. The trigger may come from outside or from inside the body. A few of these, involving the nervous and immune systems, are represented in Figure 1.

I strongly urge psychologists, psychiatrists, and all behavioral scientists to totally give up the use of the confusing and multiple-meaning word, stress. A refreshing clarity in the literature will result. Terms such as stimulus, response, and perhaps even "trigger" are much less ambiguous.

Mechanisms

Advances in research of the past 10 years and in the near future ahead of us, can bring psychoimmunology and the behavioral sciences out of the realm of folklore and into the domain of science. This occurs when we begin to examine closely the pathways involved between the trigger and the final responses, which will be physiologic, behavioral and social .

New evidence, describing in detail the interactions, the pathways and the mechanisms of NIM are coming from all disciplines of bio-science, including genetics, biochemistry, pharmacology, physiology, anatomy and immunology. Figure 2 suggests the interactions among these and other fields of science.

To the reader who wishes to examine these mechanisms in more detail than given in the cartoon (Figure 1), I refer you to the symposium volumes (NIM Workshops) listed above, which contain, in addition to their hundreds of papers, many thousands of references to the current scientific literature. Additional thousands of references to mechanisms can be found in the review books: Metalnikov, 1934; Dolin and Dolina, 1972; Korneva et al., 1978, 1985; Ader, 1981; Fabris, et al., 1983; Locke, et al., 1983; Locke et al., 1985; Guillemin et al., 1985; Frederickson et al., 1986; Janković et al., 1987; Spector, 1989; and others. In preparation for press (1989) is a new review by one of the great living pioneers in the field, B. D. Janković, with more than 600 literature references. Even with this great flow of new information, most of the research in detailing the mechanisms of NIM still lies ahead.

To conclude this brief review, a few words should be said about an area of research which provides some of the most compelling evidence for the influence of behavior upon immune response, i.e.: conditioning.

Conditioning of Immunity

Much of what I say here is taken from my recent review on this subject (Spector, 1987) and may serve as a guide for this fascinating field.

A stimulus ("unconditioned stimulus," or US, also called an "internal stimulus") that, by itself, can provoke host-defense (including immune)responses is paired with a "neutral" stimulus. Later, the neutral stimulus may either, by itself in the total

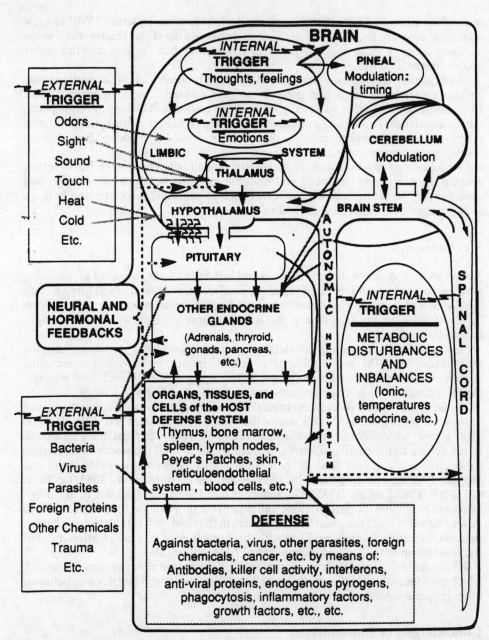

Figure 1

Neuroimmunomodulation: signaling and defense activation. External and internal triggers, circuits and feedback Pathways (in part)

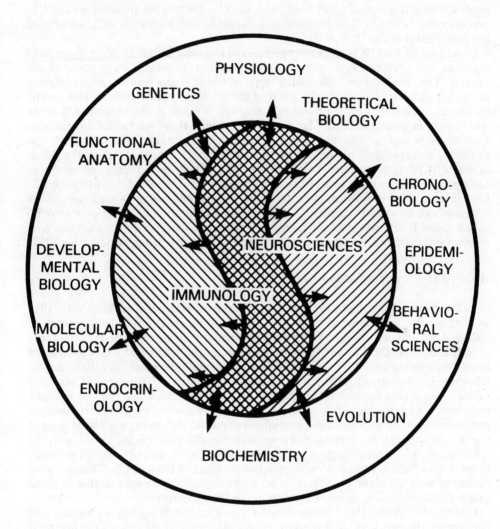

Figure 2. Neuroimmunomodulation: an expanding conceptual universe. (Modified and reprinted with permission from vol. 1, No. 1 of the *NIM Newsletter*, 1969.)

absence of the US., modify the host defense response, or, when paired with the US, increase or decrease the response that would be generated by the US alone. When a neutral stimulus is paired many times with the US, the neutral stimulus is called, in conditioning jargon, a "conditioned" (i.e., conditioning) stimulus (CS, also called the "external stimulus").

Conditioning may be considered one form of learning, although often it occurs in humans, and presumably in other animals, without conscious perception of the process. The "classical" or "Pavlovian" type of conditioning involves many pairings of the CS with the US, and finally a test of the CS alone, which then is shown to be no longer "neutral", i.e., it provokes a response similar is one that the US alone would elicit in a naive animal. There are other criteria that Ivan Pavlov and modern Pavlovians would use to test when "classical conditioning" has occurred: for example, susceptibility of the learned response to "extinction" when the CS is repeatedly presented alone without the US. I will not discuss all of these technicalities here, except to mention that there are those who feel that when the US-CS pairing is done only once, even when the animal then learns" a response, either it should not be called "classical" or "Pavlovian" conditioning at all or it may be called "one-trial" association learning." In any case, even such (one-trial association) experiments, whatever thay be called, provide strong evidence for NIM.

A Bit of History Here May be Helpful.

Luk'yanenko, in excellent 1961 review, cites the experiment of Makukahin in 1911 as perhaps the first showing "conditioned leucocytic reactions." These were not followed up, and according to Luk'yanenko, "could not be interpreted satisfactorily at that time." At the Pasteur Institute in Paris, in the 1920s and 1930s a series of ingenious experiments were conducted by S. I. ,Metal'nikov and his colleagues, V. Chorine, I. Nicolau, O. Antinescu-Dimitriu, and others. Using guinea pigs and rabbits, employing Pavlovian techniques, they demonstrated that various immune responses could be conditioned. Injections of various bacteria or bacteria-derived compounds (as the unconditional stimuli) were paired repeatedly with scratching of the skin or application of the skin of a warmed metallic plate (as the CS). Later, the CS alone evoked large changes in white blood count in (hemagluttinating) antibody titers. Other experiments followed, using other types of US and CS. Changes were produced by a CS alone in various other responses that were measurable in those times: cellular reaction, level of hemolysin, and phagocytosis.

During the 1930s, there were many reports in the literature extending and confirming the work of Metal'nikov et al., and in several cases denying their reproducibility and validity. Then, after a silent decade, came a long series of papers, many from the Soviet Union, especially from A. O. Dolin (the successor to Pavlov at Leningrad) and his colleagues and students, including especially Krylov, Flerov, and Luk'yanenko (Dolin et. al., 1952, 1960). Successes were claimed in conditioning of both specific and nonspecific immune reactions. Both immunosuppression and immunoenhancement were reported, Among the experminental animals were mice, rats, guinea pigs, rabbits, dogs, oxen, monkeys and humans. Some of the antigenic substances included: virus; foreign red blood cells; albumin; malarial parasites and other whole organisms; vaccines; extracts from salmonellae, dysentery, typhoid, paratyphoid, and diphtheria bacilli, E. coli, and staphylococci.

There is not enough space here to give all the details of these fascinating experiments. The most comprehensive review to data is that of Luk'yanenko.

For a broad perspective on the history of conditioning and NIM, additional sources are Metal'nikov's 1934 book and the chapter on conditioning in Dolin and Dolina (1972). In 1981, Ader reevaluated some of this older literature, and made a contribution by statistically analyzing the data from a number of these reports. In the context of a general theoretical physiologic approach, this subject is discussed, along with other evidence of NIM from many fields, in Spector (1980).

After a second hiatus of many years in which almost no data were published, new interest in the conditioning of immune responses was generated by the publication of Ader and Cohen's study on immunosuppression (1975). Their results were met with skepticism, but confirmation came quickly from several independent sources. Soon another wave of experimental reports appeared, from the United States, Canada, Germany, and elsewhere. Some of these were reported at the first two International Workshops on Neuroimmunomodulation (Spector *et al.*, 1985, 1989; Janković, *et al.*, 1987).

About 19 years ago, while I was visiting professor of physiology in Lyon, France, our lab had a visit from Prof. Elena Korneva of Leningrad, and we heard about her experiments with hypothalamic lesions and stimulation and the resulting changes in circulating antibodies. It occured to me that, since we were already conditioning other autonomic nervous system and hypothalamic functions, we should be able to condition immune responses as well. I thought that I had a brilliant new idea, but a search of the literature soon revealed that Metal'nikov (and perhaps even Pavlov) has scooped me by almost a half a century. I decided nonetheless to pursue this further. Before trying new conditioning experiments, I wanted to get a better grasp of the physiologic mechanisms involved in the complex interrelationships among the immune, endocrine, and nervous systems, so that when I returned to the United States, I started a series of experiments designed to pinpoint some hypothalamic or other central nervous system nuclei that are directly involved with immune functions. This work has been reviewed elsewhere (Spector, 1980). Eventually, I came back to the idea of conditioning: no one had even attempted to condition interferon (IFN) responses. In collaboration with various students and colleagues, I attempted several new techniques of "classical" conditioning. I am grateful for the very kind support of Sam Baron, who without any tangible reward, even in the form of published papers, for many years continued to do the laborious bioassays of hundreds, of serum samples for IFN. The results were tantalizing, but never so consistent as to be worth publishing.

Looking for a simple neutral CS, I discussed the problem once more with the dean of American "conditioners," Neal Miller, who suggested the odor of camphor as a CS that had worked well in other experiments. At about the same time I had the good fortune to team up with a couple of highly experienced and competent immunologists, Ray Hiramoto and Vithal Ghanta, who had an ongoing setup for assaying natural killer (NK) cell activity. Employing a classical Pavlovian technique, we then set about to try again to condition IFN responses as well as the next step, NK responses. In this experiment we were joined by Brent Solvason. Figure 3 is a cartoon of the procedure.

Table 1 shows the treatment of the various control and experimental groups. For this experiment we used only a slightly-above-threshold dose of poly I:C as the unconditioned stimulus. Because the effect of a single low dose of poly I:C tends to wear off in about three days, we decided to use a three-day interval between each of the nine conditioning sessions.

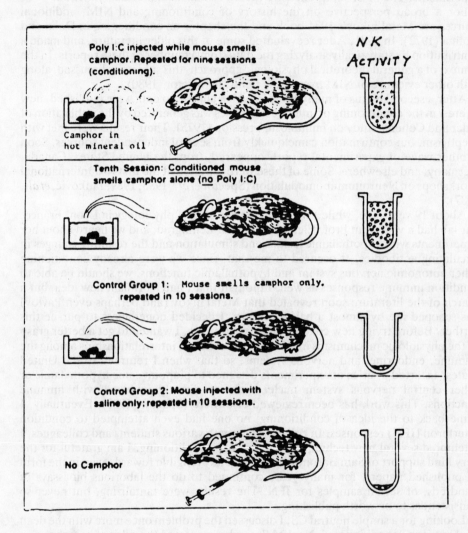

Three other control groups, with various other combinations and permutations, are not shown here.

Figure 3. Enhancement of host-defense system by classical conditioning. I am indebted to an anonymous cartoonist on the staff of the *Globe and Mail* of Toronto, Canada (January 14, 1985) for the idea for this illustration. *(Reprinted, with permission, from Spector, 1987)*

Table 1. Schedule of CS/US association trials

	Treatment	
	Association Trials Sessions 1–9 (every 72 hr)	Conditioning Test Session 10 (72 hr after Session 9)
Group 1: Saline control	Saline only No CS	Saline only No CS
Group 2: Saline + CS control	Saline + CS	Saline + CS
Group 3: Poly I:C control	POly I:C only No CS	Poly I:C only No CS
Group 4: Poly I:C, positive control	Poly I:C + CS	Poly I:C + CS
Group 5: Poly I:C, negative control	Poly I:C + CS	No treatment no CS: animals not' disturbed
Group 6: Conditioned	Poly I:C + CS	Saline + CS

ABBREVIATIONS: CS = odor of camphor; US = 20 µg Poly I:C i.p.
Reprinted in modified form, with permission, from Ghanta et al. (1985).

Our UC, poly I:C, is a synthetic polyribonucleotide that mimics the action of a virus, in that it raises IFN and NK activity, but differs from a virus in that it has no protein coat and raises little or no antibody response.

I, and my colleagues, had been using poly I:C for many years, at the suggestion of Sam Baron, in various NIM experiments, in preference to virus (which we used earlier) because of the absence of the (long-lasting, and in this case undesirable) antibody response.

Our CS, the odor of campor, was shown, in our control groups, to have no effect on NK activity. A prior search of the literature failed to reveal any other effect of camphor vapor on any other immune response.

In brief, our experiment consisted of pairing CS and US for nine consecutive sessions, repeated at three-day intervals, at the same time, place ambient temperature, and lighting conditions each time. Five different control groups (Table 1) were employed. Three days after the last association session, one group of conditioned mice was exposed to the odor of camphor. The results are shown in the cartoon (Fig. 3) and in the histogram (Fig. 4). Figure 4 shows the NK activity (measured at 50:1 effector:target cell ratio. Measurements at 100:1 and 200:1 were quite similar).

The conditioned group showed an NK activity level three times higher than the "negative control" group (conditioned but not exposed to camphor at the tenth session) and 39 times higher than the saline solution plus camphor (no Poly I:C) control groups. These results were statistically significant ($P < 0.02$ and $P < 0.0001$, respectively). Upon repeating the experiment, we obtained almost the same results, again statistically highly significant.

This was the first demonstration that NK activity could be conditioned. It was remarkable also in that it showed the possibility of a very sizeable enhancement of a

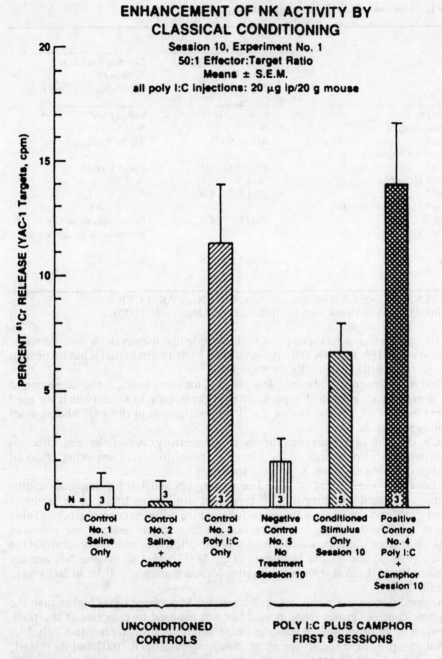

Figure 4. *(Reprinted, with permission, from Spector, 1987.)*

host-defense system in the total absence of an antigen or other US. What delighted us further was the fact, so unusual in this field of large individual variabilities, that every animal, without exception in the conditioned group, showed a rise in NK activity.

We observed, also, in this experiment, a synergistic effect of the US plus the CS (see the last bar on the right in Figure 4). An interesting historical note: Dolin and Krylov (1952) reported that the conditioned response could be many-fold greater than the response to the US alone. This was confirmed in other experiments by Berezhnykh in 1955 and Kudryasheva in 1956. Experiments in more recent times have yet to demonstrate such striking response.

Can Cancer be Reversed by Conditioning?

The experiments on conditioning are being continued and extended. Hiramoto *et al.* are combining these with studies on two cancer models in mice. We have demonstrated (Ghanta *et al.*, 1985) that conditioning can slow down the effects of cancer. Indeed, in this preliminary experiment, median survival time of the conditioned mice was longer than that of any of the several control groups, and two of the ten conditioned animals showed total and permanent regression of myeloma (MOPC 104E) tumors. Other experiments from the laboratory of Hiramoto and Ghanta employ simpler techniques of one-trial association learning, in which the NK response can be either suppressed or augmented, depending upon the nature of the US.

The doors are just being opened and the possibilities for new research and new discoveries are endless.

Neuroimmunomodulation of Immunity in Humans

The clinical applications of these findings are obviously of vast importance and offer exciting new possibilities for preventive medicine and in the treatment of many diseases, including cancer, either without the use of drugs, or least with a greatly reduced need for drugs. Often the drugs used in "treatment" today cause as many or more problems for the suffering patients than the original disease.

Luk'yanenko citied successful experiments with uses of conditioning in man. Speranskii and his followers did many experiments on dogs and then on man, in which a host of diseases were "cured" by the "pumping" technique, i.e., inserting a hypodermic needle into the subarachnoid space and pumping until the fluid turned red!! For some unknown reason, this heroic procedure and cure, widely known around the world in the 1930s seem to have vanished from the literature. See Spector, 1980, for a discussion of this strange (NIM?) phenomenon.

The time is here again to test some of our NIM concepts on humans. Using a conditioning technique, we should be able, at practically no risk to the human subject, to alter both susceptibility to disease and the course of recovery from disease.

As I have done before, I invite any of you to join me and my colleagues in several countries, in an ongoing collaborative effect to demonstrate experimentally the conditioning of NK activity and other host-defence responses in humans.

References

Ader, R. (Ed.). (1981). *Psychoneuroimmunology*. New York: Academic Press.

Ader, R, and Cohen, N. (1975). Behaviorally conditioned immuno-suppression. *Psychosomatic Medicine, 37*, 333–340.

Berezhnykh, D. V. (1955). On the question of conditioned reflex restoration of immunogenesis. *Bjulletin eksperimental 'noj Biologii i Mediciny, 40*, 49–52.

Cannon, W. B. (1936). *The wisdom of the body*. New York: Norton.

Dolin, A. O., and Dolina, C. A. (1972). *Patologilia vysshei nervnoi deyatel'nosti* (Pathology of higher nervous functions). Moskow: Vysshaya Shkola.

Dolin, A. O., and Krylov, B. N. (1952). Role of the brain in the organism's immune reaction. *Zhurnal Vysshei Nervnoi Deyatel imeni J. P. Pavlova, 2 (4)*, 547–560.

Dolin, A. O., Krylov, B. N., Luk'yanenko, V. I., and Flerov, B. A. (1960). New experimental data on conditioned reflex reproduction and suppression of immune and allergic reactions. *Zhurnal Vysshei Nervnoi Deyatel imeni J. P. Pavlova, 10*, 832–841.

Fabris, N., Garaci, E., Hadden, J., and Mitchison, N (Eds.). 1983). *Immunoregulation*. New York: Plenum.

Frederickson, R. C. A., Hendrie, H. C., Hingtgen, J. N., and Aprison, M. H. (Eds.). (1986). *Neuroregulation of autonomic, endocrine and immune systems*. Boston: Martinis Nijhoff.

Ghanta, V., Hiramoto, R., Solvason, B., and Spector, N H. (1985). Neural and environmental influences on neoplasia and conditioning of NK activity. *Journal of Immunology, 135*, 848s–852s.

Ghanta, V., Hiramoto, R., Solvason, B., and Spector, N. H. (1987). Influence of conditioned natural immunity on tumor growth. In B. D. Janković, B. M. Marković, and N. H. Spector (Eds.), Neuroimmune interactions. *Annals of the New York Academy of Sciences* (Vol. 496, pp. 637–646).

Goetzl, E., and Spector, N. H. (Eds.). (1989). *Neuro-immune networks: Physiology and disease*. New York: Alan Liss.

Guillemin, R., Cohn, M. and Melnechuk, T. (1985). *Neural modulation of immunity*. New York: Raven.

Janković, B. D., Marković, B., and Spector, N. H. (Eds). (1987). Neuroimmune interactions. *Annals of the New York Academy of Sciences* (Vol. 496).

Janković, B. D., and Spector, N. H. (1986). Lesions and Stimulation of the nervous system: Effects upon the immune system. In N. K. Plotnikoff, R. E. Faith, A. J. Murgo, and R. A. Good (Eds.), *Enkephalins and Endorphins: Stress and the immune system* (pp. 189–220). New York: Plenum.

Korneva, A. E., Klimenko, V. M., and Shkinek (1985). *Neurohumoral regulation of immune homeostasis* (Trans. and Ed. by S. A. Corson and E. O. Corson). Chicago: University of Chicago Press (Original work published 1978).

Locke, S. E., and Hornig-Rohan, M. (1983). *Mind and immunity. An annotated bibliography, 1976–1982*. New York: Institute for the Advancement of Health.

Locke, S. E. et al. (Eds,). (1985). *Foundations of psychoneuroimmunology*. New York: Aldine Publ. Co.

Luk'yanenko, V. I. (1961). The problem of conditioned-reflex regulation of immunologic reactions. *Akademia Nauk SSSR Uspekhi Sovremenoj Biologii, 51 (2)*, 170–187.

Mason, J. W. (1975). A historical view of the stress field. *Journal of Human Stress, 1 (19)*, 6–12 *(Part II in Vol. 1, issue No. 2.)*.

Metal'nikov, S. (1934). *Role de systeme nerveux et des facteurs biologiques et psychiques dans l'immunite*. Paris: Masson. (Translation in English by N. H. Spector. In preparation).

Milsum, J. H. (1985). A model of the eustress system for health/illness. *Behavioral Science, 30 (4)*, 179–186.

Pierpaoli, W., and Spector, N. H. (Eds.). (1988). Interventions in aging and cancer and NIM. *Annals of the New York Academy of Sciences* (Vol, 521).

Selye, H. (1950). *The physiology and pathology of exposure to stress*. Montreal: Acta.

Selye, H. (1956). *The stress of life*. New York: McGraw Hill.

Selye, H. (1974). *Stress without distress*. New York: Harper and Row.

Selye, H. (1975a). Stress and distress. *Comprehensive Therapy, 1 (8)*, 9–13.

Selye, H. (1975b). Confusion and controversy in the stress field. *Journal of Human Stress, 1(2)*, 37–44.

Solvason, H. B., Ghanta, V., Hiramoto, R., and Spector, N. H. (1985). Natural killer cell activity augmented by classical (Pavlovian) conditioning. In N. H. Spector et al. (Eds.), *Neuroimmunomodulation: Proceedings of the First International Workshop on NIM*. Bethesda, M. D.: International Working Group on NIM (Second edition published by Gordon and Breach, Glasgow, 1988).

Speranskii, A. D. (1934). *A basis of the theory of medicine* (Trans. and Ed. by C. P. Dutt). New York: International Publishers (Original work published 1934).

Spector, N. H. (1980). The central state of the hypothalamus in health and disease: Old and new concepts. In P. Morgane and J. Panksepp (Eds.), *Physiology of the Hypothalamus*. New York: Dekker.

Spector, N. H. (1983). Anatomical and physiological connections between the central nervous and the immune systems: Neuroimmunomodulation. In N. Fabris, E. Garaci, J. Hadden and N. Mitchison (Eds.), *Immunoregulation* (pp. 231–258). New York: Plenum.

Spector, N. H. et al. (Eds.). (1985). *Neuroimmunomodulation: Proceedings of the First International Workshop on NIM*. Bethesda, M. D.: International Working Group on NIM (Second edition published by Gordon & Breach, Glasgow, 1988).

Spector, N. H. (1986). Interactions among the nervous, immune and endocrine systems. In R. C. A. Frederickson, H. C. Hendrie, J. N. Hingtgen, and M. H. Aprison (Eds.), *Neuroregulation of autonomic, endocrine and immune systems*. Boston: Martinis Nijhoff.

Spector, N. H. (1987). Old and new strategies in the conditioning of immune responses. In B. D. Janković, B. M. Marković, and N. H. Spector (Eds.), Neuroimmune interactions. *Annals of the New York Academy of Science* (Vol. 496, pp. 522–531).

Spector, N. H. (1988). Rambunctious remarks: Perspectives in research on cancer, aging and immunity. In W. Pierpaoli, and N. H. Spector (Eds.), Interventions in Aging and Cancer and NIM. *Annals of the New York Academy of Sciences* (Vol. 521, pp. 323–335).

Spector, N. H. (in press). *The art and science of health and healing*. New York: W. W. Norton.

On Methods and Models in Research on Psychoneuroimmunology and HIV/AIDS

Lydia Temoshok

Scientists have been particularly excited about applying the methods and findings from the wider field of psychoneuroimmunology (cf. Ader, 1985; Ader, Felten, and Cohen, 1990) to biopsychosocial research in the area of Human Immunodeficiency Virus Type 1 (HIV-1), which causes the set of diseases referred to as AIDS (Acquired Immunodeficiency Syndrome). HIV disease appears to be an important area for psychoneuroimmunologic inquiry because it (a) is immunologically resisted and mediated, (b) involves immunologically exacerbated opportunistic infections and cancers, and (c) has autoimmune features. The background, rationale, and a summary of current research in this area have been summarized recently by Solomon, Kemeny and Temoshok (1990).

In addition to the temptations and advantages of using HIV as a model for psychoneuroimmunologic (PNI) research, there are a number of methodologic problems, some unique to HIV and some common to the wider field of PNI research, which must be addressed. I will comment first on some of these problems before discussing some logical and methodological issues requiring further articulation of the biopsychosocial model in terms of psychosocial and biological processes, which have arisen from our own research in this area.

Methodologic Issues in PNI Research on HIV/AIDS

Issues Involving Immunologic Measures

Many behavioral scientists believe that immunology is a more exact science than is actually the case. However, it may be said that the field, in general, suffers from a lack of information about the normal oscillation of immune parameters. There are untested assumptions involved in using and interpreting the meaning of immune measures using peripheral blood. There is debate about whether absolute numbers or percentages of different cell subsets are the more useful measure, or whether only functional tests have any meaning. There are limitations involved in both enumeration and functional assays. Unfortunately, there are no adequate measures to approximate the immune system's functioning *as a system*; i.e., keeping a homeostatic balance, responding appropriately to antigenic challenges, and so forth.

Even if there were clarity on these issues, selection of relevant measures that have a relationship to disease progression and outcome is a major challenge. Ideally, these measures would have casual or contributory significance and not be merely "marker" variables. After appropriate measures are selected, there are a number of sources of variability that must be held to a minimum: (a) technical variability (differences in laboratory technicians, reagents, equipment, etc.), (b) inter-laboratory variability, (c) within-run and run-to-run variability in a single laboratory, (d) temporal variability (how soon measurements are made after samples are obtained; time of day samples are obtained), and (e) assay variation. Behavioral scientists who must rely on outside laboratories, rather than work collaboratively with immunologists in their own settings, need to be particularly aware of these potential sources of variability, which can completely obscure any variation attributable to psychosocial factors.

Issues Arising from the Nature of HIV Disease.

While HIV/AIDS strikes the enthusiastic behavioral researcher as an ideal model of psychoimmunologic research, HIV infection and progression are extremely complex and still poorly understood phenomena. In contrast to some of the cancer models used in psychoimmunologic research, HIV presents a situation in which psychologic, neurologic, and immunologic changes occur as *central*, rather than as resultant or adjunctive, aspects of the disease process. A major problem in being able to relate psychosocial factors to disease progression is that the time of infection is usually unknown, and neither symptom development nor immunologic status is a good estimate of this. Other complications for researchers who are trying to decipher any potential contributory role for psychosocial factors include: (a) medications – – prescribed, experimental. "alternative," and self-administered, as well as vitamins; (b) illness type and severity (e.g., there are immunologic as well as psychosocial and demographic differences between persons with AIDS who have Kaposi's sarcoma and those with *Pneumocystis carinii* pneumonia as their primary diagnosis; (c) viral co-factors, such as Epstein Barr virus, or Cytomegalovirus, which may accompany, potentiate, and/or exacerbate HIV and its immunologic consequences, and (d) behaviors such as drug use, alcohol use, and sexual intercourse, which have immunologic consequences independent of their potential for HIV transmission.

Issues Involving Psychosocial Measures

Selecting relevant psychosocial measures is at least if not more difficult than choosing immunologic measures. Ideally, measures should have published reliability, validity, and norms, and have been used in at least one other psycho-immunologic study (of any kind). One problem is that because of the nature of HIV disease and its epidemiology, some standard tests are not appropriate for certain affected populations. For example, standard stress surveys are inadequate for assessing the stressors of an inner-city black adolescent, a gay man who has had 25 of his friends die from AIDS, or an intravenous drug user, among others.

Special Problems Related to Specific Subject Populations

Much of the early research (starting 1983) on psychosocial factors in HIV/AIDS was conducted using white, well-educated homosexual men in big cities – San Francisco, New York, and Los Angeles. It is likely that little of this is generalizable to other groups whose behaviors or sociodemographic situations place them at risk for HIV infection or transmission: bisexual men, IV drug users, partners of bisexual men or IV drug users, hemophiliacs, children of HIV-infected mothers, adolescents, Blacks, and Hispanics. Before attempting to ascertain the role of psychosocial factors in

HIV/AIDS progression or immunology, researchers must understand something about the sociology, epidemiology, virology, and immunology of HIV in a given risk group.

Data Analysis: The Problem of Individual Differences

A predictive model works if it is able to predict an event, on average, more of the time than not (obviously it works better if it can predict approaching 100%). A causal model works if it is able to specify precisely the times, conditions, and/or individuals under which the cause-effect linkages are 100%. In other words, if X causes Z only in the context of Y, then the precise causal model would be stated: "X in the presence of Y causes Z, not "X causes Z 80% of the time" (assuming Y is the situation 80% of the time).

The predominant use of certain statistical methods tends to bias us in terms of only being able to investigate relationships in terms of predictive rather than causal relationships. For example, different results were obtained when we examined our data on relationships among psychosocial and immunologic variables in men with AIDS using (a) between subjects correlation (collapsing immunologic and psychosocial variables across 6 weeks of measures), and (b) within subjects correlations (for each subject across 6 time points). It turns out that that for some immunologic-psychologic variables, one cluster of individuals showed one pattern, e.g., a strong positive correlation, while another cluster showed a different one, e.g., a negative correlation. The effects of these opposite patterns would cancel each other out in the between subjects correlations (cf. Temoshok & Jenkins, 1988).

Based on these experiences, we would recommend that researchers consider using less traditional analytic techniques such as within subject correlations, cluster and pattern analysis, and so forth, which may reveal subtleties of psychoimmunologic relationships and important individual differences in the nature of the direction, strength, and frequency of psychosocial-immunologic interactions that may be obscured by more traditional analytic methods.

Interpretation of Results: The Problem of Discrepant Findings

If X and Y are strongly and significantly correlated in one study, but the findings are in the opposite direction in another study, this may suggest that the relationships are non-linear. This possibility is often obscured, however, when the findings occur in separate rather than in the same study, because in the former situation, subject and other methodologic differences – – or the mere "explanation" of nonreplicability/ unstable findings – – are more salient.

In an intensive psychoimmunologic pilot study of 18 men with frank AIDS, in whom both psychosocial and immunologic measures were obtained weekly for 6 weeks (Solomon, Temoshok, O'Leary, & Zich, 1987), the following pattern of correlations was found: standard self-report measures of psychosocial distress (e.g., anxiety, depression, fatigue-intertia) were generally significantly correlated in the positive direction (controlling for type of AIDS-related illness and time since AIDS diagnosis) with absolute numbers of different T-cell subsets, including CD4 cells (Temoshok et al., 1987, June). However, significant correlations were *negative* for many of the same pairs of distress and immunologic variable in a study of 104 symptomatic seropositive men who could be said to have AIDS-related Complex or ARC (Temoshok et al., 1988, June).

One explanation to reconcile these ARC findings with the seemingly contradictory findings in the first AIDS study is to consider psychologic, neuropsychologic, and immunologic variables in terms of a process model of psychological reactions to HIV disease progression. At the initial testing point of our second study of men with ARC, the men were all newly diagnosed with HIV-related symptoms, in contrast to the men with AIDS in the first study, who had been diagnosed with AIDS for at least several months and up to 4 years. Our previous study of men with both AIDS and ARC showed that men with ARC were actually more distressed than those with AIDS (Temoshok, Mandel, Moulton, Solomon, & Zich, 1986, May). Another study comparing HIV seropositive but asymptomatic men with those who had ARC or AIDS suggested that the development and recognition of HIV-related symptoms is the most psychosocially distressing event in the HIV disease trajectory (Moulton Stempel, Bacchetti, Temoshok, & Moss, 1989). Thus, different psychosocial reactions to different points of the HIV disease trajectory could contribute to the differences between our studies of men with ARC and men with AIDS. However, in order to produce a satisfactory explanation of the differences in the *psychoimmunologic* relationships, we may need to take into account another process, the disease process itself, as well as the host's physiological responses, which will be discussed below.

It is, of course, impossible to determine causal relationships from correlational data. There are at least two alternatives to the psychosomatic hypothesis that psychcial distress affects immune functioning: (a) psychosocial distress may result from viral activation, which in turn stimulates various immunologic responses (the somatopsychic hypothesis); or (b) psychosocial distress and immunologic up-regulation may both be a function of viral activation, and/or of clinical symptoms (the third factor hypothesis).

Keeping these caveats in mind, but still attempting to see whether our data would be at least consistent with the psychosomatic hypothesis, we could speculate that the positive correlations between distress and immune cell numbers and function in men with ARC may represent the immune system's attempt to respond to or possibly to compensate for the immunologic challenge posed by HIV infection. Thus, one way to interpret the contrasting and puzzling results across the two studies is to pose the hypothesis that the hypothetical effects of psychosocial distress on the immune system may be up or down-regulating *depending on the ability of the immune system to respond to biologic or psychosocial challenges* (Temoshok, Solomon, Jenkins, and Sweet, 1989, January). Thus, for men with ARC, who have relatively well functioning immune systems characteristic of an earlier point in the HIV disease process, the response to distress may be immunologic up-regulation (yielding a positive correlation between distress and immune cell numbers); whereas, the relatively depleted and malfunctioning immune systems of men with AIDS are only able to down-regulate in the face of stress (yielding a negative correlation between distress and immune cell numbers). These interactions would produce, theoretically, a U-shaped nonlinear function if the AIDS and ARC data were combined into a single graph, and ability of the immune system to respond in an up-regulatory manner were plotted against degree of psychosocial distress.

Such an interpretation varies from such "standard" psychoimmunologic assumptions as, for example, that an increase in certain immune subsets means "immune enhancement" which is always "good;" or that a decrease in immune numbers means "immune suppression" which is always "bad". However, our experience in conducting psychoimmunologic HIV research suggests that when interpreting the meaning of psychoimmunologic relationships, it is important to consider what is "adaptive" or "maladaptive" for the system as a whole.

General Design Issues: Models and Paradigms

It is perhaps a simplistic but often overlooked truism that what emerges in a predictive model is a function of its ingredients. While fewer and more homogenous ingredients may produce an elegantly simple model, such a model may not work well when additional or different ingredients are included. As a behavioral scientist investigating psychosocial factors that may be involved in the progression of HIV disease, I have for many years embraced the *biopsychosocial model* of health and illness as an extension and elaboration of the traditional biomedical model. Unfortunately, the biopsychosocial model is acknowledged more in theory than in practice.

One possible explanation for this comes from a number of social psychological experiments showing that people often act in ways far more consistent with beliefs in unitary causation, or as if causal candidates competed with one another in a zero-sum game (Nisbett & Ross, 1980). When it comes to causes, people tend to embrace whatever looks like parsimony. For example, we have been taught and rewarded to think this way in designing scientific experiments. Single cause-effect models have some practical advantages: they are economical, efficient, decrease information overload, and enable us to act (instead of remaining lost in thought as we contemplate multiple contingencies).

If biology can explain most of the variance, statistically, in disease cause, course, and treatment, why contemplate a biopsychosocial model? One reason is accuracy, and a scientific motivation to approximate "the truth." Most events are multiply determined. Awareness of multiple influences can lead to the development of multiple interventions. When the main intervention developed from a single cause-effect model proves ineffective or unacceptable for a given person, alternatives are available. More importantly, the additional interventions may bolster the effectiveness of the primary intervention. Such interventions are complementary not competitive. At times, augmenting treatment effects may spell the difference between recovery and decline. For example, many oncologists are aware that "hope" and "social support" can significantly affect medical outcomes in their patients. The traditional medical model is also compatible with multiple interventions, and multicasual etiological formulations, as it recognizes such phenomena as drug and pathogen interactions. But the medical model traditionally restricts itself to one of intervention: biology. The biopsychosocial model legitimizes two additional domains of influence: the psychological and the social (both interpersonal and sociopolitical).

Why All this Discussion is not Merely Academic

If the "true" situation is : more X predicts increases in Z (a negative event), more Y causes decreases in Z, and more X causes increases in Y through a feedback mechanism, then if you do something to decrease X, thinking it will decrease Z, you will instead increase Z (because the decreased X will stimulate decreases in Y which will then cause more Z). This only appears to be a paradoxial occurrence to the extent prediction and cause are confused. The clinical value of prediction is informational. Being able to predict Z from X may be very useful, for example, in making accurate prognostic statements about the course of a disease, or in prescribing a medicine that will provide symptomatic relief in 90% of patients, or 90% of the time. Understanding *cause*, however, is probably crucial in developing an effective prevention or cure. To base an intervention, particularly a powerful medical one, on prediction alone is risky because one may interfere with complex causal processes, and may inadvertently cause or exacerbate a negative event.

There is much we do not understand about how the immune system works *as a system* (cf. Temoshok, 1988). We know still less about how the immune system works when it is reacting to HIV-1 and its associated infections. Effective means of preventing and treating HIV infection are dependent upon understanding causal connections and mechanisms in HIV infection, progression, and biopsychosocial responses. To do this, we must be able to recognize and respond to the methodologic challenges posed by psychoneuroimmunologic HIV/AIDS research, and to be willing to consider and employ multidimensional models of health and illness.

References

Ader, R. (Ed.), (1981). *Psychoneuroimmunology*. New York: Academic Press.

Ader, R., Felten, D.L. and Cohen, N. (Ed), *Psychoneuroimmunology II*. (1990). Orlando, FL: Academic Press.

Moulton, J. M., Stempel, R., Bacchetti, P., Moss, A., and Temoshok, L. (in press). Psychological consequences of HIV test notification: Results of a one-year longitudinal study from the San Francisco General Hospital cohort. *Journal of Acquired Immune Deficiency Syndromes*.

Nisbett, R. E., and Ross, L. (1980). *Human inference: Strategies and shortcoming of social judgement*. Englewood Cliffs, N. J: Prentice-Hall, Inc.

Solomon, G.F.F., Kemeny, M. and L. Temoshok, (1990). Psychoneuroimmunologic aspects of Human Immunodeficiency Virus infection. In R. Ader, D. L. Felten, and N. Cohen (Eds.), *Psychoneuroimmunology II*. Orlando, FL: Academic Press.

Temoshok, L. (1988). *Report on the First Research Workshop on Psychoneuroimmunology and HIV disease*. Washington, D. C.: National Institute of Mental Health.

Temoshok, L., Mandel, J. S., Moulton, J. M., Solomon, G. F. and Zich, J. (1986). *A longitudinal psychosocial study of AIDS and ARC in San Francisco: Preliminary results*. Paper presented at the Annual Meeting of the American Psychiatric Association. Washington. D. C.

Temoshok, L., Solomon, G. F., Jenkins, S.R. and Sweet, D. M. (1989) *Psychoimmunologic studies of men with AIDS and ARC*. Paper presented at the Annual Meeting of the American Association for the Advancement of Science. San Franscisco, CA.

Temoshok, L., Solomon, G. F., Sweet, D. M., Jenkins, S.R., Zich, J., Straits, K., Pivar, I. and Moulton, J. M. and Stites, D. P. (1988). *A psychoimmunologic study of men with ARC*. Paper presented at the IV International Conference on AIDS. Stockholm, Sweden.

Temoshok, L., Zich, J., Solomon, G. F. and Stites, D. P. (1987) *An intensive psychoimmunologic study of long-surviving persons with AIDS*. Paper presented at the III International Conference on AIDS. Washington, D. C.

Section 2

Health Promotion and Primary Prevention

The Importance of Psychosocial Interventions in Primary Health Care

René F. W. Diekstra and Mary A. Jansen

Introduction

The role of psychology and of many psychologists in the health field has been undergoing a gradual but important change over the last decade or so. Traditionally, psychologists have participated in teaching, research and practice in the health system, but primarily in collaboration with or under the auspices of psychiatrists. Like psychiatrists, most psychologists have defined their role as that of speciality care for mental health service delivery (Wright & Burns, 1986). The specialist role of psychologists has generally caused them to provide mental health care only for mental health problems. This orientation has had two important consequences. First of all, psychologists used to see and still see only a very small portion of the total number of people in need of mental health advice or treatment. Second, physical complaints or distress resulting from psychological or social factors, even when recognized as such, have usually been considered reasons to consult a general or family physician, not a psychologist, since in most places the health system works from general to specialized care. Reports from a number of countries indicate indeed that family physicians (Hosman, 1983; Shepherd, 1980) or pediatricians (American Academy of Pediatrics, 1978) are much more often consulted for mental and behavioural problems than psychologists or other specialized mental health workers. Since physicians generally are not well-equiped to assess, treat and prevent mental health problems, most patients consulting them for such problems (or for physical conditions they themselves have caused are often not adequately served or are even not taken seriously. This in turn reinforces already prevailing ideas that many mental health complaints are not treatable, not important enough to be presented as reasons for treatment, or simply disappear as time goes by.

It is only recently that psychologists have explored and propagated the application of their instrumentarium for general health. This is reflected in concepts like psychological medicine, behavioural medicine and health psychology. Increased effort in basic and applied research in areas such as effects of behaviour on body processes, the effects of physical abnormalities on behavior, illness behaviour, sick role behaviour, health care processes and treatment settings and devices have and still do reveal the utmost importance of a mental health and behavioural component in general health care (Hamburg, Elliott & Parson, 1982).

This development has coincided with a growing awareness among political and health policy bodies, both national and international, that existing health care systems, including traditional mental health care, have failed to provide for the health needs of most people, are too costly and are themselves a cause for a considerable burden of ill-health and disease. The main reason for this is that these systems are mostly centralized, hospital-based, specialist-focused, disease-oriented and delivered by medical personnel in a one-to-one "up-down" doctor-patient relationship. They are also predominantly reactive systems, waiting for people to become ill and then treating them or nursing them until the acute episode of the illness passes. Or they take it for granted that people will become chronically ill and provide them with medical care for the rest of their lives (WHO, 1978).

The shift in the health service structure under way in many countries, like in the United States, is towards decentralized care, with greater emphasis on health maintenance and health promotion, with active involvement of the community and the family, to be undertaken primarily by non-specialized general health workers collaborating with personnel in governmental and non-governmental sectors (e. g. self-help organizations) and only secondarily by speciality care workers.

This change in policy is epitomized in the program called Health for All by the Year 2000 (WHO, 1981) that the World Health Organization and its member states have adopted as their present and future health strategy. The implication of the Health for All strategy with its emphasis on primary health care (PHC), also in the area of mental health, will have important consequences for the role of psychology as a discipline and for psychologists as professionals in the health field (Diekstra, 1987).

The first and foremost consequence is that psychology and psychologists, in order to continue to play a significant role in health care, will have to "generalize". Psychological knowledge and skills should be adapted to the primary health care setting.

Health for All

Only a few years ago, in 1977, WHO's policy-making body, the World Health Assembly, made a momentous decision. It decided that the main social targets of governments and WHO in the coming decades should be the attainment by all people of the world by the year 2000 of a level of health that will permit them to lead a socially and economically productive life. This is popularly known as Health for All by the Year 2000 (WHO, 1981).

Behaviour and Health

If we try to sum up the implications that HFA/2000 has in general and for the related professional groups, the following picture emerges. People, including health personnel and their elected representatives, should work together to promote health, prevent disease, alleviate unavoidable disease and disability, improve the process of being born and growing up, insure that all are healthy enough to work productively and to participate in the social life of the community, and finally, facilitate growing old gracefully and dying in dignity.

The underlying assumption in all these aspects of HFA/2000 is that there is a very intimate relationship between between people's behaviour, their lifestyles, and their level of health. The impact of behaviour on the burden of illness and mortality is reflected in the fact that nonadherence to hygiene and safety prescriptions, alcohol and drug abuse, smoking, nonadherence to proven medical regimes, bad eating habits and lack of skills for coping with stress are disproportionately present among persons who are ill or die prematurely, that is, before the usual life expectancy (Hamburg, Elliott & Parson, 1982).

In developing countries the main causes of illness are malnutrition (including energy malnutrition and vitamin A deficiency blindness), malaria, acute respiratory infections, diarrhoea, leprosy, tuberculosis and common infectious diseases of childhood. Many of these illnesses are contracted, or one could even say, caused by people's behaviour. For example, in developing countries, about 200 million people are infected by parasites that cause schistomiasis, a disease that can cause very severe disability and death. To as many as 600 million people schistosomiasis represents a constant threat. It has been established that it is people's behaviour, urinating and defecating in water that is also used for swimming, fishing, farming, washing and bathing, that actually causes schistosomiasis.

Much of the disease and disability that people in the industrialized countries have is caused by overeating, overdrinking, overdriving cars, overdriving themselves, overdrugging themselves, overpolluting the air, overpolluting the water and oversedentary living in towns. No wonder that there is so much cardiovascular disease, cancer and accidents in these countries.

The question then arises, what answers are there to such diverse problems as these? They obviously cannot be dealt with adequately by a classical medical care model, that is, by waiting for people to become ill and then treating them or nursing them until the acute episode of the illness passes, or taking it for granted that people with become chronically ill and providing them with medical care for the rest of their lives.

Towards a New Model of Health Care

Is it at all possible, one could ask, to identify a universal model that could be adapted to different circumstances? An international conference, held in Alma Ata in 1978 declared that Health for All could be attained through health systems based on what is called primary health care. According to the statement that was formulated in the Alma Ata declaration, health systems based on primary health care or with an emphasis on primary health care have the following characteristics (WHO, 1978) First of all, they reflect the social, economic and political characterists of the country, state or community in question. Secondly, they give priority of those most in need. Furthermore, they address the main health problems in the community. Fourth, they provide promotive, curative and rehabilitative services. They involve other related sectors such as agriculture and animal husbandry, food, industry and most importantly, education. They use health technology that is appropriate; appropriate meaning – and implication that is essential for the role psychology will play in primary health care – that wherever possible social and behavioural alternatives for medical technical measures should be used as widely as possible. The Declaration of Alma Ata also defined eight essential elements that primary health care should include. Within the framework of this chapter, the first one is the most essential, namely: "Primary health care includes: education concerning prevailing health problems and methods of preventing and controlling them." This element, which in abbreviated form can be labelled health promotion or promotion of lifestyles or behaviour patterns that are conducive to good health, really is the antithesis of the classical medical care model

Promotion of Health

What does health promotion imply? It is an evolving concept. Some of the main components of health promotion according to WHO at this time are:

- fostering healthy lifestyles;
- fostering social, economic and environmental conditions conductive to health;
- trying to attain these two by raising awareness about health matters in individuals and communities;
- by enabling people to cope with their and their family's health problems both general and mental health problems; and
- by encouraging social support or the the use of social support.

Further, health promotion implies judicious taxation that promotes health. It also implies producing and consuming food and drink conducive to health. It emphasizes adequate and appropriate exercise. It emphasizes teaching people to use adequate and healthy sleeping patterns. It emphasizes that people are educated and work in conformity with their physical and mental capacity. It emphasizes suitable living arrangements in terms of housing and social support within reach. It emphasizes the improvement of the physical, psychological and social environment of people.

Health-Damaging Lifestyles

There exists enough scientific evidence on the effects of certain types of behaviour to classify them as well-established and unambigous forms of risk behaviour, such as excessive smoking, alcohol use in excess, misuse of medical and mood-altering drugs, inadequate eating patterns, lack of physical exercise, dangerous driving, violent behaviour and inadequate or deficient stress management skills. The negative health effects of these behaviours are in fact so well studied and – at least in principle – generally agreed upon that both large-scale intervention programmes and primary health care individually-oriented programmes are called for which aim at reducing their occurence. Several recent WHO documents explicitly state that the psychological sciences have to make a significant contribution here, such as:

- analysis of the subjective meaning and of the functions which these forms of behaviour serve for the individual or social group (e.g. youth cultures) concerned;
- identification of the social forces which tend (directly or indirectly) to stabilize and encourage these forms of risk behaviour;
- development, testing and comparison of different intervention strategies aimed both at the risk-taking individuals and at the social forces which foster such risk-taking;
- assistance in providing these interventions at all levels of care, in particular, primary health care;
- evaluation of all intervention programmes.

Other Types of Risk Behaviour

The forms of risk behaviour just mentioned explain only a part of the variants of behaviour-related health outcomes. Health education and disease intervention research and programmes tend to concentrate on these forms, probably because only individuals seem to be involved and because attempts to reduce the health risks can be directed toward individuals rather than social institutions or persons in authority. As a result, the concept of risk behaviour is in danger of being narrowed down to "misbehaviour", like excessive smoking and alcohol drinking. There are other forms of suspected risk behaviour, but current knowledge and general acceptance is perhaps not sufficient to start intervention programmes. The available knowledge in psychology though is sufficient to justify major efforts directed at the suspected health-damaging effects of some widespread and socially-accepted lifestyles. Among these are those listed in Table 1.

Table 1 *Risk behaviours and health damaging lifestyles*

Situation	Description
(a) Occupational	1. Chronic stress from structural and social conflicts in the work situation.
	2. Stress resulting from excessive time pressure.
	3. Highly competitive work situations which lead to overly aggressive behaviour, over-ambition and pressure to achieve.
	4. Shift work and unstable employment or unemployment.
	5. Alcoholism which may both result from these stressors and contribute to, or exacerbate them.
(b) Gender role	1. Chronic stress resulting from the inferior social status of women.
	2. Chronic stress resulting from the continued expectation of emotional suppression in men.
	3. Role strain arising from dual expectations most frequently seen in women in family and organizational roles.
(c) Socialization	1. Stress resulting from rapid social change including urbanization and modernization.
	2. Stress resulting from rapid technological change including computerization, job conversion or elimination due to technical advances.
	3. Stress resulting from consolidation mergers in the corporate world resulting in a need for mobility and disruption of family ties.
(d) Iatrogenic	1. Risk factors introduced by the health system itself such as poor doctor/patient communication resulting in mis-diagnosis.
	2. Over prescription of harmful or addictive drugs.
	3. Stress resulting from health care systems and professionals which encourage the passive "patient-role" with no opportunity to impact on one's own care.
	4. Impersonalization and an emphasis on technological aspects of health care.

(see also Hammonds & Scheirer, 1984, for a complete review).

Health-Enhancing Lifestyles

Enhancing lifestyles that promote, maintain or improve the health status of individuals and the population in general is clearly an important aspect of the HFA/

2000 strategy. Unfortunately, the concept of positive health is presently neither clearly defined nor well-studied empirically. If the very promising approach of supporting a healthy lifestyle is to be pursued, there is an urgent need for a much greater influence of psychological knowledge in studies and programmes directed towards establishing the positive health effects of lifestyles or elements of lifestyles. Research findings so far, especially by psychologists (Steptoe & Mathews, 1984) point to several aspects of lifestyles which probably contribute to maintenance of good health:

- sufficient income and adequate command of the work and domestic situation;
- adequate psychological and behavioural mechanisms for coping with emerging problems;
- social integration and sufficient social support in times of crisis;
- self-esteem and feelings of sufficient internal control over one's life;
- beliefs which emphasize personal influence on health and well-being.

On all these aspects psychologists have much to offer both in terms of research and strategies and methods for fostering such lifestyle aspects, and in the exploration of ways of spreading such health-enhancing lifestyles in the general population and among those in control.

Introduction of Changes of Lifestyle

Inherent in the lifestyle approach and therefore inherent in the primary health care emphasis within HFA/2000, the intention is to introduce change in prevailing lifestyles: to spread health-enhancing, and to reduce health-damaging lifestyles. From a behavioural point of view, the attempt to introduce a healthy lifestyle as a normal way of life to society poses some general problems which have consequences for the content and the provision of care. For a balance has to be found between a legitimate intent to influence other people's way of life to their own benefit on the one hand, and on the other, the basic right of these same people to choose their own way of life and define for themselves what is beneficial. This balance can obviously be established only if the "objects" of the intervention have an equal say in the planning and realization of the intervention programme.

The methodologies for such a participative approach which has to be considered as a basis for any primary health care programme are at present unsatisfactory, need further development and will be dependent upon a massive influence of psychological knowledge from research and in terms of developing and providing of health care interventions. Furthermore, if the intervention programmes focus exclusively on the well-established forms of risk behaviour – they can easily lead to moralistic attitudes (e.g. blaming the victim) and this imposes an additional burden on individuals already at increased risk.

Finally, promoting healthy lifestyles as a normal way of life has to safeguard against "healthism": establishing an ideal of a healthy, socially fully-integrated, psychologically well-balanced individual as a social norm. Before and after the year 2000 physical and emotional suffering, loneliness, poverty and misery, illness and dying will remain part of the human condition: if the ideal healthy person were established as a norm, this could help many people to adopt health-enhancing life-styles.

Another area of neglect thus far has been the development of individual health promotion in the form of counseling individuals who are starting their career as a patient in the health care system on how to change their lifestyle and develop more healthy styles of life. Behavioural counseling in primary health care is still in its infancy (Carnwath & Miller, 1986).

This leads us to the importance of social support and the importance of individuals' use of skills to mobilize social networks and to make use of social relationships in times of crisis (Mechanic, 1983). The individual's capacity to mobilize social networks related to his or her present needs signals the importance of what in present day behavioural science is called the coping repertoire or the coping styles of individuals and of groups. Since chronic conflict and stress have to be considered as major factors influencing behaviour-related health outcomes, adequate coping capacities of individuals are obviously an important element of health-enhancing lifestyles. The current state of scientific knowledge in psychology indicates that there is sufficient evidence, for example, based on studies of coping with chronic disease such as cancer, to prove the relevance of the concept. However, many questions about the differential effects need decisive answers.

Mental Health in Health Care

The mental health component of health care comprises the following quite distinct, but unfortunately often confused, areas, as described in Table 2:

Table 2 *The role of psychologists and mental health in general health care*

Emphasis	Examples
(a) Practical relevance of psychological skills in health care	1. Improving the functioning of general health sciences. 2. Supporting overall socio-economic development. 3. Enhancing the quality of life. 4. Clinical psychological interventions in general health care. 5. Promoting mental and emotional health as a positive life goal.
(b) Traditional mental health skills	1. Activities involved in the diagnosis, treatment, and rehabilitaion of mental and neurological disorders. 2. Activities to prevent the development of mental and neurological disorders.

The first group have seldom formed part of the tasks actually assigned to health care workers. But they are essential PHC skills. These aspects can be partially the responsibility of primary (mental) health care workers, but also require the involvement of specialists. If psychology is to serve both areas appropriately then it follows logically that the emphasis in the training of psychologists has to shift towards the training of mental health generalists for PHC and away from mental health/psychotheraphy specialists, without however discarding the latter.

On Appropriate Care

One of the most evident implications of the mental health component in the Health for All strategy is the introduction of psychosocial and behavioural analysis and intervention as part of the activity of primary health care workers. This requires a massive influx of skills and knowledge from scientific and professional psychology.

But how is this going to happen? It is apparent that in most countries much greater emphasis is given to physical than to mental problems in both the training and practice of those involved in primary health care. The most cursory examination of primary health care manuals and textbooks makes this apparent. This stands in clear contrast to the also broadly accepted and acknowledged fact that mental health problems are widely prevalent, constituting a distressing burden in the population, are very often brought to the attention of primary care practitioners, but are often not identified and are very frequently inadequately assessed and treated. This statement holds true for most communities despite considerable differences in the organization and delivery of primary health care. For example, in some countries such as France, the vast majority of doctors in primary health care work single-handedly, whereas in the United Kingdom the majority of general practitioners collaborate in partnership (i.e. groups of cooperating doctors) or interdisciplinary teams, usually comprised of social workers and nurses. In other countries such as the United States, patients may have a family physician but are also able to directly call on specialists such as pediatricians or gynacologists who have a specific responsibility for the category of patients within the area of expertise. Research suggests that in countries where primary health care depends on physicians, such as is the case in most parts of the world, as a group these practitioners presently lack the interest and expertise to respond to the psychological and mental health problems of their patients. There would appear to be two main avenues open to improving this unsatisfactory situation, each of which carries profound organizational, practical and research implications.

(a) The primary health care worker is guided and trained to reorient his or her way of dealing with help seekers in such a way as to include mental health care in his or her practice. This necessarily implies the need to improve knowledge and skills to ensure that necessary tasks can be carried out economically and effectively; it also implies that psychological techniques for widespread dissemination, techniques that are simple and easily applicable, be developed and tested. Health care practitioners do not perceive themselves to be the right people to deal with these problems. When faced with such problems, they usually feel inadequate and may respond with lack of sympathy or inappropriate advice. Comprehensive primary health care as meant by the Alma Ata Declaration and as meant in the WHO programme of Health for All by the Year 2000 can only be realized if there is considerable reorientation in basic and additional training of doctors, nurses and other primary health care workers. However, sufficient evidence attesting to the feasibility of this has not yet been gathered, anywhere in the world.

(b) The second avenue is essentially based on the view that it is impossible for a primary health care worker to combine in one and the same person the necessary and sufficient knowledge and skills for dealing with both the physical and psychological or mental health complaints or problems of patients. The logical consequence of this point of view is that on the primary health care level, there should be direct access and availability of generalists both in physical health care and in psychological health care. This in turn implies that primary health care should be carried out by a combination of different disciplines, of which psychology is one. The suggestion here is that psychologists as practitioners have an important role to play in primary health care, a viewpoint that has been advocated for more than a decade (Broadhurst, 1972). Indeed, in a number of countries in Europe, for example, England and the Netherlands, it is estimated that one in five to seven psychologists are already working with general practitioners.

When one asks which of the two avenues described here is generally to be preferred, the answer can only be that this is not the right question to ask. First of all, not enough research has been done thus far to allow a clear choice between the two alternatives. And secondly, the choice depends, among other things, on the cultural, social and financial situation that is present in a specific community or state. Furthermore, it might well be that both approaches are not as contradictory or mutually exclusive as they seem at first glance. It might very well turn out that the particular contributions that a psychologist could make in primary health care and to each primary medicine speciality may be different in different communities and (sub)cultures.

The Role of Psychologists with Regard to Primary Health Care

One conclusion from the foregoing is that there are different ways in which psychologists can contribute to primary health care. These are (see also Marzillier & Hall, 1987):

(a) providing a diagnostic and treatment service;
(b) acting as consultants and teachers to other professionals;
(c) acting as referrers to and quality assessors of specialty mental health services;
(d) carrying out research; and
(e) setting up, carrying out and evaluating prevention and health promotion programmes.

Clearly the difference between the two approaches described in the previous paragraphs is mainly in relation to the role described under (a). Therefore in the remainder of this paper we will mainly address important aspects of the role of psychologists in primary health care as providers of diagnostic and treatment service.

Problems Amenable to Interventions by Psychologists in Primary Health Care

An important question to be asked is: What kind of problems are amenable to interventions by psychologists in primary health care? In a survey of general practitioners in the United Kingdom the most common problems deemed particularly suitable for referral to psychologists were (in order): phobias, chronic anxiety, obsessional disorders, smoking problems, drinking problems, psychosexual problems and interpersonal problems (Marzillier & Hall, 1987). The GPs also rated a therapeutic role in primary health care as by far the most useful role for psychologists. According to the authors the answer to the questions: What sort of problems would be most effectively dealt with by psychologists in primary health care? can be answered by referring to the categories of problem areas that Kincey (1974) has described (Table 3).

Characteristics of Primary Health Care Psychology

Although without any doubt most psychologist practitioners would agree that they have special competence in these areas, it has to be pointed out that dealing with such problems within primarily health care requires specific adaptations and skills which

Table 3 *Psychosocial interventions categories of psychological problems amenable to primary psychological intervention (adaped from Kincey, 1974)*

Category	Description
(a) Problems of anxiety and stress	Generalized anxiety, panic attacks, phobias, obsessional ideas or rituals, stress-induced or aggravated illnesses, e.g. migraine, asthma, cardiovascular disease.
(b) Habit disorders	Various habitual behaviors that lead to personal distress, ill-health or social problems, e.g. smoking, obesity, bulimia, problem drinking, enuresis, encopresis, drug addiction.
(c) Educational, occupational difficulties or decisions	Choice of transition points throughout life span, e.g. leaving school, change of job, retirement. Problems that arise in the educational-occupational context, e.g. study problems, lack of confidence and social skills.
(d) Interpersonal-social-marital problems	Problems arising from relationship with others, e.g. shyness, unassertiveness, marital discord, psychosexual problems, antisocial and aggressive behaviour.
(e) Psychological adjustment to physical illness and other significant life events	Adjustment to psychological aspects of illness and hospitalization. Adjustment to chronic disability, childbirth, accident, terminal illness, death.

psychologists trained traditionally usually do not have. Typically, primary mental health care differs from traditional psychological service in three ways: more clients are seen, less time is spent with each and clients generally have less debilitating forms of disorder, implying usually a more rapid turnover of clients and briefer consultations as well as other forms of short-term care. The problem is, however, as Wright and Burns (1986) also stated, that psychologists' exclusive commitment to traditional approaches often prevents them from developing training and research resources for the most ubiquitous problems and the most frequently-used methods for responding to them. However, when psychology really strives for an important and essential role in primary health care as envisioned in HFA/2000 it will of necessity have to reorient itself in this respect, implying that one is willing to give up or modify some of the traditional approaches and viewpoints and look for more effective, shorter and simpler ways of dealing with behavioural and emotional problems. A clear example of this is the wide diversion in the psychological literature on what can be called short-term interventions (Strupp & Binder, 1984). Under this term some authors see treatments that might amount to 20 sessions of 50 minutes each within the period of 6 to 12 months. Other authors define as short term, treatments that do not exceed five sessions of 50 minutes each or even shorter duration. Within the framework of primary health care the first definition of short term is clearly unacceptable. One could also argue that the second definition of five sessions of 50 minutes or less should even be closely scrutinized and not accepted without discussion. As a matter of fact, some of the studies that have looked into the effectiveness of psychological treatment, that is treatment by psychologists on the primary health care level, have revealed that even shorter treatments can be effective (Rosen & Wiens, 1979). Robson, France and Bland (1984) assigned 429 patients randomly either to a treatment group consisting of psychological treatment from one of four psychologists working in general practice or to a control group which consisted of management by a general practitioner. Treatment was up to a maximum of 10 weeks and averaged 3.6 sessions with 2-½ hours of psychologist's time. The results of the study showed favourable reactions to psychological treatment. Patients treated by the psychologist showed significantly greater improvement in their presenting problems than control patients immediately after treatment and up to 24 weeks follow-up. They made significantly fewer visits to the GPs during treatment and up to 24 weeks follow-up and received significantly less psychotrophic medication during treatment and up to one year follow up. Control patients improved steadily over time, but at a lesser rate than those treated by a psychologist.

An explanation, at least partial, for these findings is that individuals who are in emotional distress are as a group also significantly higher utilizers of all general medical services. Once their emotional distress is adequately dealt with through psychological or psychosocial methods, the utilization of services tends to decrease. During the period in which these emotionally-distressed persons are receiving psychological services, however, there is not yet any evidence of a reduction of total costs of health care, The explanation for that is that even effective psychological service delivery is, at best, generally being substituted for other less appropriate and unnecessary general medical expenditures. Only after completion of psychological services do significant declines in medical service utilization, the so-called medical offset phenomenon, occur (Mumford, Schlesinger, Glass, et al., 1984). These declines tend to remain constant during the following years up to five years following termination of psychological intervention, without additional intervention being required.

The Use of Psychological Interventions to Improve Physical Health

Since the early 1970s psychologists (and particularly health psychologists) have been regularly and extensively exploring clinical interventions with patients who have obvious health problems.

Summarizing the present state of knowledge on the basis of available literature, VandenBos and DeLeon (1988) conclude that with patients suffering from four categories of *chronic disease* (diabetes, asthma, hypertension and ischaemic heart disease), a minimum amount of outpatient psychological care (one counseling session) is not associated with lower medical costs, whereas a slightly longer (and thus seemingly more appropriate) period of outpatient psychological care (two to six sessions) is associated with a medical offset effect and, further, there is an increasing effect. This increasing effect can appropriately be labelled a "dose-response effect", meaning that more psychological intervention sessions lead to a stronger medical offset effect. A second conclusion is that primary source of cost-savings that produces the medical offset effect is associated with lowered inpatient utilization and hospital expenses.

Mumford, Schlesinger and Glass (1982) reviewed the literature on the effect of psychological intervention on recovery from *surgery* and *heart attack*. They used the term psychological intervention to cover a broad range of activities performed by psychologists, psychiatrists, surgeons, nurses, and others intended to provide information or emotional support to patients suffering disabling illness or facing surgery. These activities ranged from special programmes to simple additions to or modifications of required medical procedures. These authors were able to identify 34 controlled experimental studies that tested the effects of providing psychological support as an adjunct to medically-required care to patients facing surgery or recovery from heart attack. In each study, the data on the intervention group were compared to that of a control group not provided with the special intervention. The review concludes that in 85% of the reported findings positive advantages can be observed for psychological interventions with surgical patients and heart attack victims. The strongest effects are found for speed of recovery, (e.g. two days fewer in hospital) and fewer post-hospitalization complications.

Such findings demonstrate the relevance of behavioural science knowledge and skills to health care, both on more specialized and on the primary levels. What one cannot directly conclude from these findings is that delivery of services using such knowledge and skills can of necessity only be done by psychologists themselves, a conclusion that, unfortunately, for obvious reasons is too hastily drawn by psychologists themselves (see VandenBos & DeLeon, 1988).

Conclusions

Of decisive importance for the future of psychology as a discipline within the health sector will be its ability to establish an accepted role within primary health care. This necessarily implies within the discipline itself a well-defined and visible distinction between psychological knowledge and skills relevant to general or primary mental health care provision and psychological knowledge and skills relevant to speciality mental health care. Research and training should account for this distinction.

An important part will be the development, evaluation and provision of very short-term and simple methods of assessment, treatment and prevention for the primary level (see Carnwath & Miller 1986 for a laudable, though incomplete effort). By the same token, specialized psychological services should be designed and marketed more for a wide variety of patients and offer a variety of treatment approaches rather than simply psychotherapy. This is not to say that long-term psychodynamically-or personality-oriented psychotherapy has no place at all in health care. But it is just one of the many tools that psychology has to offer and one of relatively minor importance within the emerging health care systems.

Under such a model psychologists as practitioners could have a number of roles, depending upon national health care systems, cultural factors and financial resources.

The most encompassing role would be that of the primary health care psychologist, who would deal both diagnostically and therapeutically with psychosocial and behavioural problems on the primary health care level in much the same way that general practitioners or general physicians in a number of countries deal with physical problems and illnesses.

This, however, is certainly not the only, nor necessarily the most desirable role that psychologists/practitioners could play within a primary health care system. Psychologists, themselves specialized mental health care practitioners, could have an important contribution to the primary health care level by skill sharing with primary health care workers, by supervising them and by monitoring and evaluating their interventions with regard to psychological and behavioural problems.

Yet another possible role is that of the psychologist/practitioner who would be involved on the primary health care level primarily with the development and evaluation of preventive strategies or programmes, such as by educating or training individuals, families or communities on health-enhancing or health-promoting behaviours.

Common to all three roles is that psychologists would be seen as offering a more preventive approach and the public would be more likely to have access to psychological services. Third-party reimbursement systems could probably be convinced more easily to support such programmes for their shorter, more appealing nature in contrast to the uncertainties of the long-term psychotherapeutic approach which is now what is often thought of when one thinks of mental health benefits.

It is important to note that psychologists, whatever their role on the primary health care level, have to be specially trained as such and that relevant training programmes, firmly based on scientifc evidence, have yet to be developed, although some efforts are under way (Cummings, 1986).

A danger waiting just around the corner is a schism between generalists in the field. In medicine it has been a vintaged tradition that the money and the status is where the specialists are. Since both are important incentives, PHC doctors tend to give up their work and move into specialist private practices. In light of the fact that psychology has an important role to play within primary health care both in the best interests of the public and psychology as a profession, it would seem that universities and professional organizations of psychology while developing training and research programmes in primary health care psychology should avoid that same mistake. The unfortunate consequence of this mistake is that the more complicated, technological and expensive the treatment is that the doctor provides and the smaller the number of patients that profit from this treatment, the higher the status and salary.

The future role of psychology as a science and a professional discipline will very much depend on its success in developing psychosocial and behavioural interventions that are generally applicable in health care and could serve as alternatives for medical technology and in developing training methods for health care workers to apply these interventions. If psychology succeeds in carrying out the task delineated in the first part of the previous sentence it will certainly be itself an important provider of those health care services. Maher's (1983) words express this same idea in a timely way: "Procedures and people whose services ultimately tend to reduce the bottom line for medical care will have a serious role to play in the health care delivery system".

The views expressed in this article are those of the authors and do not necessarily reflect those of their organization

References

American Academy of Pediatrics. (1978). *The Task Force of Pediatric Education*. Chicago: Author.

Broadhurst, A. (1972). Clinical psychology and the general practitioner. *British Medical Journal, 1*, 793–795.

Carnwath, T., and Miller, D. (1986). *Behavioural Psychotherapy in Primary Care: a Practice Manual*. London: Academic Press.

Cummings, N. (1986). The dismantling of our health system: Strategies for the survival of psychological practice. *American Psychologist, 41*, 426–431.

Diekstra, R. (1987). The relevance of psychology and psychologists to Health For All/2000. In: H. Dent (Ed.) *Clinical Psychology: Research and Developments*. London: Croom Helm, p. 14–24.

Hamburg, D. A., Elliott, G R., and Parson, D. L. (Eds.). (1982). *Health and Behavior: Frontiers of Research in the Biobehavioral Sciences*. Washington: National Academy Press.

Hammonds, B. L., and Scheirer, C. J. (Eds.) (1984). *Psychology and Health. The Master Lectures Series*. Washington: American Psychological Association.

Hosman, C. M. H. (1983). *Hulpzoeken bij Psychosociale problemen* (Helpseeking in case of psychosocial problems), Lisse: Swets & Zeitlinger.

Kincey, J. A. (1974). General practise and clinical psychology – some arguments for a closer liaison. *Journal of the Royal College of General Practitioners, 24*, 882–888.

Lipowski, Z. Y. (1988). Somatization: The concept and its clinical application: *American Journal of Psychiatry, 145*, 11, 1350–1378.

Maher, B. (1983). The education of health psychologists: Quality counts – numbers are dangerous. *Health Psychology, 2* (Supplement), 37–47.

Marzillier, J. S., and Hall, J. (1987). *What is Clinical Psychology?* Oxford: Oxford University Press.

Mechanic, D. (Ed.). (1983). *Handbook of Health , Health Care and the Health Professions*. New York: Free Press.

Mumford, E., Schesinger, H., and Glass, G. (1982). The effects of psychological intervention on recovery from surgery and heart attacks: An analysis of the literature. *American Journal of Public Health, 72*, 141–151.

Mumford, E., Schlesinger, H., Glass, G., Patrick, C., and Cuerdon, T. (1984). A new look at evidence about reduced cost of medical utilization following mental treatment. *American Journal of Psychiatry, 141*, 1145–1158.

Robson, M. H., France, R., and Bland, M. (1984). Clinical psychologists in primary care: Controlled, clinical and economic evaluation. *British Medical Journal, 28*, 1805–1808.

Rosen, J., and Wiens, A. (1979). Changes in medical problems and use of medical services following psychological intervention. *American Psychologist, 34*, 420–431.

Roskies, E., and Avard, J. (1982). Teaching health managers to control their coronary-prone (Type A) behavior. In: K. R. Blankenstein and J. Polivy (Eds.). *Self-control and self-modification of emotional behavior*. New York: Plenum Press.

Shepherd, M. (1980). Mental health as an integral part of primary medical care. *Journal of the Royal College of General Practitioners, 30*, 657–664.

Steptoe, A., and Mathews, A. (Eds.) (1984). *Health Care and Human Behaviour*. London: Academic Press.

Strupp, H. H., and Binder, J. L. (1984). *Psychotherapy in a New Key*. New York: Basic Books.

VandenBos, G. R., and DeLeon, P. H. (1988) Use of psychotherapy to improve physical health. *Psychotherapy, 25*, 335–343.

World Health Organization. (1978). *Primary Health Care: Alma Ata 1978*. Geneva: World Health Organization.

World Health Organization. (1981). *Global Strategy for Health for All by the Year 2000.* Geneva: World Health Organization.

Wright, L., and Burns, B. J. (1986). Primary mental health care: A "find" for psychology? *Professional Psychology, 17*, 6, 560–564.

Health Promotion and Health Education in Relation to Non-Communicable Diseases: Present Findings From Belgian Studies

France Kittel, G. De Backer, M. Dramaix and M. Kornitzer

Introduction

Presently, it is widely accepted that the most important non-communicable diseases and incidents regarding fatal issues such as cancer, road accidents, and especially cardiovascular diseases, are largely due to harmful behaviours. These behaviours include: unbalanced diet (fat, fiber, salt, sugar), smoking, alcohol, and sedentary life, which in turn influence risk factors such as relative weight, serum lipids and blood pressure.

Moreover, the literature contains sufficient evidence showing that these behaviours are related to psychosocial factors (e. g. social class, gender, culture etc.) as are the diseases themselves.

Behavioural change, which not only aims at changing risk factors, but also the incidence of the disease, is also supposedly linked to psychosocial factors.

In order to test this hypothesis, results obtained from the Belgian Heart Disease Prevention Project were analysed.

The Belgian Heart Disease Prevention Project – B. H. D. P. P. (N=19, 409), part of the WHO European Collaborative Group – W.H.O.E.C.G. (WHO European Collaborative Group, 1974), in which, in addition to Belgium, Great Britain, Italy, Poland and Spain participated (N=60, 881), is a controlled randomized multifactorial intervention trial which was initiated in the early seventies.

Design and Methodology

The design and methodology of this trial, a summary of which is given below, are described extensively in an earlier article (De Backer et al., 1977).

This randomized controlled trial was carried out over a period of 6 years in 30 factories. The factories were paired off and assigned to a control (N=10, 900) or to an intervention group (N=8, 509). The subject were males aged 40–59 years.

Prevalence data were obtained for the total intervention group (N=7, 398) and for 10% of the control group (N=901). At baseline examination, bio-clinical measures such as weight, height, blood pressure, cholestrol, smoking, and age were taken. Social characteristics such as culture (French- and Dutch- speaking subjects), occupational level (executives, white- and blue-collar workers), marital status (married, unmarried) were determined. Psychological dimensions, essentially type A and neuroticism, were assessed.

The final examination, after 6 years, comprised the same measures for both the total intervention and control group.

The intervention consisted of advice related to:

- Diet (reducing fat intake, especially saturated fats) in order to diminish cholesterol.
- Cigarette smoking cessation.
- Weight reduction (if subjects were more than 15% overweight).
- Taking daily exercise (if subjects had a sedentary life).
- Control of hypertension (if subjects had a systolic blood pressure ≥ 160) but only by diet (reducing salt and weight) and referral to the general practitioner for medication prescription.

The control group did not receive the intervention programme. The intervention group was subdivided into two sub-groups: the high-risk subjects, who were in the upper quintiles of a global risk score, and the low-risk subjects, who were in the 4 lower quintiles of the same global risk score.

The low-risk group received booklets concerning risk factors and how to deal with them, a letter was sent to their general practitioner informing him of their results, anti-smoking conferences were organized, posters were placed on the walls of the factories where they worked, and dietary advice was given to the canteens.

The high-risk subjects in the intervention group received the same programme in addition to individualized, face-to-face advice (twice a year the two first years, once a year the four remaining years).

After the 6 years' follow-up, an additional 4 years of mortality follow-up was performed.

Results of the present paper were analyzed as follows:

For the prevalence data, two new variables, derived from the risk factors, were calculated:

Body Mass Index (=BMI): Height / (Weight)^2
Multiple Logistic Function (=MLF):
$1 / 1 \times e^{-(\alpha + \beta_i x_i)}$

Where $\alpha =$ constant.
$\beta_i =$ coefficients.
$x_i =$ risk factors.

The generally accepted risk factors are: age, Body Mass Index (BMI), cholesterol, systolic blood pressure and amount of cigarettes smoked.

The five coefficients are those derived from A. Key's prospective Seven Counties Study.

The MLF gives a coronary risk profile or the probability of developing a coronary event within 5 years.

Data with respect to the following were analyzed after 6 years:
1. Mortality and incidence of morbidity.
    A % net difference was calculated

$$\% \text{ net difference} = \frac{C - I}{I} \times 100$$

Where I = Intervention
    C = Control

2. Evolution of risk factors.
    A mean data was calculated for the total low risk (=LR) and high risk

subjects (=HR)

Delta = Final – Initial value = F – Io

% net change was calculated also for these groups

$$\% \text{ net change} = \frac{I(F - Io) - C(F - Io)}{Io}$$

Finally, data were analyzed after 10 years in terms of mortality; therefore a % net difference in cumulative incidence was calculated.

$$\% \text{ net difference} = \text{cumulative incidence} \frac{(I - C)}{C}$$

Results

After 6 years' follow-up, the results with respect to mortality and morbidity were in favour of the intervention group. To be more precise, % net difference total mortality was: 17.5% ($p \leq 05$), for coronary mortality: 20.8% (not significant), for coronary incidence (Fatal CHD and non fatal MI): 24.5% ($p \leq .05$) and for fatal MI: 26.1% ($p \leq .05$).

Table 1 shows the evolution of risk factors after 6 years in terms of the observed mean delta in the various subgroups. The greater increase in coronary risk – expressed through the MLF – in the control group, which did not receive the intervention programme, is particularly pronounced in the high risk subgroup.

Table 1: *Evolution of risk factors after 6 years: Comparison of mean delta, of risk factors and MLF*

SUB-GROUP	GROUP	BMI	CHOL	CIG	SBP	MLF
Total	Intervention	0.28	-7.5	-1.5	3.5	0.0116
(LR+HR)		**	**		*	
N = 5677	Control	0.39	2.6	-1.1	1.6	0.0128
Low risk	Intervention	0.35	2.5	-0.7	4.7	0.0112
					*	
N = 4284	Control	0.46	5.2	-0.7	2.9	0.0114
High risk	Intervention	-0.03	-14.0	-3.7	-1.2	0.0133
		**	**			(0.07)
N = 1087	Control	0.39	-6.4	-2.1	-3.2	0.0171

Delta: Final-Initial Value

**$p \leq 0.01$

* $p \leq 0.05$

If we consider the four risk factors separately, it appears that mass-media advice – given to the low risk subjects – was only successful in lowering serum cholestrol.

Confirmation of this finding can be seen in Table 2, which presents the % net change of the risk factors after 6 years. For blood pressure control, no type of intervention proved to be effective. In addition, we can see more clearly that the cigarette smoking, mass media advice – given to the low risk subjects – had no effect, while the individualised counselling – given to the high risk subjects – had a beneficial impact.

Table 2: *Evolution of risk factors after 6 years: % net change of risk factors and MLF*

SUB-GROUP	BMI	CHOL	CIG	SBP	MLF
Total	−0.7	−1.5	−2.2	+1.4	−7.3
Low risk	−0.4	−1.2	0	+1.4	−1.5
High risk	−1.6	−2.9	−7.5	+1.3	−12.7

$$\% \text{ Net change} = \frac{I(F\text{-}Io) - C(F\text{-}Io)}{I(Io)}$$

I: Intervention Group
C: Control Group
F: Final Value
Io: Initial Value

In order to determine the potential links between psychosocial factors and risk factor change, covariance analyses were performed using the four risk factors and the MLF as dependent variables. The independent variables introduced were: the group (or type of intervention), psychosocial variables, the covariate, being the initial variable of each risk factor or MLF, respectively.

Table 3 illustrates the results obtained from the 10 analyses. Several results can be observed.

The initial value of all risk factors and the MLF (covariable) was significant in all analyses.

The intervention by mass media (low-risk subjects) was favourable for lowering cholesterol but for the other risk factors has either no effect (smoking and BMI) or negative effect (blood pressure).

Looking closer at the data it appears that in particular subgroups there was an interaction of psychosocial variables with the mass-media intervention.

For BMI, the mass-media intervention was beneficial for Dutch-speaking subjects, while in the French-speaking subgroup, control subjects were better off.

For cigarette smoking globally, when compared to the French-speaking subgroup, it was found that the Dutch diminished their consumption. In the intervention group, blue collar workers diminished the amount of cigarettes they smoked a little more, and in the control group the executives behaved better. Among married subjects no difference was found between the Dutch- and French-speaking subgroups. Among

Table 3: *Evolution of risk factors after 6 years: Covariance analysis of delta of risk factors and MLF*

	BMI		CHOL		CIG		SBP		MLF	
	LR	HR	LR	HR	LR	HR	LR	HR	LR	HR
COVARIABLE	xxx	xxx	xxx	xxx	xxx	xxx	xxx	xxx	xxx	xxx
Main Effects										
Group (I/C)		x	x	xx				xx	xxx	
Age	xxx			xx		xx		xxx	xxx	xxx
Cult. (D/F)			x			xx		xx	xx	
Prof. (E/W C/BC)	xxx									
Marital St (M/U)										x
Interaction										
Group × Cult.	x				x					
Age × Cult.		x								
Group × Prof.						xx				
Cult. × Marital St.						x				
Age × Prof.									xxx	
Age × Marital St.										x

Delta: Final-Initial Value; xxx: p≤0.001; xx: p≤ 0.01; x: p≤0.05
I: Intervention; C: Control; LR: Low-Risk; HR: High-Risk; D: Dutch; F: French; E: Executives; WC: White-Collar workers; BC: Blue-Collar workers; M: Married; U: Unmarried.

unmarried subjects, however, it was found that the French-speaking subgroup in contrast to the Dutch, who remained constant, increased its cigarette consumption over time.

For the MLF, evolution in the three first age groups was similar, but in the 55–59 age group, the evolution of the coronary risk profile was less favourable in the lower professional class. Moreover, for the two first age groups no difference by marital status could be seen in the MLF's evolution, but from the age of 50, unmarried subjects showed a less favourable evolution.

The intervention by face-to-face counseling (high-risk subjects), on the other hand, was significantly favourable for weight, cholesterol and reduction in the amount of cigarettes smoked, and nearly significant for coronary risk profile (determind by the MLF). Moreover, psychosocial variables no longer appeared to have a detrimental effect on the change of the risk factors: socioprofessional, cultural and familial differences in evolution, vanished.

After 10 years' follow-up, 4 years after completion of the intervention programmes, no differences were found between the control and intervention group with respect to mortality and morbidity (De Backer et al., 1988). A slight difference subsisted in favour of the intervention group for the total mortality, but not for cardiovascular and coronary mortality. When superimposing the curves of mortality and MLF, a remarkable congruence emerged for the first 6 years.

Discussion

After 6 years, the observed differences with respect to mortality and morbidity in favour of the intervention group (Kornitzer et al., 1983) were parallel with the observed differences in coronary risk profile. This latter result was, most probably, due to the individualized face-to-face intervention, as the difference was more pronounced in the high-risk subjects (Kittel, 1984).

Psychosocial variables are associated with the change in risk factors and coronary risk profile when a minimal intervention programme is applied, namely with mass-media techniques. But the results show clearly that whenever individualized techniques are used, all subgroups benefit equally from the intervention programme, erasing the psychosocial inequalities in terms of risk evolution (Kittel, 1984;1986).

After 10 years' follow-up, 4 years after completion of the intervention programmes, the difference in mortality and morbidity in favour of the intervention group disappeared (De Backer et al., 1988). Moreover, the fit between the curves of mortality and MLF for the first 6 years leads to the reasonable hypothesis that at the end of the follow-up the risk factors went up again in the intervention group. From this the following can be deduced: changes in risk profile obtained through intervention programmes are rapidly followed by changes in mortality and morbidity, but this applies in both directions. In other words, in order to achieve a long-lasting preventive effect, risk reduction by intervention programmes should be maintained.

Conclusions

As stopping the intervention means returning to the previous situation, long-term impact will only be achieved by means of a "continuous climate of prevention".

However, this type of intervention is also costly in the long run. On the other hand, the absence of intervention is also costly, not only in terms of money but in terms of human lives, quality of life, work hours ... .

Moreover, little or no action (e.g. mass-media) is ethically undefensible, as less socially favoured groups will then develop more illnesses.

Therefore, action has to be undertaken which is not restricted to classic health education towards prevention of cardiovascular or even noncommunicable diseases or incidents, but enlarged to health promotion with a positive health concept, where everybody is concerned and participates.

Practically, for research design, these findings imply that the following requirements should be met.
- interventions should be performed for the various risk factors at different population levels: for some risk factors and/or sub-groups at the community level, and for other risk factors and/or high-risk groups at the individual level.
- With respect to previous recommendations, various means of intervention should be used: mass-media, group or individual techniques.
- Not only risk factors or groups should be taken into consideration, but also protective factors (e.g. social support and network, physical fitness ...) and protected groups (e.g higher-educated subjects, pre-menopausal women ...).
- New psychological risk factors should be looked for (e.g. hostility, working conditions and organizational situations...).

Ideally, the following recommendation should be followed:

– The general population, including younger and older subjects, women, unemployed or retired, opinion leaders, key persons, health personnel, associations, lay-groups, family, peers ..., should be integrated in intervention studies. In turn, attention should be paid to the combination of different methods and strategies, varying with the target population, type of behaviour to change, stage of behaviour, taking into account the dynamics (evolution in time) and interactions of the factors. The programmes should be applied in different settings: school, family, groups in order to favour synergism. Moreover, the global environment of the target in terms of social, enconomical, medical and behavioural variables should be analyzed, and the functioning of health services and resources considered. Finally, the agricultural, industrial and technological framework wherein the programmes have to be delivered should be looked for, this by trying to influence them with the aim of optimizing all existing and potential resources.

References

Backer, G. de, Kornitzer, M., Thilly, C., and Depoorter, A. M. (1977). The Belgian Multifactor Preventive Trial in CVD. Design and methodology. *Heart Bulletin. 8*, 143–146.

Backer, G. de, Kornitzer, M., Dramaix, M., Kittel, F., Thilly, C., Graffer, M., and Vuylsteek, K. (1988). The Belgian Heart Disease Prevention Project: 10-year mortality follow-up. *European Heart Journal, 9*, 238–242.

Kittel, F. (1984). Approche psychosociale de la prévalence et de l'incidence des affections coronariennes. (A psychosocial approach of prevalence and incidence of coronary heart diseases). Project Belge de Prevention des Affections Cardio-vasculaires. These de doctorat en Santé Publique, Université Libre Bruxelles.

Kittel, F. (1986). Type A and other psychosocial factors in relation to coronary heart disease. In Schmidt, T. H., Dembroski, T. M., and Blumchen, G. (Eds.), *Biological and psychological factors in cardiovascular disease* (pp. 63–85). Berlin: Springer.

Kornitzer, M., Backer, G. de, Dramaix, M., Kittel, F., Thilly, C., and Graffar, M. (1983). Belgian Heart Disease Prevention Project: Incidence and mortality results. *Lancet I*, 1066 –1070.

WHO European Collaborative Group (1974). An international controlled trial in the multifactorial prevention of coronary heart disease. *International Journal of Epidemiology, 3*, 219–224.

Self-Efficacy, Protection Motivation and Health Behaviour

Erik Taal, Erwin Seydel, and Oene Wiegman

In health psychology several models and theories have been developed with more or less success to explain, predict and change behaviour. Bandura (1977) introduced the concept of self-efficacy in his social-learning theory. He postulated that people's perceptions of their capabilities affect their behaviour, motivation, thought patterns and their emotional reactions in critical situations. Self-efficacy refers to beliefs in one's capabilities to successfully execute the behaviour required to produce a certain desired outcome.

Research has shown the importance of self-efficacy in relation to health. Self-efficacy expectations play an important role in smoking cessation (DiClemente, Prochaska & Gibertini, 1985; Strecher, Becker, Kirscht, Eraker & Graham-Tomasi, 1985) and patient compliance with medical regimens (Klepac, Dowling & Hange, 1982). High self-efficacy expectations lead to adequate coping behaviour and anxiety reduction during unpleasant medical procedures (Bandura, 1986; Turk, Meichenbaum & Genest, 1983) and quicker recovery from heart attacks (Taylor, Bandura, Ewart, Miller & DeBusk, 1985). Self-efficacy also contributes significantly to the control of rheumatoid arthritis (RA). In a recent study we found that the more RA patients considered themselves capable of controlling their own disease (self-efficacy), the better they judged their own health status, i.e. pain, disability, anxiety and depression (Taal & Seydel, 1988). In other studies with arthritis patients, similar relations were found (Lorig, Chastain, Ung, Shoor & Holman, 1989. O'Leary, 1985; Shoor & Holman, 1985).

A model often used to explain preventive health behaviour is the health belief model (HBM)(Becker, 1974). This model provides a straightforward framework to explain health behaviour. However, HBM neglects the explicit role of personal mastery as described in Bandura's social-learning theory. Rogers (1983) developed the protection motivation theory (PMT), which incorporates the HBM-factors but also makes use of Bandura's concept of self-efficacy. according to Rogers' model, protection motivation, and subsequently the adaptive or coping response, is evoked when (a) the threat to health is severe (severity), (b) the individual feels vulnerable (susceptibility), (c) the adaptive response is believed to be an effective means for averting the threat (response-efficacy), and (d) the person is confident in his or her ability to successfully complete the adaptive response (self-efficacy).

This study sought to determine the predictive value of the factors comprising the PMT, i.e. beliefs concerning severity, susceptibility, response-efficacy, and self-efficacy with respect to behavioural intentions, reported behaviour and also actual behaviour related to the prevention of cancer.

113

Method

Subjects

Subjects were 266 men and women who had applied to participate in a study which was described in a newspaper advertisement as a study on educational television programmes. In the experimental groups the participants were exposed to information on cancer. The control group saw a programme on an unrelated topic. To measure behavioural intentions and reported behaviour, some days before exposure to the programmes, all subjects completed a mailed questionnaire. In order to ascertain actual behaviour the subjects were given the opportunity to order two information leaflets from the Dutch Cancer Society (DCS), one leaflet about general cancer prevention and one about breast self-examination, using an orderform which had been handed out after viewing the programme.

Data of 10 cancer patients were not analyzed. The remaining sample consisted of 124 men and 132 women with a mean age of 38 years, ranging from 19 to 73 years.

Variables

Behavioural Intentions. Questions were asked concerning intentions to:

– Go and see a doctor upon detecting a complaint associated with the seven warning signs of cancer.

– Do breast-self-examinations (BSE) every month.

– Check one's own body to detect cancer signs in time.

– Have a pap test made every three years for the early detection of cervical cancer.

Seven-point scales were used ranging from *definitely not* to *most certainly*.

Reported Behaviour. For the last three topics mentioned above the subjects were also asked if they already performed these behaviours.

Actual Behaviour. Measurement of actual behaviour concerned the actual ordering of the two leaflets.

Severity and Susceptibility. Perceived severity was measured by two questions: "I think cancer is more serious than any other illness I know", and "In spite of advances in medical science, cancer is still as serious as it ever was". Perceived susceptibility was also measured by two questions: "It is quite probable that I will at some time contract some form of cancer", and "The chance that someone of my age in similar circumstances will contract cancer is quite high". Answers were ratings on 7-point scales ranging from *totally disagree* to *totally agree*.

Response-Efficacy and Self-Efficacy. For every behaviour response efficacy was measured with a 7-point scale ranging from *most unlikely* to *very probable*. Questions were formulated as follows: ".... can lead to early detection of cancer". Self-efficacy was also measured with one 7-point scale for every behaviour ranging from *totally disagree* to *totally agree*. Questions were formulated as follows:"It is difficult for me to ...."

Results

Behavioural Intentions

Table 1 shows the results of multiple regression analysis on behavioural intention. The main contribution to the predictive value of the PMT comes from self-efficacy and response-efficacy. Beliefs concerning severity and susceptibility are not adequate predictors of behavioural intentions. An exception was the assessment of severity by women, in relation to going to see the doctor in time (r=0.31), and in relation to breast self-examination (r=0.29).

Table 1 *Multiple regression analysis on behavioural intentions*

		MR	R^2	simple r	Beta
Go and see a doctor					
-men(n=113)	Response-efficacy	0.52	0.27	0.52	0.48**
-women (n=126)	Response-efficacy	0.46	0.21	0.46	0.36**
	Self-efficacy	0.55	0.30	0.38	0.30**
	Severity	0.58	0.34	0.31	0.20*
Breast self examination					
-women (n=125)	Self-efficacy	0.59	0.35	0.59	0.52**
	Response-efficacy	0.67	0.45	0.41	0.31**
	Severity	0.69	0.48	0.29	0.17*
Check own body					
-men (n=113)	Response-efficacy	0.34	0.12	0.35	0.30**
	Self-efficacy	0.41	0.17	0.29	0.22*
-women (n=122	Self-efficacy	0.35	0.12	0.35	0.35**
	Response-efficacy	0.43	0.19	0.30	0.24*
Pap test					
-women (n=126)	self-efficacy	0.44	0.19	0.44	0.38**
	Response-efficacy	0.49	0.24	0.32	0.21*

*p<0.05;**p<0.01;(only significant predictors are listed)

Reported Behaviour

With respect to reported behaviour, response-efficacy and self-efficacy also had good predictive value (Table 2). For the pap test however, severity and susceptibility also accounted for a considerable proportion of the variance. It was remarkable that the correlation between perceived severity and the pap test was negative (r=−0.13), implicating that the women who considered cancer to be a serious illness reported having had a pap test least often.

Actual Behaviour

The question of the predictive value of PMT can best be answered on the basis of the hardest criterion, the actual ordering of leaflets from the DCS. As mentioned earlier, protection motivation factors were measured before viewing the programmes. An

Table 2 *Multiple regression analysis on reported and actual behaviour*

		MR	R^2	simple r	Beta
Reported behaviour					
Breast self-examination					
-women (n=127)	Self-efficacy	0.49	0.24	0.49	0.47**
	Response-efficacy	0.52	0.27	0.25	0.16*
Check own body					
-men(n=115)	Self-efficacy	0.29	0.08	0.29	0.28**
	Response-efficacy	0.30	0.09	0.13	0.05*
-women (n=123)	Response-efficacy	0.40	0.16	0.40	0.38**
	Self-efficacy	0.46	0.21	0.27	0.23**
Pap test					
-women (n=125)	Self-efficacy	0.43	0.18	0.42	0.38**
	Susceptibility	0.48	0.23	0.25	0.22**
	Severity	0.50	0.25	-0.13	-0.16*
Actual behaviour (ordering leaflets)					
Leaflet 1: General cancer prevention					
-men(n=117)	Self-efficacy	0.22	0.05	0.22	0.22*
-women (n=123)	Response-efficacy	0.32	0.11	0.32	0.31**
Leaflet 2: Breast self-examination					
-women (n=116)	Response-efficacy	0.24	0.06	0.25	0.25**
	Self-efficacy	0.31	0.09	0.20	0.18*
	Severity	0.34	0.11	0.15	0.20*

*p0.05;**p<0.01; (Only significant predictors are reported)

extra factor included in the analysis was exposure to the health education message. For women, response-efficacy was an important predictor for ordering the leaflet about general cancer prevention, whereas for men, self-efficacy was a good predictor. The remaining variables made no further contribution (see Table 2). regarding the ordering of the leaflet on breast self-examination, it appeared that not only response-efficacy and self-efficacy, but also the assessment of severity, made a significant contribution to the ordering of the leaflet. The factor health education made no contribution in this respect.

Discussion

In health education the perception of threat, i.e. perceived severity and susceptibility, is often seen as a factor that should be strengthened to change health behaviour. However, this study shows that perceived severity and susceptibility are not sufficient predictors of preventive behaviour. Self-efficacy and response-efficacy are more important predictors of preventive health behaviour. This has also been indicated in other studies within the framework of PMT, where the greatest and most consistent relations were found between response-efficacy and self-efficacy and behavioural intention (Rogers, 1983; Rogers & Deckner, 1975; Mewborn & Rogers, 1979; Leventhal, Meyer & Guttman, 1980). In an extensive review of research on the HBM, Janz and Becker (1984) also stressed the predictive value of the efficacy component. Further, Hochbaum proposed to modify the HBM by pointing out the central role of the efficacy dimension in preventive behaviour (Hochbaum, 1983).

Some restriction must be made in generalizing the results of this study to the whole Dutch population, because the sample we used comprises people who voluntarily applied to take part in a study on educational television programmes.

Contrary to what would be expected, in one case we found a negative correlation between perceived severity and having a pap test. Comparable negative correlations between perceived severity and behaviour have also been reported elsewhere (Weinsenberg, Kegeles & Lund, 1980; Kegeles & Lund, 1982). An explanation for this negative correlation may be that women who consider cancer as a severe threat may perceive physical examinations, like a pap test, as even more threatening and so adopt a more defensive avoidance style of coping. Also Leventhal's (1970) review of the literature on fear communications suggests that if a person feels threatened he is less receptive to behavioural recommendations which are in themselves threatening.

Self-efficacy and response-efficacy were good predictors of the actual ordering of leaflets. For women the most important predictor of ordering the leaflet about general cancer prevention was response-efficacy, whereas for men the best predictor was self-efficacy. If this points at a systematic difference between men and women is questionable. It might be speculated that men are more inclined to rely on expectancies about their own efficacy, i.e. their assessment of their own capabilities, than women, reflecting the status position of women in our society. However, for women, self-efficacy is also an important predictor for ordering the leaflet on breast self-examination. This implies that there is no unambiguous systematic difference between men and women in this respect. However, in certain areas there may well be such differences; this is an issue for further investigation.

This study leads to the general conclusion that the factors from the HBM, i.e. severity, susceptibility and response-efficacy, are not adequate predictors of preventive behaviour in relation to cancer. Self-efficacy is a factor that should be included. We can state the PMT is able to provide a better prediction of behavioural intention and actual behaviour that the HBM. So, for the prediction of preventive behaviour related to cancer, PMT is to be preferred. One should not conclude that perceived severity and susceptibility are unimportant factors in the adoption of preventive behaviour. Without the notion of a certain severity or susceptibility, an individual will not be likely to behave in a preventive way to reduce the threat.

However, perceived severity and susceptibility in themselves are insufficient motivators for preventive behaviour. In an applied context health education should also include specific behavioural instructions which may enhance self-efficacy expectancies. This will facilitate the successfull performance of the recommended behaviour.

This study was supported by the Dutch Cancer Society

References

Bandura, A. (1977). Self-efficacy: Toward a unifying theory of behavioral change. *Psychological Review, 84*, 191–215.

Bandura, A. (1986). Self-efficacy mechanism in physiological activation and health promoting behavior. In J. Madden IV, S. Matthysse, and J. Barchas (Eds.), *Adaptation, learning and affect*. New York: Raven Press.

Becker, M. H. (Ed.).(1974). The health belief model and personal health behavior. *Health Education Monographs, 2*, 326–473.

DiClemente, C. C., Prochaska, J. O., and Gibertini, M. (1985). Self-efficacy and the stages of self-change of smoking. *Cognitive Therapy and Research, 9*, 181–200.

Hochbaum, G. M. (1983). *The health belief model revisited*, paper for the symposium The Health Belief Model After Three Decades, at the Annual Meetings of the APHA, Dallas, TX, November 14.

Janz, N. K., and Becker, M. H. (1984) The health belief model. *Health Education Quarterly, 11*, 27–47.

Kegeles, S. S., and Lund, A. K. (1982) Adolescents' Health Beliefs and Acceptance of a Novel Preventive Dental Activity: Replication and Extension. *Health Education Quarterly, 9*, 192–208.

Klepac, R. K., Dowling, J., and Hange, G. (1982). Characteristics of clients seeking therapy for the reduction of dental avoidance: Reactions to pain. *Journal of Behaviour Therapy and Experimental Psychiatry, 13*, 293–300.

Leventhal, H. (1970) Findings and theory in the study of fear communications. In: L. Berkowitz (Ed.), *Advances in experimental social psychology* (Vol. 5). New York: Academic Press.

Leventhal, H., Meyer, D., and Guttmann, M. (1980). The role of theory in the study of compliance to high blood pressure regimens. In R. Haynes, and M. Mattson (Eds.), *Patient compliance to prescribed antihypertensive medication regimens: A report to the National Heart, Lung, and Blood Institute*, (NIH Publ. No. 81-2102). Bethesda, Md.: U.S. Department of Health and Human Services.

Lorig, K., Chastain, R., Ung, E., Shoor, S., and Holman, H. R. (1989). Development and evaluation of a scale to measure perceived self-efficacy in people with arthritis. *Arthritis and Rheumatism, 32*, 37–44.

Mewborn, C. R, and Rogers, R. W. (1979) Effects of threatening and reassuring components of fear appeals on psychological and verbal measures of emotion and attitudes. *Journal of Experimental Social Psychology, 15*, 242–253.

O'Leary, A. (1985). *Psychological factors in rheumatoid arthritis pain and immune function: A self- efficacy approach*. Unpublished doctoral dissertation, Stanford University, Stanford, CA.

Rogers, R. W. (1983). Cognitive and Physiological Processes in Fear Appeals and Attitude Change: A revised theory of Protection Motivation. In J. T. Cacioppo, and R. E. Petty (Eds.), *Social psychophysiology: a sourcebook*. New York: The Guilford Press.

Rogers, R. W., and Deckner, C. W. (1975) Effects of fear appeals and physiological arousal upon emotions, attitudes, and cigarette smoking. *Journal of Personality and Social Psychology, 32*, 222–230.

Shoor, S. M., and Holman, H. R. (1984). Development of an instrument to explore psychological mediators of outcome in chronic arthritis. *Transactions of the Association of American Physicians, 97*, 325–331.

Strecher, V.J., Becker, M. H., Kirscht, J. P., Eraker, S. A., and Graham-Tomasi, R. P. (1985). Psychosocial aspects of changes in cigarette-smoking behaviour. *Patient Education and Counselling, 7*,249–262.

Taal, E., and Seydel, E. (1988). *Patient Education for patients with rheumatoid arthritis*. Paper presented at the XIII World Conference on Health Education. Houston, TX, USA.

Taylor, C. B., Bandura, A., Ewart, C. K., Miller, N. H., and DeBusk, R. F. (1985). Exercise testing to enhance wives' confidence in their husbands' capabilities soon after clinically uncomplicated acute myocardial infarction. *American Journal of Cardiology, 55,* 635–638.

Turk, D., Meichenbaum, D., and Genest, M. (1983). *Cognitive therapy of pain.* New York: Guilford Press.

Weisenberg, M., Kegeles, S. S., and Lund, A. K. (1980). Children's Health Beliefs and Acceptance of a Dental Preventive Activity. *Journal of Health and Social Behavior, 21,* 59–74.

The Effectiveness of Health Education at the Workplace

Gerjo Kok, Ruud Jonkers and P. Liedekerken

Health education at the workplace is a relatively new but very promising field for health educators. In this chapter we will first give an overview of systematically planned health education as a part of health promotion. Secondly we will review the effectiveness of health education at the workplace and suggest the characteristics of the workplace that would increase the potential of health education, *if* planned systematically. It is important to note that health education interventions at the workplace are not only focussed on individual behavior change, but on organizational change as well. We shall illustrate the propositions with examples from both occupational health and safety as well as health promotion interventions.

Planned Health education

Planned health education consists of a planning phase and an evaluation phase, (see Figure 1).

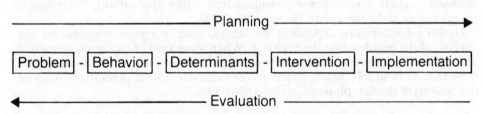

Figure 1. Planned health education, *(Based on Green & Lewis, 1986)*

In the planning phase five questions have to be answered:
1. What is the health problem?
2. What is the behavior related to the health problem?
3. What are the determinants of that behavior?
4. What intervention is possible to change that behavior?
5. How can that intervention be implemented?

In the evaluation phase five comparable questions have to be answered:
6. Has the implementation been conducted as planned?
7. Was the intervention realized as planned?
8. Have the determinants been changed?
9. Has the behavior changed?
10. Has the problem decreased?

An example of the potential application of this model with respect to hearing impairment and the use of ear protectors might present the following planning questions

1. Problem: Hearing impairment in employees
2. Behavior: The non-use of ear protectors
3. Determinants: Lack of possibilities for communication between employees when using ear protectors, increasing the potential danger of accidents
4. Intervention: The intervention combines both structural and motivational approaches, for example, the availability of some ear protectors combined with possibilities for communication, and instructions for use.
5. Implementation: Organizational change initiatives in order to adjust safety regulations and some combination of control and feedback from the manager or supervisor.

The questions to be asked during the evaluation phase might be:

6. Implementation: Have regulations been adjusted, did the manager exercise control and did he give feedback (for instance about the decrease of hearing impairment)?
7. Intervention: Did the employees receive the new ear protectors and did they understand how to use them correctly?
8. Determinants: Are the employees convinced communication is possible while they are using ear protectors?
9. Behavior: Are more employees using ear protectors:?
10. Problem: Are there fewer cases of hearing impairment (after some time)?

This is a hypothetical example. As far as we know, there is no complete example of the systematic application of all ten questions in the field of health education at the workplace. There are, however, examples from other applications, for instance, energy saving at the workplace (Siero et al., 1989).

Health educators are dependent on others, such as epidemiologists, for the analysis of the problem and the behavior. When some kind of consensus is reached about those two phases and about the kinds of behaviors that are undesirable and those that are desirable, health educators (or social scientists in general) can focus on the analysis of the determinants of those behaviors.

Determinants of Behavior

The analysis of the determinants of behavior is based on social psychological theory development. Figure 2 presents a model of behavior determinants integrating the work of Fishbein and Ajzen (1975) and Bandura (1985).

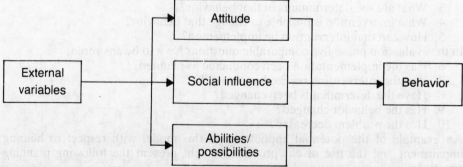

Figure 2. Determinants of behavior (see also Ajzen & Madden, 1986; deVries et al, 1988.)

Behavior is determined by three variables: attitude, social influence and abilities/ possibilities. An attitude is the weighing of all the advantages and disadvantages of the behavior. It is important to note that health considerations are mostly *not* very salient. It is a common pitfall for health educators, managers, politicians, etc. to focus on the health disadvantages of the undesired behavior; people themselves have other reasons, for instance, the lack of communication while using ear protectors.

Social influence is the effect that others have on the behavior of the person: colleagues, family, chief, friends, public persons, etc. The influence can be direct in the sense that others expect us to behave in an certain way, or it can be indirect in the sense that others behave in a certain way (modeling).

Abilities/possibilities concern the person's ability to perform the desired behavior (Bandura's "personal efficacy"). There may be personal barriers (lack of abilities) or circumstantial barriers (adequate ear protectors not available). The literature on health education and social psychology reveals a growing interest in this third determinant as a very important reason why people do not behave in the desired way, even if they know about the dangers of their undesired behavior (e.g. Strecher et al., 1986). Research focusses on the determinants of personal efficacy, using, for instance, attribution theory (Eiser & van der Pligt, 1988; Weiner, 1986).

External variables are all other variables (like demographic, personality, organizational characteristics) that may have an effect on the behavior. That effect is supposed to be mediated by the three determinanats.

The model of behavior determinants is a framework that has to be specified for each combination of desired and undesired behavior. For some behaviors those analyses have already been done. For instance, with respect to quitting smoking, we know that the decision to quit is determined by health complaints and social pressure (attitude and social influence), while success in quitting over time is determined by people's ability to cope with negative emotional and positive social situations (Schwartz, 1986; Marlatt & Gordon, 1986).

Interventions: Health Promotion

After analyzing the problem, the behavior and the determinants, the choice of an intervention is not necessarily limited to health education interventions. Figure 3 illustrates a model of health promotion with three goals and three strategies.

Health Promotion	Primary prevention	Early detection	Patient care
Health education			
Facilities			
Regulations			

Figure 3. The Health Promotion Matrix

We will illustrate the matrix with examples about hypertension. Hypertension can be prevented by quitting smoking, a better diet, an improved ability to cope with stress, etc. Early detection of hypertension can be organized by screening programs at the workplace and patient care can be achieved by improving medicine compliance in hypertensive patients. These three goals can be reached with education, facilities and regulations: quitting smoking, for instance, by the availability of a Stop Smoking Course for employees (facility), on a voluntary basis (education) or forced by means of a rule that forbids smoking at the workplace (regulation). Health education is based on the personal motivation of the receiver; regulations are based on protecting the health of employees often by using sanctions and control. Facilities promote the desired behavior and are mostly organised by the management or the government, but at the same time mostly used on a voluntary basis. For instance, a company can offer low fat food in the employee's restaurant, combined with education about the health effects of high and low fat food. A company can organize screening programs for hypertension, with regulations about participating, but also with education about ways to prevent or decrease hypertension.

The choice for the optimal intervention is a difficult one and is determined not only by rational considerations about effectiveness of interventions, but also by considerations about economic aspects, public relations, political feasibility, etc. (see for instance Milio, 1985; de Leeuw, 1988). In the remainder of this chapter we will focus on health education as one possible effective strategy, which does not exclude organizational change as part of the health educators' role.

Interventions: Health education

Health education is based on motivation. In health education we try to change people's behavior by changing the three determinants of behavior: attitude, social influence and abilities/possibilities, by means of communciation. For instance, with respect to quitting smoking, we convince people about the risks of passive smoking to the health of their colleagues (attitude), we help them with organizing social support for quitting (social influence), and we provide them with ways to overcome urges and cravings (possibilities).

Because of its communicative nature effective health education depends on the interaction between educator and target person or target group (McGuire, 1985; Kok, 1988). Therefore the first phase in health education is the attention phase: do people listen to you and do they understand what you mean? Educators differ in background, life style, etc. from target groups, and mutual understanding should not be taken for granted.

Getting attention and changing determinants are necessary but not sufficient for behavior change. Health education is only then effective, when the desired behavior has become a new habit: the desired behavioral change is maintained. Such a behavioral maintenance is not easy to reach. It might be easy to get people to try the new behavior: it is much more difficult to get people to maintain that behavior. Of considerable importance in this respect is the question whether the observed effects of the behavior change or some other kind of feedback are rewarding. Basically however, most behavioral changes in health education do not have direct or short term rewarding effects. Most forms of natural feedback are not rewarding; for instance, people who stop smoking feel bad at first, sometimes gain weight and may have conflicts with their family and colleagues. Such lack of rewards, or even negative effects, can lead to lapse and even relapse. Health educators have to provide some kind of organized rewarding feedback, for instance an increase in physical fitness that can be shown by a test every three months. In a company a decrease in absenteeism or an increase in productivity as a result of a health promotion program could be shown. This form of feedback will be especially effective with people who feel committed to the company.

Health education in practice is a challenging activity, which we cannot describe in any satisfactory way here. Examples of health education at the workplace are given by Parkinson et al. (1982). We will now focus on research about its effectiveness.

Effectiveness Studies on Health Education at the Workplace

1. Occupational safety and the prevention of accidents: These programs appear to be successful. Different educational methods have been used, focussing on prompting (Laner & Sell, 1960), overcoming resistance and social control (Zohar et al., 1980), information and feedback (Hopkins, 1981; Komaki et al., 1980).
2. Quitting smoking: The participation rate is low, but the effect is high, compared with the same programs outside the workplace (Kornitzer et al., 1980). Smokers have more health problems and the increase in health and in productivity as a result of quitting seems high (Fielding, 1982; 1984; Kristein, 1982).
3. Fitness, a popular issue in health education at the workplace: Again, the participation rate is low, but the effect is high, compared with the same programs outside the workplace (Cox et al., 1981; Fielding, 1982; Shephard et al., 1982). Participants show less absenteeism, less turnover, and less days at the hospital. Participants also show an increase in physical fitness (Bjurstrom et al., 1978; Blair et al., 1987).
4. Hypertension: Hypertension programs at the workplace are more successful than the same programs outside the workplace (Fielding, 1982; 1984; Logan et al., 1981). Carefully planned anti-hypertension programs lead to a decrease in absenteeism (Alderman & Davis, 1976; Alderman et al., 1980; Alderman & Malcker, 1981; Novelli & Siska, 1982).
5. Mental health/stress reduction: at this moment these programs seem to be promising; the designs of the effectiveness studies have not been very adequate so far (Murphy, 1985). Mental health education programs seem to have positive effects on satisfaction and morale (Cox et al., 1981; Shephard, 1983). Stress reduction programs could have high potential; Collings (1984) reports an impressive decrease in stress indicators.
6. Absenteeism, not only a health problem but also a company problem: health education programs result in a decrease of absenteeism (Brennau, 1982; Cohen & Murphy, 1985; Fielding, 1982; Reed et al., 1985), and are in that respect cost-effective.
7. Life-style programs that are directed at a combination of health behaviors (weight, smoking, fitness, etc.): at this moment life-style programs seem to be the most promising (Fielding, 1982; Love et al., 1981). Programs are directed at "positive health" (Bly et al., 1987; Nathan, 1984), or at the prevention of cardiovascular diseases (Kornitzer et al., 1980; Rose et al., 1980), and seem to be cost-effective.

In sum, health education programs at the worksite do have potentially positive effects. Adequate research designs with longitudinal measures are still missing, but in a number of cases the results of acceptable research give ground for optimism. The first goal of the programs is health, but a second, important goal, cost-effectiveness, seems feasible. Parkinson et al. (1982) suggest five conditions that have to be fulfilled to achieve success (see Figure 1):
* careful analysis of the problem, the behavior, and the determinants
* clear and operational endgoals and subgoals
* careful analysis of the intervention setting and of the feasibility of the goal
* a careful development of an intervention, based on the first three issues
* a precise decision about the implementation, the material and immaterial means that are needed, with respect to both education and facilities and possible regulations.

Other authors stress the importance of personal rewards and personal efficacy (Davis et al., 1984), the participation of the target group (Cohen & Murphy, 1985; Alderman et al., 1980), the participation and commitment of management (Smith et al., 1978), and the structural character of health education programs (Cohen & Murphy, 1985; Dupont & Basen, 1982).

Conclusions

On the whole, we need better research, at least from a scientific point of view (most managers seem to be convinced already). We have seen that there is some variation in effectiveness, depending on the kind of health problem and the related behavior. Health education programs at the workplace seem to be able to motivate people to behave healthier by overcoming resistance, social control, training and feedback.

Changes are achieved in attitude (advantages and disadvantages of desired and undesired behavior), in social influence (pressure and control by colleagues and chief), and in abilities/ possibilities (training to be able to perform the desired behavior, feedback).

Why is health education so effective when conducted at the workplace? Probably because of the "attention" advantage, the social netweork, and the "group" effect on efficacy. Firstly, workplace health education programs can achieve an enormous amount of attention, and a well organized campaign will reach every employee. Secondly, the social network plays an important role in the success or failure of a health education program. At the workplace the social network can be modilized in favour of the program. Thirdly, methods to increase personal efficacy make use of groups, because of the interchange of ideas, suggestions, and advice that help people to prevent relapse. The workplace is thus an ideal situation for relapse prevention.

These observations are completely in line with recent developments in health education that emphasize the effectiveness of the community based approaches.

Community programs share the following characteristics: use of the social network, directed at life-style, multi-intervention strategies, multi-media methods, and participation of the target group (Farguhar, 1984). The workplace can be seen as a community.

More research is needed on the cost-effectiveness of the programs and on the conditions in which the programs can be most effective. We also need studies on process-evaluation in order to develop protocols about intervention development and implementation.

Health education at the workplace is a very promising field. If planned systematically, programs can be (health) effective and cost-effective. Health education has been shown to be beneficial not only for the individual employee, but for the company as well. These shared benefits explain the growing enthusiasm in the workplace for health education.

References

Ajzen, I. and Madden, T. J. (1986). Prediction of goal-directed behavior: attitudes, intentions and perceived behavioral control. *Journal of Experimental Social Psychology, 22*, 453–474.

Alderman, M. H. and Davis, T. K. (1976). Hypertension control at the worksite. *Journal of Occupational Medicine, 18*, 793–796.

Alderman, M. H., Green, L. W. and Flynn, B. S. (1980). Hypertension control programs in occupational settings. *Public Health Reports, 95*, 158–163.

Alderman, M. H. and Melcker, L. A. (1981). A company instituted program to improve blood pressure control in primary control in primary care. *Israël Journal of Medical Science, 17*, 122–128.

Bandura, A. (1986). *Social foundations of thought and action; a social cognitive theory.* Prentice Hall: Englewood Cliffs, N. J.

Bjurstrom, L. A. and Alexion, N. G. (1978). A program of heart-disease intervention for public employees. *Journal of Occupational Medicine, 20*, 521–531.

Blair, S. N., Piserchia, P. V., Wilbur, C. S. and Crowder, J. H. (1987). Interventiemodel voor conditieverbetering van werknemers in verschillende bedrijven. *Journal of the American Medical Association (Dutch Edition), 3*, 97–103.

Bly, J. L., Jones, R. C. and Richardson. J. E. (1987). Effect van bedrijfsgezondheidsprogramma's op kosten en gebruik medische voorzieningen. *Journal of the American Medical Association (Dutch edition), 3*, 91–96.

Brennau, A. J. J. (1982). Health Promotion: What's in it for business and industry? *Health Education Quarterly, 9*, 9–19.

Cohen, A. and Murphy, L. (1985). Indicators and measures of health promotion/health protection at the workplace. US Dept. of health and human services. Public Health Service. Centers for Disease Control. National Institute for Occupational Safety and Health. Cincinatti, Ohio.

Collings, G. H. (1984). Stress and the workplace. In J. D. Matarazzo, S. M. Weiss, J. A. Herd, N. E. Miller and S. M. Weiss (Eds.), *Behavioral health* (p. 1079–1086). New York: Wiley.

Cox, M., Shephard, R. J. and Renzland, P. (1982). Fitness program reduces health care costs. *Dimensions*, 14–15.

Davis, K. E., Jackson, K. L., Kronenfeld, J. J. and Blair, S. E. (1984). Intention to participate in worksite health promotion activities: a model of risk factors and psychosocial variables. *Health Education Quarterly, 11*, 361–378.

Dupont, R. L. and Basen, M. M. (1982). Control of alcohol and drugs in industry, in R. S. Parkinson, (Ed.) *Managing Health Promotion in the workplace* (p. 194–216). Palo Alto: Mayfield.

Eiser, J. R. and Pligt, J. van der (1988). *Attitudes and decisions.* London: Routledge.

Farquhar, J. W., Maccoby, N. and Solomon, D. S. (1984). Community applications of behavioral medicine. In W. D. Gentry (Ed.), Handbook of behavioral medicine (p. 437–478). New York: Guilford.

Fielding, J. E. (1982). Effectiveness of employee health improvement programs. *Journal of Occupational Medicine, 24*, 907–916.

Fielding, J. E. (1984). Health promotion and disease prevention at the worksite. *Annual Review of Public Health, 5*, 237–265.

Fishbein, M. and Ajzen, I. (1975). *Belief, attitude, intention, and behavior: An introduction to theory and research.* Reading, Mass.: Addison-Wesley.

Green, L. W. and Lewis, F. M. (1986). *Measurement and evaluation in health education and health promotion.* Palo Alto: Mayfield.

Hopkins, B. L. (1981). Behavioral procedures for reducing worker exposure to carcinogens. NIOSH Contract. Rept. Z 10–77–0042, NIOSH Cincinatti, Ohio.

Kok, G. (1988). Health motivation: Health education from a social psychological point of view. In S. Maes, C. D. Spielberger, P. B. Defares and I. G. Sarason (Eds.), *Topics in health psychology* (p.295–300). New York: Wiley.

Komaki, J., Barwich, K. D. and Scott, L. R. (1978). A behavioral approach to occupational safety: pinpointing and reinforcing safe performance in a food manufacturing plant. *Journal of Applied Psychology, 63*, 434–445..

Kornitzer, M., DeBacker, G., Dramaix, M. and Kittel, F. (1980). The Belgian heart disease prevention project. *Circulation, 61*, 18–25.

Kristein, M. M. (1982). The economics of health promotion at the worksite. *Health Education Quarterly, 9*, 27–36.

Laner, S. and Sell, R. G. (1960). An experiment on the effect of specially designed safety posters. *Occupational Psychology, 34, 153–169.*

Leeuw, E. de (1989). *The sane revolution; backgrounds, scope, prospects.* Assen, Neth.: Van Gorcum.

Logan. A., Milne, B., Achber, C. (1981). Cost-effectiveness of worksite hypertension treatment program. *Hypertension, 3*, 211–219.

Love, M., Morphis, L. and Page, P. (1981). Model for employee wellness project. *Journal of the American College Heart Association,* Feb, 171–173.

Marlatt, G. A. and Gordon, J. R. (1985). *Relapse prevention; maintenance strategies in the treatment of addictive behaviors.* New York: Guilford.

McGuire, W. J. (1985). Attitudes and attitude change. In G. Lindsay and E. Aranson (Eds.), *Handbook of social psychology*, 3rd edition, vol. 2 (p. 233– 346). New York: Random House.

Milio, N. (1986). *Promoting health through public policy.* Ottawa: Canadian Public Health Association.

Murphy, L. R. (1985). Evaluation of worksite stress management. *Corporate Commentary, 1*, 24–31.

Nathan, P. E. (1984). Johnson & Johnson live for life: a comprehensive positive lifestyle change program. In J. D. Matarazzo, Sh. M. Weiss, J. A. Herd, N. E. Miller and St. M. Weiss (Eds.), *Behavioral health* (p. 1064–1070). New York: Wiley.

Novelli, W. D. and Ziska, D. (1982). Health Promotion in the workplace: an overview. *Health Education Quarterly, 9*, 20–26.

Parkinson, R. S. and Associates (1982). *Managing health promotion in the workplace; guidelines for implementation and evaluation.* Palo Alto, Cal.: Mayfield.

Reed, R. W., Mulvaney, D., Bellingham, R. and Huber, K. C. (1985). *Health Promotion Service evaluation and impact study.* Indianapolis: Blue Cross and Blue Shield of Indiana.

Rose, G., Heller, R. F., Tunstall-Pedoe, H. and Christie, D. G. E. (1980). Heart disease prevention project: a randomized control trial in industry. *British Medical Journal, 280*, 747–751.

Schwartz, J. L. (1987). Review and evaluation of smoking cessation methods: the United States and Canada, 1978–1985, U. S. department of Health and Human Services, Public Health Service, National Institutes of Health, Bethesda, Maryland.

Shephard, R. J., Cox, M. and Corsey, P. (1981). Fitness program participation: its effects on worker performance. *Journal of Occupational Medicine, 23*, 359–363.

Shephard, R. J., (1983). Employee health and fitness: the state of the art. *Preventive Medicine, 12*, 644–653.

Smith, M. J., Cohen, H. H., Cohen, A, and Cleveland, R. J. (1978). Characteristics of succesful safety programs. *Journal of Safety Research, 10*, 5–15.

Siero, S., Boon, M. E., Kok, G. J. and Siero, F. (in press). Modification of driving behavior in large transport organization: a field experiment. *Journal of Applied Psychology.*

Strecher, V. J., De Vellis, B. M., Becker, M. H. and Rosenstock, I. M. (1986). The role of self efficacy in achieving health behavior change. *Health Education Quarterly, 13*, 73–92.

Vries, H. de, Dijkstra, M. and Kuhlman, P. (1988). Self efficacy: The third factor besides attitude and subjective norm as predicate of behavioral intention. *Health Education Research, 3*, 272–282.

Weiner, B. (1986). *An attributional theory of motivation and emotion.* New York: Springer.

Zohar, D., Cohen, A. and Azar, N. (1980). Promoting increased use of ear protectors in noise through feedback. *Human Factors, 22*, 69–79.

Prevention in The Workplace: An Integrative Cooperation Task

Gerhard Murza

Changes in the Understanding of Health and Prevention

Recently there have been fundamental changes in the way prevention is viewed. The subject of health is becoming increasingly important in sociopolitical discussions, in public service and trade, as well as for the individual. Within this context, prevention has increasingly taken on a new meaning. Although its intent is still to prevent the onset of illness, the underlying concept of health has been given new accent. In the 1970's there was a change in the traditional view from a polar health – illness scale to an orientation that emphasized the significance of emotional, somatic and social aspects for prevention. Nowadays there is emphasis on positive feedback and experiences made possible by a healthy lifestyle, the idea being to encourage conscious alterations in individual lifestyles. Health is depicted as a way of life that is positive and fun. This trend can also be seen in the Federal Republic of Germany. "Wellness" or health, the new fitness, has found a lot of followers, especially in the United States and in Japan. It is a philosophy of life that brings together the joy of living and rules of health. Interest has focused on the use of proper diet and fitness in connection with stress-reducing programs in order to bring about the experience of well-being and emotional harmony (Ardell, 1985; Mullen, 1986; Greenberg, 1985; Lautenschläger, Hamm & Lagerstroem, 1987).

On the other hand, much interest is still directed at the classical view of prevention. In particular, the human cardiovascular system will continue to be the primary target of health campaigns (Laaser, Murza, Gerdal & Borgers, 1988). As before, morbidity and mortality rates affect health-policy decisions, and results of intervention research suggest that the so-called risk factors for cardiovascular diseases will continue to play a role in the future (Löwel & Keil, 1988; Mannebach, Gleichmann & Gleichmann 1985).

Preventive projects, however, are increasingly based on aspects of social theories and the social sciences have a growing influence on preventive planning and practice. Social marketing models of cooperation, organization and communication are being used more and more as the basis for planned modifications in health-related attitudes and the behavior of target groups (Troschke, 1985; Murza & Laaser, 1985; Laaser, 1986; AOK, 1981).

Cooperative prevention as a basis for health promotion programs at the workplace

In recent years the principle of cooperation has come to be regarded as a component of actual prevention. The cooperation of groups, organizations and institutions is an essential element in political decisions (GMK, 1982) and in comprehensive scientific studies, both in the Federal Republic of Germany and in other countries (DHP, 1988; Farquhar, Maccoby & Wood, 1983; Elder, McGraw & Lasater, 1987; Gutwiller, Junod & Schweizer, 1985).

The term "cooperative prevention" is often understood to be an alternative to "community prevention" (Laaser, 1986; DHP, 1988; Buchholz, 1981). Both concepts are in accordance with community-oriented programs, scientific studies and pragmatic municipal and district projects.

It appears that, in the future, more emphasis will be laid on congruence between target groups and health-related offers, and acceptance by these groups of health measures. In general, traditional health education has often failed to produce healthy lifestyles in large parts of the population. Many people do not avail themselves of medical checkups or other health-related possibilities.

– There are indications, for example, that participants in screening programs do not match the general population with regard to age and sex. The same problems have been reported in community-oriented studies (Heuermann & Murza, 1987; Parisch, Catford & Howsen, 1987).

– According to a recent survey (Infratest, 1987), managers live more healthily and feel healthier than other groups.

– Mortality rates for ischemic diseases reveal a disadvantage for lower social classes (Gutzwiller, 1988).

– Employees whose worksite is characterized by bad working conditions and/or limited participation in decision making more frequently display behavioral risks (e.g. smoking, alcohol consumption, stress) (Kotthoff, 1986).

These and similar results have directed attention to working people. This field of intervention is included within the theoretical concept of community-oriented prevention; in practice, however, projects in industrial settings are rare.

In contrast to Scandinavian countries or the United States, prevention in the workplace is not very popular in the Federal Republic of Germany, where prevention is regarded more in terms of safety, preventing work accidents and diseases caused by environmental pollutants.

Prevention at the worksite and prevention in the community can only be understood as a cooperative challenge (Pelletier, 1986; Wilbur, Hartwell & Piserchia, 1986) and is demonstrated by many worksite programs in the United States. Pilot projects show that it is possible to transfer these experiences to the situation in the Federal Republic of Germany.

At the very outset of planning a worksite program, it is necessary to secure the agreement and sustained support of management, labor union representatives, company physicians and the company insurance office. In large companies existing social work staffs, psychologists, company sport clubs and health service directors should also be included.

At first glance, cooperation would seem to be plausible, but one must bear in mind that the afore-mentioned groups have very different interests. Improving productivity, increasing performance, promoting work satisfaction, reducing illness or accidents, improving work conditions or even securing a good image are only a few aspects, some of which may proved to be barriers to a company health committee.

One other aspect deserves mention. In contrast to health education, the concept of health promotion is extended to include approaches to individual behavior as well as modifications to certain structural aspects in the company. Educational measures pertaining to the individual employee are just as qualified as those oriented toward organizational factors such as work design or work climate.

From this point of view, program planning should be described as comprehensive efforts to incorporate many single health-habit interventions into an integrated program. In this respect the key to accepted worksite programs is dealing with sophisticated communication strategies that utilize proven prevention methods to create health policy within the company.

Criteria of a Worksite Prevention Program

The institute for Social Medicine (IDIS) has developed a comprehensive service consisting of consultants, media, exhibitions, organizational know-how and technical equipment in order to support the planning, realization and evaluation of workplace prevention programs in the West German state of Northrhine-Westfalia. One cooperation partner is the "Landesverband der Betriebskrankenkassen NRW" (State Association of Company Insurance Programs in Northrhine-Westfalia). Nine companies are currently taking part in pilot projects.

The following criteria can be used to describe the program, based on the previously-described concept of health promotion and cooperative prevention:

The Focal Point: Positive Health

The goal of all efforts is to develop health-related attitudes and habits as components of the individual's lifestyle. Healthy behavior is encouraged, and alternatives to risk behavior are outlined.

Communication

Program planners are encouraged to make use of a wide variety of communication strategies; these include individual counseling, public relations in health affairs and modifications to current supplies and needs. Screening, educational courses and activities contribute to a philosophy of wellness.

Cooperation

A prerequisite for effective cooperation is to incorporate management officials, labor union representatives, and company health insurance executives into a health promotion committee.

Modules as Program Design

Each individual activity is a unit which can be selected at will. The worksite program can therefore be designed to accomodate personal and financial resources.

ALL EMPLOYEES ARE ENCOURAGED TO PARTICIPATE

Every employee can take part in the prevention program, and family members are also invited to participate.

VISUAL COMMUNICATION

The slogan which accompanies all parts of the program can be translated as "Have a Heart for your Heart" (see Figure 1).

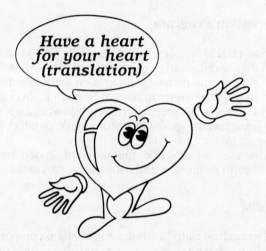

Figure 1. The cartoon heart of the prevention program.

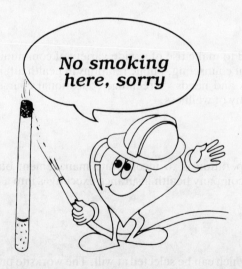

Figure 2. The cartoon of the non-smoking campaign.

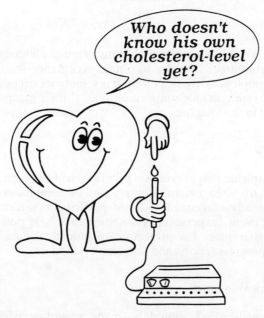

Figure 3. The cartoon of the cholesterol screening

A pilot study showed that this cartoon scored high on sympathy and recognition; in addition, the figure can be used for communicative purposes. To deliver different messages the design of the heart can be varied, as shown in Figures 2 and 3. This cartoon heart is found on all of the announcements, posters, brochures, leaflets, exhibitions and other material. Interview results show that the cartoon heart evokes positive valences (König & Murza, 1988).

Planning and Preparation

The specific schedule shows that a lot of planning processes must take place, decisions and agreements have to be reached and preparations have to be made. Several key aspects are summarized in the following paragraphs.

Commitment

Carrying out a prevention program requires commitment and support on the part of upper management and the company board of directors. The first step in convincing cooperation members is precise presentation of the goals, program arrangements and evaluation methods.

Objectives

Objectives must be described precisely. Plans should aim at continuing the program over several years. Long-term planning is a prerequisite for securing financial resources, surveying health-related habits and evaluating progress.

Planning Group

Experience has shown the value of establishing a formal planning group, such as a company health committee. In order to obtain acceptance for the program, it is essential to secure employees' participation. It is sometimes necessary to limit length of attendance (e.g. one year) for some employees, if their manpower involvement cannot be tolerated in the long run.

Protection of Data

There can be no suspicion that prevention programs will deliver health-related data on the employees to management. For reasons of compliance and evaluation, however, it is often advantageous to address participants directly and organize a follow-up. In any event, experience has shown that is it possible to reach an agreement which guarantees the protection of individual data and still permits follow-up studies, progress reports and outcome evaluations.

Specification of the Worksite

To begin with, specifications should be made regarding personnel structure, employees' health status and working methods. Outline form can be used to describe decentralization, shifts, automation and other stress-inducing circumstances.

Realization

To begin planning, the health committee will be given an outline of twelve proposed program units (see Table 1). The actual execution of the program is supported by IDIS. Checklists, information material and equipment are available for most of these models.

Table 1. *Schedule for a prevention program in the workplace*

1. Watch your weight and blood pressure.
2. Health forum.
3. Quit smoking. Smoke-free workplace.
4. Who doesn't know his own cholesterol level yet?
5. Dietary counseling for everyone.
6. Start the New Year with good resolutions.
7. Two times a year: Check your blood pressure.
8. Canteen project: Herbs and spices instead of salt.
9. Relaxation and exercise at the workplace.
10. Am I eating the right foods?
11. Coping with stress.
12. Test it again: Blood pressure, weight and chlosterol.

This schedule (see Table 1) has the following model characteristics:
– It enforces the idea of regularly setting health priorities
– It underlines the fact that there are strong links between different areas in health
  promotion
– It implies that this may be the beginning of continuous worksite prevention, and
  extensions to this program
– It takes both individual and structural prevention aspects into account
– It encourages the individual to take responsibility for his own health

Outlook

Following a pilot study completed in 1987, IDIS intends to support further worksite
programs in Northrhine-Westfalia. Previous experience with community-oriented
projects has helped in developing screening methods, educational material and
organizational know-how (Murza & Schapeit, 1985; Murza, Laaser & Annuss, 1988;
IDIS, 1988). Meanwhile, chlosterol screening is possible. During the pilot study
cholesterol screening was carried out with the employees of six companies and three
administration offices in Bielefeld (Federal Republic of Germany), a total of about
8500 employees. The participation rate was approximately 85%, 24% of the
employees already knew their own cholesterol levels. Cholesterol screening should,
in the future, be increasingly regarded as a prevention strategy. Relationships
between tests and dietary counselling will be explored. With regard to chlosterol
distribution within the general population, another study showed that 27% of the
employees involved in the study had cholesterol levels above 250 mg/dl. 6% availed
themselves of the opportunity to participate in dietary consultations.

The possibilities of fitness screening as a motivation vehicle to get the employees
in contact with local sport associations will be analyzed.

References

AOK. (1988). *Grundlagenbericht zur Aktion Gesundheit* [Report of a health campaign]. Velbert: AOK für den Kreis Mettmann.

Ardell, D. B. (1985). The history and future of wellness. *Health Values, 9*, 37–57.

Buchholz, L. (1981). Das Modell "Kommunale Prävention" (Local prevention as a model). *Prävention, 4*, 105–107.

DHP. (1988). *Studienhandbuch der Deutschen Herz-Kreislauf-Präventionsstudie* (Manual of the german cardiovascular prevention study). Bonn: WIAD.

Elder, J. P., McGraw, S. A., and Lasater, I (1987). Gemeindenahe Prävention von Herz-Kreislauf-Krankheiten in den USA – Die Pawtucket-Studie (Community prevention of cardiovascular diseases in USA). *Prävention, 10*, 107–111.

Farquhar, J. W., Maccoby, N., and Wood, D. P. (1983). *Education and community studies: Vol. 3. Investive methods in public health*. Oxford: Pergamon Press.

GMK. (1982). Entschließung der 50. Konferenz der für das Gesundheitswesen zuständigen Minister und Senatoren der Länder (Declaration of the 50. conference of ministers of health). *Prävention, 2*, 63.

Greenberg, J. S. (1985). Health and wellness: a conceptual differentiation. *Journal of School Health, 55*, 403–406.

Gutzwiller, F., Junod, B., and Schweizer, W. (1985). *Wirksamkeit der gemeindeorientierten Prävention kardiovaskulärer Krankheiten* (Efficiency of community prevention of cardiovascular diseases). Bern: Huber.

Gutzwiller, F. (1988). Herz-Kreislauf-Krankheiten: Ein medizinisches und soziales Problem (Cardiovascular diseases: a medical and social problem). *Sozial-und Präventivmedizin, 33*, 6–9.

Heuermann, S., and Murza, G. (1987). Bluthochdruck – weit verbreitet? (To the incidence of hypertension). *Prävention, 10*, 99–102.

IDIS. (1988). *Gesunde Städte. Aktuelle Literatur zum "Gesunde-Städte-Projekt" der Weltgesundheitsorganisation* (Healthy cities – a bibliography of a WHO-project). Bielefeld: Author.

Infratest (1987). Manager-Verhaltensstudie (Manger behavior-study). Unpublished manuscript.

König, U., and Murza, G. (1988) *Umfrage zur Wiedererkennung und Akzeptanz der visuellen Komponente eines Herz-Kreislauf-Präventionsprogramms* (Recognition and acceptance of visual elements of a cardiovascular prevention program). Unpublished manuscript.

Kotthof, H. (1986). *Betriebliche Personalpolitik im Umgang mit gesundheitlichen Beeinträchtigungen* (Impairment and personal policy as a management problem). Saarbrücken: Arbeitskammer des Saarlandes.

Laaser, U. (1986). Die Deutsche Herz-Kreislauf-Präventionsstudie: Das Modell einer kooperativen Prävention (The german cardiovascular prevention study: A model of cooperative prevention). In C. Halhuber and K. Traencker (Eds.), *Die Koronare Herzkrankheit – eine Herausforderung an Gesellschaft und Politik* (pp. 212–232). Erlangen: Perimed.

Laaser, U., Murza, G., Gerdel, W., and Borgers, D. (1988). Strategien zur Prävention von Herz-Kreislauf-Krankheiten (Prevention-strategies of cardiovascular diseases). *Sozial- und Präventivmedizin, 33*, 226–232.

Lautenschläger, F., Hamm, M., and Lagerstroem, D. (1987). *Wellness, die neue Fitness* (Wellness, the new fitness). München: Goldmann.

Löwel,H., and Keil, U.(1985). Morbidity and mortality of myocardial infarction in the monica-study area Augsburg in 1985. *Sozial- und Präventivmedizin, 33*, 17–21.

Mannebach, H., Gleichmann, S., and Gleichmann, U. (1982). Risikofaktoren-Modifikation: Stand der Interventionsforschung (Up-date of interventive research). *Prävention, 5*, 72–79.

Mullen, K. D. (1986). Wellness: The missing concept in health promotion programming for adults. *Health Values, 10*, 34–37.

Murza, G., and Laaser, U. (1985). Kooperation auf dem Prüfstand der Praxis-Umfrage bei den Gesundheitsämtern in Nordrhein-Westfalen zur Existenz von Arbeitsgemeinschaften für Gesundheitsförderung (Cooperation as a challenge to everyday-business of health promotion). *Zeitschrift für öffentliches Gesundheitswesen, 50*, 151–154.

Murza, G., Laaser, U., and Annuss, R. (1988). Cholesterinscreening im Rahmen präventiver Strategien (Cholesterol-screening as a prevention strategy). *Sozial-und Präventivmedizin, 33*, 51–55.

Murza, G., and Schapeit, M. (1985). *Kommunale Prävention. Gesundheitsaktion Oberbergischer Kreis* (Community-orientated prevention – health campaign im Oberbergischen Kreis). Bielefeld: IDIS.

Parish, R., Catford. J. C., and Howsen, H. (1987). Promoting health through collaboration with industry and commerce. The development of the welsh heart programme. In Akademie für öffentliches Gesundheitswesen (Ed.), *Gemeindebezogene Gesundheitsvorsorge und Gesundheitsförderung: Vol. 15.* Düsseldorf: Akademie für öffentliches Gesundheitswesen.

Pelletier, K. R. (1986). Healthy people in healthy places: Health promotion programs in the workplace. In M. F. Cataldo and T. J. Coates (Eds.), *Health and industry: A behavioral medicine perspective* (pp. 351–372). New York: Wiley.

Troschke, J. (1985). Die soziale Prozeßevaluation der deutschen Herz-Kreislauf-Präventionsstudie (DHP) I (The social process-evaluation of the german cardiovascular prevention study). *Prävention, 8*, 35–42.

Wilbur, C. S., Hartwell, T. D., and Piserchia, P. V. (1986). The Johnson and Johnson "Live for life"-program: Its organization and evaluation plan. In M. F. Cataldo and T. J. Coates (Eds.), *Health and industry: A behavioral medicine perspective* (pp. 338–350). New York: Wiley.

Marketing Health and Changing Behaviour

Arild Raaheim

Health Marketing – Some Introductory Remarks

A great many of the industrialised nations suffer from high mortality caused by unhealthy behaviour. We eat too much fat food, we drink too much alcohol and use other stimulants like tobacco to excess. As a result, we spend vast sums of money treating a number of 'self-inflicted' diseases. In comparison very little has, traditionally, been spent on prevention of diseases and on health promotion. It is, e.g. estimated that the American medical care system provided the public with $287 billion worth of goods and services in 1982. Of this only 4% was spent on prevention of diseases and on health promotion. Furthermore, it is estimated that 48% of U.S. mortality (1975) is due to unhealthy behaviour or lifestyle (O'Donell & Ainsworth, 1984).

As the connection between lifestyle habits and disease has become clearer, and also since it is obvious that much money might be saved if more were done in terms of prevention of disease, the marketing of healthier behaviour and positive lifestyle habits is today very much in focus. A number of programs have been designed to help people change their unhealthy behaviour and lifestyle. Likewise, many campaigns focusing on the relationship between lifestyle habits and health have been introduced. As one has come to accept the costs attributed to specific lifestyle habits – e.g. smoking – efforts have been made to induce better health habits both at the individual level, at the worksite and at a community level (Leventhal & Cleary, 1980; Jarvis, 1983; Fielding, 1982, 1984; Lichtenstein & Mermelstein, 1984; Windsor & Bartlett, 1984).

In 1971 the term 'social marketing' was introduced to describe the use of marketing principles and techniques to advance a social cause, idea or behaviour (Frederiksen, Solomon & Brehony, 1984). As consumers of an endless variety of products, we have come to accept the existence of advertisers, public relations people and market analysers. Admittedly such bodies affect our opinions of various products and thus exert a very direct influence on our choice of product. If this holds true for household goods, may not the same be true for social causes? What makes the 'selling' of health information any different from any other selling and buying, one asked.

Before starting a discussion of how to change peoples health behaviour, we ought probably first to acknowledge that such marketing, at least to some extent, is a bit self-contradictory. A person who enjoys smoking does not necessarily see a life without tobacco as a better, more promising and healthier life. He may, consequently, not buy our arguments as he already considers himself to be in possession of what we have to offer. If we, in spite of this fact, succeed in convincing

141

the person to stop smoking, it would probably only be achieved after having 'attacked' him to make him feel bad about himself. In order to become "healthier" and to lead a "better life" – as *we* define these concepts – the individual must first feel to be in the need of a change. If he stops smoking, we have no guarantee that he actually feels good as a result of this.

We have, then, a situation where we must convince the individuals who belong to our target group that what they do, feel or think is wrong, and that by following our advice they will be better off. If or when they are convinced, we have to make sure that they do indeed change their behaviour. It ought not come as a surprise to anyone that changes in personal health habits do not occur overnight, but will come about quite slowly (if indeed at all). But is this a truth necessarily shared by those who campaign for changes in personal health behaviour? The way some campaigns are introduced to the public, one may well ask. Sometimes one is left with the impression that those running the campaigns generally assume that people actually will change, once they are reminded of some negative consequences of their behaviour – in other words, that this is a necessary but also a sufficient reason for change to take place. It seems to be an assumption based upon the idea that the human being is a rational creature, and as such always relates to information in a matter-of-fact sort of way. This does not mean that health experts do not accept the general idea that humans may behave in an irrational manner, and that they often act in contrast to what they know is the correct or sensible thing to do. However, it seems that such an insight sometimes is lost when it comes to the planning and presenting of health information, or more importantly; when it comes to the question of the effects one thinks the information will have upon the audience. There is, of course, nothing wrong in expecting your information to have a particular effect on the audience. When one informs someone who smokes of the dangers involved, one may expect that he or she understands what is being said. One may expect that he or she recognises that what is being said is the truth, and that he or she, as a consequence, will behave in accordance with this, say that they will stop smoking. The fact is, however, that neither of these expectations may come true, and so we must be open to alternatives. One alternative is, of course, that the information will have no direct, observable effect. Another alternative might be that the information leads to some direct changes, but not to the kind you had wished for or seen as the most favourable ones.

The fact that human behaviour is often unpredictable is not always sufficiently taken care of by those planning a health campaign. The way some campaigns are introduced makes one believe that those in charge take it for granted that everyone looks upon the information in the same way, and that the information either leads to the expected change or to no change at all. In making such an assumption, one neglects the audience. We may, therefore, as has also been pointed out by others, have difficulties in explaining exactly how the information affects the audience and why the information does not lead to the expected change (Kaplan, 1984). If, on the other hand, we accept that humans are irrational, and at the same time acknowledge that health information may be perceived in different ways, we might perhaps plan and present the information in a different way, thus being able to affect the audience much more effectively.

When one is planning a health campaign it is important to bear in mind the type of audience one is addressing. To most people this seems self-evident and hardly worth mentioning. In any case, the fact remains that some planners are quite negligent as to their target population. This is e.g. revealed by the way the information ('the message') is presented; by the language used and the way it is introduced. In marketing health and trying to change the behaviour and attitude of a particular target population, one has, furthermore, to be aware of the distinctive characteristics of the arena. What does the arena – the marketplace – look like, and what are the "change-potentials'?

The Marketplace

The term marketplace may have more than one meaning. On the one hand it may refer to the physical-geographical and economic environment in which the individual lives. In this respect a particular attitude or a particular type of behaviour may prove to have or to have had in the past some significant adaptive function. On the other hand, the term may refer to the social environment of the individual. Although it may give rise to some minor problems, one may try to separate the one from the other. In what follows, 'marketplace' will be take to mean 'the social environment of the individual'.

Now, as used here, 'social environment' has many connotations. Besides referring to what is normally understood – i.e. the factors that constitute the individual's conscious experience of reality – social environment refers to the things that determine a person's actual position in different organisations or work settings, and his feelings, thoughts and actions within different organisational settings. It also refers to the more informal parts of our daily life; how what we do is governed by formal as well as informal norms and rules. In short, 'social environment' comprises both what might be called the open and the hidden 'norm-culture'.

If we take a closer look at the more limited work-setting, it becomes clear that the social environment of any individual is related to, and to some extent influenced by, the administrative and technical-economic environment typical of the worksite. But even if this is true, the chances are that many important decisions are made either directly or indirectly through the influence of a hidden norm-culture.

To have some knowledge of the marketplace and to be aware of some of the main 'market forces' governing the behaviour of a particular target population, is important to everyone who wishes to achieve a change of attitudes through the use of information. An external party that stays on the outside and is reluctant to seek such information, or is blind to the existence of such norm-cultures, will probably have little chance of success when it come to anything but minor changes in the way people behave. One may, at first, experience what seems to be real changes, only to learn at a later stage that these were only apparent changes, or changes that took place at a surface level.

One may also find that whether or not the information is perceived as relevant, and leads to any changes, is highly dependent on the behaviour of one significant member of the organisation. This individual may, as a consequence of his rank or position within the organisation, have the authority to enforce his decisions on others. Or, as is sometimes found, his actions may be followed by others out of silent respect, because of his long experience, or due to some other virtue ascribed to him. When propagandistic information fails to have an effect, then, the reason may be that the informers fail to get through to such an influential member of a group or organisation.

When collecting data on work environment and lifestyle habits among employees at
a Norwegian ferroalloy plant, I found that the response rate varied very much from
one division to another. Whereas nearly everyone answered the questionnaire in
some of the divisions, other divisions had a response rate close to zero. A repeated
request was sent out but this did not have much effect. As a final effort I paid a visit
to all divisions. On these visits not only the foremen were approached (they had
previously been requested to distribute the questionnaire and to ask the people
working in their own division to fill them in), but a number of other people were also
seen. What was found during these visits ought probably not to have come as a
surprise, but it did. In some divisions the foreman had little to say on matters which
were not directly related to doing the job. In one case the response rate was raised
from 0 to 60% as I managed to persuade one of the older employees to fill in the
questionnaire, not being aware of this person's importance as an informal leader.
What happened was not his asking the others to fill in their questionnaire. The mere
fact that he himself filled it in made most of the others do the same (Raaheim, 1987,
1989).

There is, probably, more than one lesson to be learned from this. Theory and
practice are seldom the same. We may know all there is to know about informal
leadership and group processes in theory, but when it comes to practice we
sometimes behave in ways contrary to such knowledge. Equally important is
probably the lesson that different groups and organisations have their own informal
structure and norm-culture influencing the behaviour of their members.

As part of the study mentioned above, employees were offered participation in a
smoking cessation program at the worksite (Raaheim & Myklebust, 1988; Raaheim,
1989). The employees had previously been asked to state their opinion as to their
participation were such a program to be set up. Forty-nine made a positive response.
Of these, 30 signed up for a meeting where information about the program was to be
presented. Only 13 turned up. Of these, 10 took part in the program. Whereas all 10
stopped smoking at the date agreed upon, only two were abstinent at a three month
follow-up. Not a very promising result, but then again, one very similar to what has
been found before (Ockene, Nutall, Benfari, Hurwitz & Ockene, 1981; Hall, Rugg,
Tunstall & Jones, 1984; Ossip-Klein & Bigelow, 1986). In our own case, however,
the relapse is very rapid. Most likely this has something to do with the setting – the
marketplace – in which our participants find themselves. Smoking is more than just
lighting a cigarette. Smoking is a ritual, and by taking part in this you demonstrate
that you are part of a special group (e.g. blue collars). Lighting a cigarette becomes
a symbol of solidarity, and as the pressure from outside increases (health warnings),
such symbolism becomes even more important. Quitting smoking is, therefore, not
an easy thing to do, and indeed not a personal matter. It is in fact an act of treason.
By putting your tobacco on the shelf you not only let go your group membership.
You also make clear that you are more able, more conscious or maybe even more
considerate than the rest. Clearly a provocative act, and one which the group
disapproves of and tries to prevent. There are, in other words, barriers preventing
you from taking action to change your behaviour. These barriers exist within you but
they are, at the same time, inseparable from the opinions of the people belonging to
the same group. Any decision of yours is, consequently, not uniquely your own since
it has an effect on the others as well.

The Information

The way it is defined here, the 'marketplace' also encompasses the shared experience within an organisation or a social group of what is good or bad, just or injust, positive or negative. There is, in other words, no objective criterion for deciding what is the one and what the other. Social marketing is, however, the promotion of one particular idea or value system. Sometimes this is close to or concurrent with the ideas of the target group, but sometimes it may clash and evoke very negative responses. Such responses may be triggered by a hidden message which, whether consciously placed there or not, is part of every health campaign. When, for example, we confront our target group with some information as to the hazards of cigarette smoking, we also say that those who continue to smoke after having heard what we have said, are less talented or more ignorant than the rest of us.

Now, let's say our target population is a group of teenagers, indulging in activities – including cigarette smoking – known to be health hazardous. Chances are that our information about the negative effects of cigarette smoking will have close to no effect on their smoking behaviour, unless some specific situational factor makes the information especially convincing. Teenagers are often very sensitive to the hidden message, and very much so if the information is supplied by someone distant to the youth culture. When health information fails to have an effect on this audience, part of the reason may be that those who supply the information are not seen as credible, because the hidden message lurking underneath the surface is so easily detected. When confronting one audience or another, we are up against different market forces. The forces are probably more extreme and more influencial among teenagers, probing the joys of life in a setting often asking for conformity, than will be found elsewhere. This is not to say that any attempt to get through with health information is a waste of time. But, one may add, since the marketplace never is the same from one group to another, the information needs to be differentiated accordingly.

If we take a closer look at some of our more recent national efforts in Norway, we will have a further illustration of some of the ideas presented above. During the past decade Norwegian authorities have focused much attention on the increasing number of road accidents involving young people. The problem has been looked at from different angles, and a variety of measures have been discussed and put into action. The striking thing is, however – both as far as the direct measures are concerned and with regard to the more general discussion – that much of it seems to discredit youths. Sometimes in a direct manner, but most of the time in more subtle ways, youths are portrayed as incompetent, immoral and immature. They are pictured as individuals in restless search of excitement, using alcohol and other stimuli to excess, each being perceived as a potential danger once seated behind the wheel of a car or on a motor cycle. These are attitudes that are not often expressed openly, but which constitute the hidden message that young people sense and respond to.

Looking at the different measures that have been suggested or carried out, we find that they almost exclusively concentrate on the negative aspects of what youths do. Only seldom is any attention paid to the positive aspects of alternative activities. Instead of rewarding those who drive according to the law, the focus is always on the rule breakers. One result of this is that all insurance companies have set higher rates for those under 23. In this way everyone under the age of 23 is punished economically as well as being stigmatised. Furthermore, there have been discussions about enforcing severe penalties for those who break the rules, and the neccessity of increasing the minimum age for driving. All of this when one still is hoping to create positive changes.

As it becomes clear that the different measures taken have but a minor effect, one would expect alternative measures to be discussed. Instead we find that officials and experts behave the way a doctor sometimes is seen to do, when one of his patients does not respond to medication. First he may try to increase the dose (more of the same). If this does not work, he may turn to another pill (still using the same remedy). By the time he finds out that all the patient really needed was someone to talk to, the patient may long since have gone to see somebody else.

Whether or not health information will have a persuasive effect depends not only on some characteristic or other of the audience, but also on the nature of the information and on the way it is presented. Some rely on threat communication and believe this to be the best way to achieve a behavioural change. If the information is fear arousing, is perceived as something of importance to the person, and if the person is supplied with alternatives, feels to be in control and has the personal efficacy to change, then a change of behaviour is likely to take place, the argument goes (Rogers, 1975; Beck & Lund, 1981).

Indeed a lot of if's. What if normally it turns out to be difficult to meet them all? What may the barrier be? Perhaps the information was too threatening and therefore has led to some cognitive 'blockade'? Maybe too much emphasis was put on the health threat and too little was said about the alternatives? Whatever the reason, the question remains whether the same cognitive and motivational processes can be triggered by non-threatening communication.* We know that (especially young) people often conceive of their own susceptibility to health risks to be weaker than that of their peers, and that perceived control is related to an optimitic bias associated with health hazards (Weinstein, 1982, 1984). It is also commonly accepted that information – whether it is health information or not – very often is perceived in accordance with some understanding or attitude which the person already possesses (e.g. Snyder, Tanke & Bersheid, 1977). Can it be that health information presented in the form of threats, rather than leading to a lasting change in attitude or behaviour, sometimes leads to a defensive action on the part of the individual such as to give a directly opposite effect from that intended? We may very well find that the individuals we address change their behaviour, but the question is; for how long? Chances are that the change is relatively shortlived and that the individuals in question will be back to where they started when an immediate threat is no longer felt. The information may have had an effect, but since it has such a threatening and provocative nature it may be stored in a separate cognitive 'compartment'. Following the same line of reasoning we may say that the changes that take place are ways of dealing with the increased emotional tension, and not something that comes about as a result of a genuine acceptance or conviction.

Those who believe that the best way to change people's health hazardous behaviour is to present information that may create cognitive dissonance, most probably are mistaken. One of the reasons for this is the likelihood that the people we address will not necessarily experience the information in the same way, or in the

---

* As Leventhal (1970) describes in his review of the literature on fear communication, a number of studies show a negative relationship between fear and persuasion.

way we do (Weinstein, 1983, 1984; Kirscht, 1983; Allen, 1984). In spite of the fact that those we address understand and acknowledge that what we tell them is the truth, the information we supply may in some cases only lead to an apparent inconsistency, and not a real cognitive dissonance, expected to be accompanied by some change or other.

> During a visit to one of the divisions of the ferroalloy plant mentioned earlier, I became involved in a conversation with one of the older employees. The topic under discussion was the use of safety equipment, how it had improved over the years, and how unwise it was not to use it when necessary. Mention was also made of former colleagues who were now experiencing hearing losses because they had not been using the equipment to prevent them from being exposed to heavy noise for long periods of time. And then, seconds later, our informant himself walked into the noisy production hall, to continue his work without using any equipment to protect his own hearing. Someone who was watching this person walking into the production hall – and ignorant of the conversation – might have regarded the person to be ill-informed or unaware of the dangers involved in noise exposure. On the background of our own knowledge it is, however, a clear misfit. How then, can we explain the seemingly odd behaviour? Instead of using labels like 'stupid', 'irresponsible' and the like, we ought to look for 'real' answers. One suggestion might be that the man did not, as we would have thought, experience any inconsistency. "What happens to others does not necessarily happen to me." A self-explanatory activity like this is effective because an eventual negative outcome is far into the future. Besides, the man is himself in control of the situation. To a certain extent it is probably fair to say that the man accepts the risk he is taking because he does not perceive the risk to be too high (Fischhoff, 1981; Weinstein, 1984).

Concluding Remarks

As has been argued by others, the business of health marketing and the promotion of health behaviour can only be marginally successful unless one has some ideas of the conceptions of health held by ordinary people (Burt, 1984). These conceptions may vary from one individual to the next, and may be quite different from what is guiding the efforts of those campaigning for better health behaviour. When people are reluctant to change their behaviour, and when communication fails to be persuasive, the reason may be that one has failed to get through to the audience. Not everyone is likely to share the WHO definition of health as : "..a state of complete physical, mental and social well-being and not merely the absence of disease or infirmity." Could it be that people have different opinions of what health really is, and that their behaviour agrees with their opinion, regardless of what an external party means, or what is commonly seen as healthy or unhealthy? "When physicians or health psychologists say that smoking is bad for your health, it is not me they are talking about. I know that smoking is a health hazard, - provided you smoke excessively. I only smoke 10 cigarettes a day so it is no concern of mine."

For some this is probably what happens. If in spite of everything they should feel some discomfort, it is easily mastered by trading a little health for pleasure. "What is the point of living if I cannot have some pleasure?" Instead of reducing a cognitive dissonance by putting an end to smoking, the smoker who is discomforted by some threatening information refrains from counting his daily consumption. He takes pleasure in smoking and he allows himself the pleassure. This is quite straight-forward because he believes that there are more dangerous things in life than smoking a few cigarettes a day.

As will be understood, it is a hard job indeed to achieve better health behaviour and attitudes, solely by launching an 'attack' on what people do or what they say about their own behaviour. In order to achieve some lasting effects one probably has to do something about the conceptions of health people have, or at least come to terms with what they are. Not only do we have conceptions of what is healthy and what is not. As Burt (1984) has argued, some of the most important conceptions are those we have about our own future and the way we see ourselves, either as the master of destiny or as a passive and generally pessimistic individual at the mercy of others. Both conceptions may be equally challenging for professionals working towards a betterment in public health behaviour, since both are difficult to change. A person who believes that he or she knows best, may ignore any information seen as unsuitable, whereas an individual with the latter view may prove to be extremely difficult to access.

Having their roots within the general field of cognitive dissonance theory, a number of health officials and experts have seen the use of information as a necessary and sufficient means of changing people's attitudes. If a person is presented with information which contradicts his or her previous knowledge, this is believed to lead to some sort of cognitive imbalance, and a change of attitude and/or behaviour is likely to take place as a consequence. With theory in hand, such experts thus seem to imply that human attitudes are the result of (more or less conscious) reflections on various sorts of information, and that human behaviour is a (direct) result of the specific attitude(s) that people have. Provided the information reaches its audience, and provided its nature is such that will create a sense of dissonance, some change or other will, sooner or later, be brought about, it is inferred.

There is, of course, much evidence supporting the cognitive dissonance theory. However, some questions still remain. As already argued, some information or other which is believed to create a feeling of dissonance does not always do so. A person may accept the information at an intellectual level – as it relates to others – without necessarily taking it to be something of any relevance to himself. On may, furthermore, find that individuals who do experience a cognitive dissonance, out of choice continue to behave the way they have always done. Cognitive dissonance resulting from some health-hazardous activity or other is perhaps the 'seasoning' that adds real taste to life?

The author is indebted to the Royal Norwegian council for Scientific and Industrial Research for providing financial support for this work.

References

Allen, H. M. (1984). Consumers and choice: Cost containment strategies for health care provision. *Health Psychology, 3*, 411–430.

Beck, K. H. and Lund, A. K. (1981). The effects of health threat seriousness and personal efficacy upon intentions and behaviour. *Journal of Applied Social Psychology, 11*, 401–415.

Burt, J. J. (1984). Metahealth: A challenge for the future. In Matarazzo, J. D., Weiss, Sh. M., Herd, J. A., Miller, N. A. and Weiss, St. M. (Eds.) *Behavioral Health. A Handbook of Health Enhancement and Disease Prevention* (pp. 1239–1246). New York: John Wiley and Sons.

Fielding, J. E. (1982). Effectiveness of employee health improvement programs. *Journal of Occupational Medicine, 11*, 907–916.

Fielding, J. E. (1984). Health promotion and disease prevention at the worksite. *Annual Review Public Health, 5*, 237–265.

Fischhoff, B., Lichtenstein, S., Slovic, P., Derby, S. L. and Keeney, R. L. (1981). *Acceptable Risk*. Cambridge University Press.

Frederiksen, L. W., Solomon, L. J. and Brehony, K. A. (1984). *Marketing Health Behavior. Principles, Techniques and Applications*. New York: Plenum Press.

Hall, S. M., Rugg, D., Tunstall, C. and Jones, R. T. (1984). Preventing relapse to cigarette smoking by behavioral skill training. *Journal of Consulting and Clinical Psychology, 3*, 372–382.

Jarvis, M. (1983). The treatment of cigarette dependence. *British Journal of Addiction, 78*, 125–130.

Kaplan, R. M. (1984). The connection between clinical health promotion and health status. A critical overview. *American Psychologist, 7*, 755–765.

Kirscht, J. P. (1983). Preventive health behavior: A review of research and issues. *Health Psychology, 2*, 277–301.

Leventhal, H. (1970). Findings and theory in the study of fear communications. In Berkowitz, L. *Advances in Experimental Social Psychology*. Vol 5, (pp. 149–186). New York: Academic Press.

Leventhal, H. and Cleary, P. D. (1980). The smoking problem: A review of the research and theory in behavioral risk modification. *Psychological Bulletin, 2*, 370–405.

Lichtenstein, E. and Mermelstein, R. J. (1984). A review of approaches to smoking treatment: Behavior modification strategies. In Matarazzo, J. D., Weiss, S.M., Herd, J. A., Miller, N. E. and Weiss, S. M. (Eds.) *Behavioral Health. A Handbook of Health Enhancement and Disease Prevention* (pp. 695–712). New York: John Wiley & Sons.

Ockene, J. K., Nutall, R., Benfari, R. C., Hurwitz, I. and Ockene, I. A. (1981). A psychosocial model of smoking cessation and maintenance of cessation. *Preventive Medicine, 10*, 623–638.

O'Donnell, M. P. and Ainsworth, T. (1984). *Health Promotion in the Workplace*. New York: John Wiley & Sons.

Ossip-Klein, D. J. and Bigelow, G. (Eds.)(1986). Task force 1: Classification and assessment of smoking behavior. *Health Psychology, 5* (Suppli.), 3–11.

Raaheim, A. (1987). *Arbeidsmiljø og livsstil. Undersøkelse ved Fiskaa Verk*. (Work environment and lifestyle. Research project). FAHS Publications, University of Bergen.

Raaheim, A. (1989). *Røykeavvenning på arbeidsplassen Erfaringer fra en norsk industribedrift*. (Smoking cessation at the worksite. Results from a study among employees within a Norwegian ferroalloy plant). Journal of the Norwegian Psychological Association, *12*, 843–850.

Raaheim, A. and Myklebust E. (1988). *Røykeavvenningskurs*. (A smoking cessation program). FAHS Publications, University of Bergen.

Rogers, R. W. (1975). A protection motivation theory of fear appeals and attitude change. *The Journal of Psychology, 91*, 93–114.

Snyder, M., Tanke, E. D. and Bersheid, E. (1977). Social perception and interpersonal behavior: On the self-fulfilling nature of social sterotypes. *The Journal of Personality and Social Psychology, 35*, 656-666.

Weinstein, N. D. (1982). Unrealistic optimism about susceptibility to health problems. *Journal of Behavioral Medicine, 5,* 441–460.

Weinstein, N. D. (1983) Reducing unrealistic optimism about illness susceptibility. *Health Psychology, 2,* 11–20.

Weinstein, N. D. (1984). Why it won't happen to me: Perceptions of risk factors and susceptibility. *Health psychology, 3,* 431–457.

Windsor, R. A. and Bartlett, E. E. (1984). Employee self-help smoking cessation programs: A review of the literature. *Health Education Quarterly, 4,* 349–359.

Motivation to Change Smoking Behavior: Determinants in the Contemplation Stage

Rien H. M. Breteler, Noontje H. M. Mertens and René Rombouts

Introduction

Many a smoker has exclaimed, when asked why he/she doesn't give up smoking, "I would like to, but I don't know how!". Some point to their smoking spouse as an excuse for not trying whereas others bluntly deny the health benefits of cessation. On the other hand successful quitters report that they were fed up with "being hooked on nicotine" or stress the importance of good health or "being a good example to my children".

The few lines above illustrate three dimensions which are commonly distinguished in the research of smoking cessation: pharmacological, psychological and psycho-social.

The pharmacological effects of nicotine may prompt smoking in a state of stress and anxiety because the anxiolytic effect of nicotine-induced endorphin release in the central nervous system previously has alleviated the distress (Pomerleau, 1986).

An important psychological factor in this respect is the self-efficacy-expectation (Bandura, 1977). This concept refers to the expectation of being able to perform a behavior required to reach a desired outcome (e.g., refrain from smoking). Although self-efficacy expectations appear to be related to nicotine dependence at initial cessation, it continues to be an important factor in long term maintenance of non-smoking, long after nicotine withdrawal symptoms have disappeared (McIntyre et all, in O'Leary, 1985). Psycho-social factors like social support, the presence of smokers and situational norms also play a part in maintenance of non-smoking (Shiffman, 1984).

Recent studies in the field of smoking cessation increasingly acknowledge the fact that change of smoking behavior takes place in various stages (Schlegel, Manske & Shannon, 1983; Velicer, DiClemente, Prochaska & Brandenburg, 1985). Although differing in concepts and number of stages, grossly three stages can be found in these models: (1) a stage of contemplation to change smoking behavior, (2) actual smoking cessation and (3) maintenance of non-smoking. The general issue of motivation to change is a very important topic in this view, with concrete consequences for any intervention program designed to change smoking behavior. On the other hand, DiClemente, Prochaska and Gilbertini (1985) found that the transition from the contemplative stage to the stage of actual cessation could be predicted by strong beliefs about the cons of smoking, low situational temptations to smoke and high self-efficacy expectations.

The World Health Organization's (WHO) European regional action program "Health For All by the Year 2000" states that healthy behavior should be promoted, striving for a minimum of 80% non-smokers and a 50% reduction of national tobacco consumption in the Member States (WHO, 1985). In order to achieve this target an increase of motivation is needed in the various stages of change. The current study addresses the stage of contemplation to stop smoking, testing a model that describes the effects of concepts from the various dimensions on motivation and self-efficacy expectations.

Method

Subjects

Employees of a Dutch nationwide banking company received a written questionnaire from the bank's health department. Of 2357 mailed questionnaires, 671 copies were returned. 38.3% of the respondents were smokers. The current analysis is based on 154 cigarette smokers. These respondents had missing data on maximally one variable. In this sample, 71% of the subjects are men, 29% are women and seven subjects didn't provide data for gender. Mean age is 35.8 years and mean daily cigarette consumption is 16.1.

Measures

Motivation to change smoking behavior is measured by two instruments. The intention to change is measured by six statements constituting a scale of intention to change. The lowest score on this scale (1) is attached to the statement "I want to decrease my smoking", the highest score (6) to "I want to stop smoking immediately". If a smoker checks several statements, the statement resulting in the highest value is scored. Another measure of motivation to change smoking behavior is the difference between the amount smoked and the amount preferred. We related this measure to the amount smoked, which resulted in a measure "wished decrease in cigarettes".

Self-efficacy expectations are represented by a 20-item expectancy questionnaire, which measures the perceived certainty of being able to perform various acts: observe one's smoking, gradually reduce one's smoking, refrain from smoking, and claim an anti-smoking point of view. These perceptions are measured with regard to five situations: at home with people, alone, when craving, when in a negative mood, when in a positive mood. Response categories vary from "very uncertain" (1) to "very certain" (4). Addition of the scores on items leads to an overall self-efficacy score. Cronbach's alpha of this questionnaire is 0.88.

Subjective pressure to stop smoking is measured by seven sources of incitement to quit as perceived by the smoker: partner, relatives, physician, friends, colleagues, anti-smoking commercials and bodily complaints. Scores on this measure are computed by adding the number of sources of incitement named by the subject. The internal consistency of this measure is 0.45.

Nicotine dependence is measured by means of Fagerstrom's (1978) Tolerance Questionnaire (TQ). This 8-item questionnaire measures behavioral aspects of smoking that are related to pharmacological parameters of nicotine dependence. Scores can vary from 0 to 11. Cronbach's alpha of the TQ is 0.65.

Previous attempts to stop smoking are measured by a question consisting of five categories, ranging from "no previous attempt" (1) to "more than three previous attempts" (5). Beliefs are represented by 13 statements about smoking and 15 statements about not smoking. The items, tuned positively as well as negatively were scored on a four-point scale. Scores on negatively-tuned items were subtracted from scores on positively-tuned items (leading to differential beliefs, see Fishbein, 1980). Internal consistency of beliefs about smoking is 0.47, internal consistency of beliefs about not smoking is 0.45.

Data Analysis

In accordance with our theoretical consideration the model was tested using LISREL IV (Jöreskog & Sörbom, 1978). The main reasons for the use of this statistical program are that it can handle various dependent variables simultaneously and that it allows for the distinction between instruments of measurement and their latent constructs, the latter being of more interest than the former. LISREL compares a theoretically-derived variance-covariance matrix with the observed variance-covariance matrix.

Table 1 *Variance-covariance matrix of the measured variables of the tested model (n=154).*

	1	2	3	4	5	6	7	8
1	2.268							
2	0.526	4.139						
3	0.516	0.633	2.067					
4	-1.961	0.190	0.018	-22.683				
5	1.111	0.104	0.044	-12.832	25.240			
6	0.822	0.805	0.856	- 1.824	1.608	3.259		
7	0.124	0.291	0.160	- 0.319	0.155	0.223	0.109	
8	3.332	-3.428	1.212	- 8.652	17.279	1.897	-0.429	117.281

1 = incitements to quit smoking 2 = Tolerance Questionnaire 3 = previous attempts to quit smoking 4 = beliefs about smoking 5 = beliefs about not smoking 6 = intention of behavior change 7 = proportion cut down in cigarette consumption 8 = expectancy questionnaire

The fit of the model is tested with a chi-square statistic. A large chi-square/d.f. ratio (with concomittant low p-value) signifies an unsatisfactory fit (i.e., the values in the observed variance-covariance matrix should not be attributed to the model tested). Corrections in the specifications of the model may lead to a better fit in a second run.

Results and Discussion

For theoretical reasons the relationship between subjective pressure and motivation to change was maintained in the model, leading to a satisfactory goodness-of-fit (chi square=26.4, d.f.=21, p=0.19).

The low response in this study has been attributed to two factors: 1. a reorganization in the company, which led to mistrust concerning the anonymity of

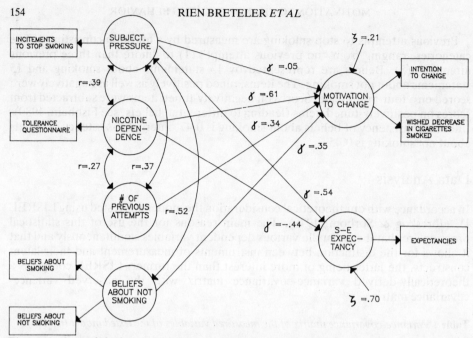

Figure 1. A model of motivation to change smoking behavior.
r= correlation coefficient   γ= standard regression coefficient   ζ = proportion of explained variance

Table 2. *Mean and standard deviation of variables, measured for a model of motivation to change smoking behavior (n=154).*

variable	mean	standard deviation
intention to change	3.0	1.8
proportion cutdown	0.6	0.3
self-efficacy expectancy	45.9	10.9
incitements to stop smoking	1.7	1.4
Tolerance Questionnaire	4.4	2.0
number of previous attempts	2.7	1.4
beliefs about smoking	−8.7	4.8
beliefs about not smoking	16.8	5.0

the data and 2. the holiday season. However, the data are in accord with internal company data on the ratio of male to female employees and with cohort analyses of the Dutch Population (van Reek, Drop & Adriaanse, 1985). Therefore, with regard to smoking we regard the sample as representative for the addressed staff.

As far as interventions are concerned we must acknowledge the limited impact of the constructs under study, as motivation and self-efficacy expectations are not synonymous with behavior. For this reason we can only speculate about findings that may be of importance. During the analyses it was found that the role of bodily complaints as a stimulus adds considerably to the explanation of the model (Mertens, Breteler & Rombouts, 1987). Whenever a smoker perceives bodily complaints as a

Table 3. *Change in the fit of a LISREL model for the motivation to change smoking behavior* ($n=154$).

Cumulatively delated relationships between construct A and B	Strength of delated relationship	Chi square	d.f.	p
A	B			
none (initial model tested)		20.1	15	0.17
previous attempts	beliefs about not smoking	0.00 20.1	16	0.22
nicotine dependence	beliefs about not smoking	−0.01 20.1	17	0.27
previous attempts	s-e expectation	0.06 20.5	18	0.31
beliefs about not smoking	s-e expectation			
s-e expectation	motivation	0.20 22.1	19	0.28
beliefs about smoking (error of measurement)	beliefs about not smoking (error of measurement)	−0.21 24.4*	20	0.22
		−0.14 26.4*	21	0.19

*: decrease in p-value, yet non-significant increase in chi-square, regarding the change in d. f.

stimulus to quit smoking, its role in motivation appears to be an important one.

Second, high subjective pressure leads both to high motivation and high self-efficacy expectations. Taking into account our operationalization, this result can be compared with the influence of social support on maintenance of non-smoking (Lichtenstein, Glasgow & Abrams, 1986).

Thirdly, nicotine dependence plays a key role in the model: high nicotine dependence leads to high motivation, yet to low self-efficacy expectations. This triangle is typical for the classical "dissonant smoker" (McKennel & Thomas, 1967).

A last remark concerns the number of previous attempts to quit smoking. Those with many previous attempts are highly motivated to change their behavior, which is in line with cognitive dissonance theory. Yet this does not mean that they expect to be efficacious. Although DiClemente, Prochaska and Gilbertini (1985) neither found a relationship between these two factors, they did report an association between the duration of the last attempt and self-efficacy. The latter is an argument for research about various cognitive representations of previous behavior and their role in self-efficacy.

Looking at these results we note that motivation may be ineffective unless self-efficacy is sufficiently high (cf. O'Leary, 1985). The finding of Brod and Hall (1984) that joiners of smoking cessation treatment have higher self-efficacy expectations than non-joiners supports this view.

Cautiously extrapolating our results to interventions, the latter should increase self-efficacy expectations, e.g. by pointing to stimulations from the social environment. Also, giving attention to bodily complaints may increase the likelihood of transition from the stage of contemplation to the action stage. Whereas our results support WHO's suggestion that non-smoking should be established as the positive social norm (WHO, 1985), incitements to stop smoking are reported relatively seldom. This may reflect the rather liberal climate of the Dutch society concerning smoking and constitutes a call for more effort by the government and the health care system to promote non-smoking as a major health behavior.

Acknowledgement

Preparation of this text was supported by grant 28–1085 from the Prevention Fund, the Hague, the Netherlands.

References

Bandura, A. (1977). Self-efficacy: Toward a unifying theory of behavioral change. *Psychological Review, 84*, 191–215.

Brod, M. I., and Hall, S. M. (1984). Joiners and non-joiners in smoking treatment: a comparison of psycho-social variables. *Addictive Behaviors, 9*, 217–221.

DiClemente, C.C., Prochaska, J. O., and Gilbertini, M. (1985). Self-efficacy and the stages of self-change of smoking. *Cognitive Therapy and Research, 9*, 181–200.

Fagerstrom, K. O. (1978). Measuring degree of physical dependence to tobacco smoking with reference to individualization of treatment. *Addictive Behaviors, 3*, 234–241.

Fishbein, M. (1980). A theory of reasoned action: some applications and implications. In H. E. Howe (Ed.), *Nebraska Symposium on Motivation* 1979 (pp. 65–116) Nebraska: University of Nebraska Press.

Jöreskog, K. G., and Sörbom, D. (1978). *Lisrel IV, analysis of linear structural relationships by the method of maximum likelihood*. Chicago, Ill.: International Educational Services.

Lichtenstein, E., Glasgow, R. E., and Abrams, D. B. (1986). Social support in smoking cessation: in search of effective interventions. *Behavior Therapy, 17*, 609–617.

McKennell, A. C., and Thomas, R. K. (1967). *Adults' and adolescents' smoking habits and attitudes*. Government social survey SS 353. London: HMSO.

Mertens, E. H. M., Breteler, M. H. M., and Rombouts, R. (1987). *LISREL analyses of a model for explanation of the motivation to change smoking behavior in patients with cardiological and/or pulmonological complaints*. Unpublished Manuscript.

O'Leary, A. (1985).Self-efficacy and health. *Behavior Research and Therapy, 23*, 437–451.

Pomerleau, O. F. (1986). The "why" of tobacco dependence: underlying reinforcing mechanisms in nicotine self-adminstration. In J. K. Ockene (Ed.), *The Pharmacological Treatment of Tobacco Dependence: Proceedings of the World Congress*. Cambridge, MA.: Institute for the Study of Smoking Behavior and Policy.

Shiffman, S. (1984). Coping with temptations to smoke. *Journal of Consulting and Clinical Psychology, 52*, 261–267.

Reek, J. van, Drop, M. J., and Adriaanse, H. (1985). Smoking cessation in the Netherlands since 1958. *Tijdschrift voor Alcohol, Drugs en andere Psychotrope stoffen, 11*, 168–173.

Schlegel, R. P., Manske, S. R., and Shannon, M. E. (1983). Butt out! Evaluation of the Canadian Armed Forces smoking cessation program. In W. F. Forbes, R.C. Frecker and D. J. Nostbakken (Eds.), *Proceedings of the Fifth World Conference on Smoking and Health*. Ontario: Canadian Council on Smoking and Health.

Velicer, W. F., DiClemente, C. C., Prochaska, J. O., and Brandenburg, N. (1985). Decisional balance measure for assessing and predicting smoking status. *Journal of Personality and Social Psychology, 48*, 1279–1280.

World Health Organization (1985). *Targets for Health for All. Targets in support of the European regional strategy for health for all*. Copenhagen: World Health Organization, Regional Office for Europe.

Section 3

Stress, Health, and Disease

The Study of Chronic Stress: A Psycho-Biological Approach

Ad Vingerhoets, Arjen Jeninga, Lea Jabaaij, Jeff Ratliff-Crain,
Peter Moleman and Louwrens Menges

Introduction

In modern behavioral stress research, one can roughly distinguish among three
research traditions: 1) epidemiological, questionnaire studies; 2) the experimental,
psychobiological approach and 3) field studies in which psychological and biological
reactions to (semi-)natural stressors are measured. Each approach has its own
strengths and weaknesses. The use of questionnaires has some well-known
disadvantages. For example, it is difficult to distinguish between (subjective)
complaints and (objective) symptoms. Laboratory research is limited because of the
ethical aspects; the stressors that can be applied have limited ecological validity, and
it is impossible to study chronic stress with humans within the laboratory. Field
studies are therefore very important because they can yield information concerning
the validity and generalizability of laboratory findings.

In the last decade, both the epidemiological approach and the experimental
approach have met with much criticism. It has been suggested that too much
attention has been paid to life events, neglecting the importance of other sources of
stress (e.g., chronic stressors, daily hassles, or role-stressors). The experimental
approach has been criticized because of its use of artificial stressors (e.g., reaction
time tasks, mental arithmetic) which often lack the emotional component that is so
characteristic of real life stressors. In addition, the value of measuring short-term
physiological reactions as predictors of the future health status has been questioned.

In the present project, we want to bridge the gap between the epidemiological
approach and the experimental approach. By combining these two approaches, both
may benefit from such an integration. The aim of the project was to independently
explore the associations between being under load and reporting psychosomatic
symptoms, on the one hand, and psychological and psychobiological variables, on
the other hand. More precisely, the focus was on the study of personality attributes,
coping variables, as well as psychological, electro-physiological, endocrinological
and immunological parameters as functions of the level of psychosocial load,
symptoms and the relationship between load and symptoms. In the project two
phases can be distinguished: 1) the questionnaire study, with the examination of the
personality and coping variables and the selection of subjects who met the
requirements for participating in the second phase as central issues, and 2) the
laboratory study to investigate the psychological and psychobiological reactions to
stressful stimulation. Here we want to describe how we designed our study and to
summarize the most important results. For details concerning the specific measuring
tools and psychobiological assessment techniques the reader is referred to the
relevant research reports (Jabaaij, Vingerhoets, Ballieux, Menges & Van Houte,
submitted; Ratliff-Crain, Vingerhoets, Baum & Menges, submitted; Vingerhoets,
Jabaaij, Tilders, Moleman & Menges, accepted for publication; Vingerhoets &
Menges, 1989a, 1989b;Vingerhoets, & Van Heck, 1990).

161

Subjects and Procedures

A central issue in the study was the composition of four groups: (1) low-load, few symptoms; (2) low-load, many symptoms; (3) high-load, few symptoms; and (4) high-load, many symptoms. In this way it is possible to study independently the effects of being exposed to stressors and reporting psychosomatic symptoms on several both psychological and biological, dependent variables. To maximize the validity of our selection procedure it was decided to measure two kinds of stressors or load: life events and daily hassles. Only when a subject had high or low scores on *both* measures was that person assigned to the high-load or low-load group. The measuring tools used were the Recently Experienced Events Questionnaire (REEQ) (Van de Willigen, Schreurs, Tellegen & Zwart, 1985) and the Everyday Problem Checklist (EPCL) (Vingerhoets, Jeninga & Menges, 1987, 1989). Symptoms were measured using the Hopkins Symptom Checklist (HSCL) (Derogatis, Lipman, Rickets, Uhlenhuth & Covi, 1974; Dutch version by Luteijn, Hamel, Bouman & Kok, 1984). The sample used for the personality and coping studies consisted of 461 males and 528 females (age range 25–50 years), whereas the subjects that participated in the laboratory study were only males (N=91) in the same age range. The questionnaire subjects were recruited on a random basis in two relatively small villages (a typically rural and a more urban) in the Province of Brabant in the Netherlands. The original sample consisted of 2500 persons. Men and women were equally represented. The age range was 25–50 years. On thousand one hundred and ninety-seven (47.9%) of them reacted positively to our invitation but due to missing data (mostly because of missing pages in the test booklets) the data of 200 individuals could not be used for the present analysis. The laboratory subjects were selected from a group of approximately 950 males who participated in a questionnaire study. This group was recruited in two ways: about 350 subjects were from the questionnaire sample, and the remaining 600 were volunteers who reacted to advertisements in papers and local magazines, and to announcements in several companies and clubs. Only males were invited to take part in this psychobiological part of the study, because we wanted to avoid the need to take into account disturbing factors such as the use of oral contraceptives and the phase of the menstrual cycle, when analysing the endocrinological and immunological data.

In the laboratory study the subjects were exposed to six short (5 to 8 min.) films and a rest condition, in which they listened to music. In the first two conditions, 'buffer' films were shown to make the subjects familiar with the experimental procedures, followed by four stressful films: (a) a driving test; (2) a woman dying at home and her funeral; (3) abdominal surgery after a car accident; and (4) rape. The first three films were chosen because previous research (Vingerhoets, 1985) had showed that they evoke both psychological and electro-physiological reactions. The rape film was added on the basis of data collected in a pilot-study, in which it appeared to evoke strong psychophysiological reactions. Two films (Driving Test and Rape) were known to lead to increased sympathetic nervous system activity, whereas the other two experimental films (Deathbed and Surgery) were previously found to evoke responses consistent with vagal stimulation. Electro-physiological recordings were made during these conditions and during one-minute periods preceding each condition. In addition, after each condition, blood samples were drawn for the analysis of immunological and endocrine parameters. Finally, the subjects completed an Adjective Checklist (ACL) containing three dimensions: (1)

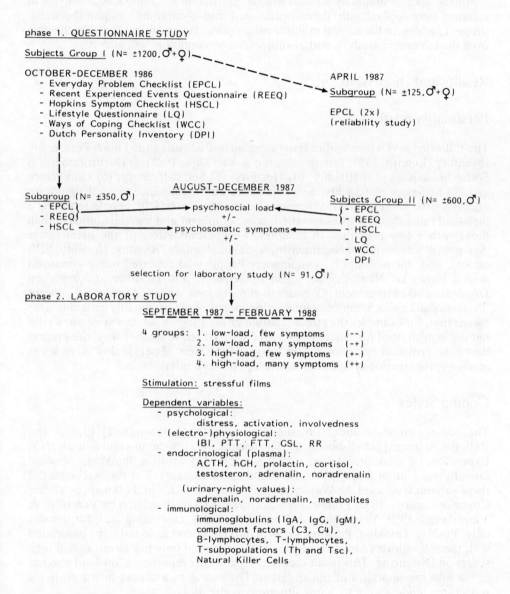

phase 1. QUESTIONNAIRE STUDY

Subjects Group I (N= ±1200, ♂+♀)

OCTOBER-DECEMBER 1986
   - Everyday Problem Checklist (EPCL)
   - Recent Experienced Events Questionnaire (REEQ)
   - Hopkins Symptom Checklist (HSCL)
   - Lifestyle Questionnaire (LQ)
   - Ways of Coping Checklist (WCC)
   - Dutch Personality Inventory (DPI)

APRIL 1987
Subgroup (N= ±125, ♂+♀)

EPCL (2x)
(reliability study)

AUGUST-DECEMBER 1987

Subgroup (N= ±350, ♂)
   - EPCL
   - REEQ
   - HSCL

→ psychosocial load ←
          +/-
→ psychosomatic symptoms ←
          +/-

Subjects Group II (N= ±600, ♂)
   - EPCL
   - REEQ
   - HSCL
   - LQ
   - WCC
   - DPI

selection for laboratory study (N= 91, ♂)

phase 2. LABORATORY STUDY

SEPTEMBER 1987 - FEBRUARY 1988

4 groups: 1. low-load, few symptoms   (--)
           2. low-load, many symptoms   (-+)
           3. high-load, few symptoms   (+-)
           4. high-load, many symptoms   (++)

Stimulation: stressful films

Dependent variables:
   - psychological:
            distress, activation, involvedness
   - (electro-)physiological:
            IBI, PTT, FTT, GSL, RR
   - endocrinological (plasma):
            ACTH, hGH, prolactin, cortisol,
            testosteron, adrenalin, noradrenalin

       (urinary-night values):
            adrenalin, noradrenalin, metabolites
   - immunological:
            immunoglobulins (IgA, IgG, IgM),
            complement factors (C3, C4),
            B-lymphocytes, T-lymphocytes,
            T-subpopulations (Th and Tsc),
            Natural Killer Cells

Figure 1.

Psychological distress; (2) De-activation; and (3) Openness-Involvedness: (for details, see Ratliff-Crain et al., submitted; Vingerhoets, 1985; Vingerhoets et al., accepted for publication). Figure 1 summarizes schematically the design of the project.

For the sake of simplicity all data will be reported in the same way. Analyses of variance were applied with 'Psychosocial load' and 'Symptoms' as main (between-subject) factors. In the case of multiple measurements per subject (i.e., for the data from the laboratory study) a within-subject factor 'condition' was added.

Results and Discussion

Personality attributes

The following seven personality traits were measured, using the Dutch Personality Inventory (Luteijn, 1974; Luteijn, Starren & Van Dijk, 1985): (1) Neuroticism; (2) Social Inadequacy; (3) Rigidity; (4) Hostility; (5) Self-sufficiency; (6) Dominance and (7) Self-esteem. Rigidity, Self-sufficiency and Dominance yielded significant effects for the main factor 'Psychosocial Load'. More precisely, people reporting a high load rated themselves as less rigid, more dominant and less self-sufficient than those with a low load did. In addition, a significant effect of the main factor 'Symptoms' was found for Neuroticism, Social Inadequacy, Rigidity, Hostility, Self-esteem, and, for males only, Dominance. People who reported many symptoms scored higher on Neuroticism, Social Inadequacy, and Hostility and lower on Dominance and Self-esteem. Contrary to expectations, we failed to find a significant 'Psychosocial Load x Symptoms' interaction for any of the personality variables. This means that, for example, the stress-resistant group ('high-load, few symptoms') did not distinguish itself for any of these variables . To put it another way, the present data have provided evidence only in favour of the view of personality variables as *mediating* the stressor-symptom relationship, not as moderating it.

Coping Styles

The coping variables under investigation were the following: (1) Planful and Rational Actions; (2) Self-blame; (3) Distancing; (4) Day-dreams and fantasies; (5) Expression of emotions/seeking social support; (6) Positive thinking, Personal Growth and Humor and (7) Wishful thinking/emotionality. For the assessment of these variables, we used the Ways of Coping Checklist (Aldwin, Folkman, Schaefer, Coyne & Lazarus, 1980; Folkman & Lazarus, 1980; Dutch version by Van Heck & Vingerhoets, 1989; Vingerhoets & Van Heck, 1990). Distancing and, for females only, Positive Thinking, Personal Growth and Humor were found to be associated with the self-reports of load. Individuals who reported only few stressors had high scores on Distancing. This result seems to suggest that reporting a low load also has to do with the appraisal of the situation. Distancing as a coping factor probably reflects the tendency *not* to define situations as stressful.

In addition, three coping factors showed strong associations with the self-report of psychosomatic symptoms: Self-blame, Day-dreams, and Fantasies and Wishful thinking/Emotionality. Subjects who report many symptoms consider themselves to be the cause of their troubles and they also report more psychological escape such as daydreams/fantasies and wishful thinking. Not only did we fail to find significant interactions for the personality variables, but also for any of these coping variables. We therefore have to conclude that the present study does not support the hypothesis that coping strategies can act as moderating variables. Again, we only found evidence in favor of the view of coping as a *mediating* factor.

Psychological Reactions to Stressful Films

When exposed to the stressful films the four groups of subjects reacted to the films in generally the same way. This conclusion is based on the failure to find a significant three-way (Psychosocial Load x Symptoms x Conditon) interaction. On the other hand, both for 'Distress' and 'De-activation' significant main effects were found for 'Symptoms'. This result means that people who report many symptoms also report more feelings of distress and more lack of energy during the experimental session than people with a low level of symptoms do. No such effect was found for the third ACL factor ('Openness/Involvedness') indicating that the former effects need not be attributed to response sets. It is concluded that these results confirm the validity of our selection procedures.

Psychobiological Variables

Because of space restrictions we will confine ourselves principally to the main effects of the ANOVAs and not go into the details of the sometimes rather complex significant interactions.

The electro-physiological variables yielded significant main effects ('Symptoms') for Inter-Beat-Interval (IBI), ECG T wave amplitude, and a trend ($p < 0.10$) for a heart rate variability measure. In short, subjects reporting many symptoms appear to have a fast and regular heart rate, and a low ECG T wave amplitude. This pattern of findings strongly suggests a relatively high sympathethetic tone on the heart.

The endocrine variables also yielded some main effects. A notable 'dissociation' of the catecholamines was found since noradrenaline appeared to be associated with 'Symptoms', whereas adrenaline yielded significant effects for the factor 'Psychosocial Load'. To put it differently, individuals reporting many symptoms had higher plasma noradrenaline concentrations than those reporting few symptoms whereas those who reported a high load had higher adrenaline levels in comparison to the low-load subjects. In addition and contrary to expectations, the plasma cortisol levels of the high-symptoms group proved to be significantly lower.

During two preceding nights we also collected the urine passed during the night and on arising in the morning for the analysis of the catecholamines. Here we saw a slightly different picture: adrenaline showed a relationship with symptom reporting. The low symptom group excreted significantly less adrenaline than the high-symptoms group.

Finally, the following immunological parameters in the blood plasma were assessed: immunoglobulins (IgA, IgG and IgM), complement factors (C3 and C4), and the percentages and absolute numbers of the following lymphocyte subsets (monoclonal antibodies within parentheses): T suppressor/cytotoxic cells (CD 8), T helper/inducer cells (CD 4), T cells (CD 3), Natural Killer Cells (Leu 7) and B cells (HLA-DR). After excluding those subjects who had diseases or used medicines that might influence their immunological state, the results of the ANOVAs indicated that: (1) subjects who reported a high level of complaints had a lower percentage of T cells, and (2) high-load subjects had lower plasma IgG concentrations. Summarizing, contrary to expectations, most of the immunological parameters under investigation did not appear to be affected by either psychosocial load or psychosomatic symptoms. Regression analysis indicated some weak, but statistically significant associations with smoking and personality variables (especially hostility and rigidity) for some of the immune parameters.

Conclusions

The main conclusions from the above-reported findings can be summarized as folllows: (1) both personality variables and coping styles act more as mediating variables than as moderating variables in the stressor-symptoms relationships; (2) reporting a high psychosocial load does not suffice as a condition to show altered psychobiological functioning; in contrast, reporting many symptoms is associated with increased sympathetic tone and, surprisingly, lower cortisol levels; (3) the structure of the immunological system is not necessarily affected by load or symptoms, in spite of apparent effects on endocrine functioning; (4) the present psychobiological results suggest that people reporting many symptoms must not be considered as mere complainers; (5) neither at the psychological level, nor at the psychobiological level did the stress-resistant individuals ('high-load, few symptoms') distinguish themselves. Caution is therefore needed when interpreting the results of studies which restrict themselves to only two groups (most often only 'high-load, few symptoms' and ' high-load, many symptoms'). The differences between groups found in such investigations must probably be attributed to 'symptom' reporting, rather than be associated with 'stress resistance'.

References

Aldwin, C., Folkman, S., Schaefer, C., Coyne, J. C. and Lazarus, R. S. (1980, August). Ways of coping: A process measure. Paper presented at the Meeting of the American Psychological Association, Los Angeles, CA.

Derogatis, L. R., Lipman, R. S., Rickets, K., Uhlenhuth, E. H. and Covi, L. (1974). The Hopkins Symptom Checklist (HSCL): A self-report symptom inventory. *Behavioral Science, 19*, 1–15.

Folkman, S. and Lazarus, R. S. (1980). An analysis of coping in a middle-aged community sample. *Journal of Health and Social Behavior, 21*, 219–239.

Jabaaij, L., Vingerhoets, A., Menges, L. J., Ballieux, R. and Van Houte A. J. (in preparation) Psychosocial load, symptoms, and immunological parameters .

Luteijh, F. (1974). *De konstructie van een persoonlijkheids- nvragenlijst [The construction of a personality inventory]*. Unpublished Thesis, University of Groningen.

Luteijn, F., Hamel, L. F., Bouman, T. K. and Kok, A. R. (1984). *HSCL Hopkins Symptom Checklist (Manual)*. Lisse: Swets and Zeitlinger.

Luteijn, F., Starren, J. and Van Dijk, J. (1985). *Handleiding bij de NPV (herziene uitgave) [NPV manual (revised edition)]*. Lisse: Swets and Zeitlinger.

Ratliff-Crain, J., Vingerhoets, A. J. J. M., Baum, A. and Menges L. J. (submitted). Electro-physiological reactions to stressful films as a function of psychosocial load and psychosomatic symptoms.

Van de Willige, G., Schreurs, P., Tellegen, B. and Zwart, F. (1985). Het meten van 'life events': de Vragenlijst Recent Meegemaakte Gebeurtenissen (VRMG) [The measurement of 'life events': the Recently Experienced Events Questionnaire (REEQ)]. *Nederlands Tijdschrift voor de Psychologie, 40*, 1–19.

Van Heck, G. L. and Vingerhoets, A. J. J. M. (1989). Copingstijlen en persoonlijkheidskenmerken [Coping styles and personality characteristics]. *Nederlands Tijd-schrift voor de Psychologie, 44*, 73–87.

Vingerhoets, A. J. J. M. (1985). *Psychosocial stress: An experimental approach. Life events, coping, and psychobiological functioning*. Lisse: Swets and Zeitlinger.

Vingerhoets, A. J. J. M., Jabaaij, L., Tilders, F. G. H., Moleman, P., and Menges, L. J. Psychosocial load and symptoms: Their relationship to psychoneuro endocrine functioning. *Psychosomatic Medicine*(accepted for publication).

Vingerhoets, A. J. J. M., Jeninga, A. J. and Menges, L. J. (1987). Chronic pain and everyday problems. *International Journal of Psychosomatics, 34*, 9–11.

Vingerhoets, A. J. J. M., Jeninga, A. J. and Menges, L. J. (1989). Het meten van chronische en alledaagse stressoren: Eerste onderzoeks-ervaringen met de Alledaagse Problemen Lijst (APL) II. [The measurement of chronic and everyday stressors: Preliminary results with the Everyday Problem Checklist (EPCL) II] *Gedrag en Gezondheid, 17*, 10–17.

Vingerhoets, A. J. J. M. and Menges, L. J. (1989, a). Psychosocial load and symptoms: An inquiry into their relationship with coping styles. *Stress Medicine, 5*, 189–194.

Vingerhoets, A. J. J. M. and Menges, L. J. (1989, b). Psychosocial load and symptoms: The realtionship with personality factors. In J. MacDonald Wallace, F. J. McGuigan and W. E. Sime (Eds.), *Stress and tension control III*. New York: Plenum Press.

Vingerhoets, A. J. J. M. and Van Heck, G. L. (1990). Gender, coping, and psychosomatic symptoms. *Psychological Medicine, 20*, 125–135.

Predictors of Individual Stress Responses in a Standardized Physical Load

Gabriele Fehm-Wolfsdorf, Peter Schwarz, Hellmuth Zenz and
Karlheinz Voigt

Hormonal stress responses may play a critical role in the onset and development of various chronic diseases. Mainly a hyperactivity of the hypothalamic-pituitary-adrenal axis resulting in hypersecretion of cortisol and catecholamines has been assumed to be a major damaging factor leading to illness as a consequence of chronic stress. Reactivity of the hypothalamic-pituitary-adrenal (HPA) system was investigated by Berger et al. (1987) in the context of the frequently observed hypercortisolism and cortisol non-suppression after dexamethasone application in psychiatric patients. The authors studied the cortisol response of 12 healthy young men to five different stress tests, and stated a broad spectrum of cortisol responses among subjects with "reactors" as well as "nonreactors". Subjective feelings of stress were not correlated with cortisol reactions (defined as difference in pre-post stress >2 μ/dl). In a preceding study by our group (Fehm-Wolfsdorf & Voigt, 1989) cortisol reactions to exhausting physical load after intake of dexamethasone showed a broad range of responses, mimicking dexamethasone non-suppression in healthy volunteers as frequently has been described for a subgroup of depressive patients. In spite of the multitude of studies on cortisol hypersecretion and dexamethasone non-suppression, inter-individual differences in cortisol response remain unexplained in patients as well as in healthy people.

The psychological characteristics of the situation (e.g. controllability and predictability) and the characteristics of the person as well as the situation-person interaction may contribute to hormone output modulation. In a standard laboratory stress situation, a physical load till exhaustion, we first studied the influence of the predictability and controllability of the situation on hormonal patterns. Results indicating a significant decline in hormonal stress responses with increasing predictability of the situation are reported elsewhere in more detail (Voigt et al., 1990). Secondly we tested whether personality factors like e.g. emotional unstability, specific coping styles, or subjective states in the situation predicted interindividual variations in hormonal output. Here we will report on the relations between individual psychological data and the corresponding endocrine reactions in the first session. How individual appraisal and experience in a given stress situation may lead to increased predictability of the situation and then modulate the endocrine stress response might be investigated in later studies with sample sizes large enough for multifactorial analyses. Another focus of this report will be the cortisol secretion which is expected to reflect individual differences in coping with the situation more clearly than e.g. prolactin or growth hormone release.

Methods

Untrained student volunteers (eight males and eight females) participated in four sessions each identical in timing, location, experimenters, and task demands. Session two to four addressed the question of the influence of familiarity with task and situation on hormonal output. After a medical examination subjects recorded their preceding sleeping and eating pattern, physical activity, and other events which could influence actual hormonal output. Then the subject had to ride a bicycle starting at one watt/kg body weight. Loading was increased by one watt/kg body weight every three minutes till the subject was exhausted. Higher payment was promised depending on the extent the subject used up his personal physiological capacity. Indeed, all subjects in each session worked at very high levels in each session as can be inferred from the blood pressure or lactate scores. Means of physiological recordings are given in Table 1.

Table 1. *Average physiological scores during exhaustive loading.*

Variable (mean and SEM)	male	female
Watt performance max	331.5/18.5	220.9/11.9
Watt/kg body weight at anaerobic level (lactate 3.5 mMol/1)	3.6/ 0.2	2.8/ 0.3
lactate, end of loading, mMol/1	9.5/ 0.6	7.6/ 0.7
O_2/kg uptake, max (ml)	55.8/ 1.5	45.2/ 3.2
O_2 uptake/percent of nominal value	113.8/ 5.5	88.8/ 5.7
pulse working capacity, HR 170bpm	3.4/ 0.2	2.5/ 0.1
breathing frequence, max/minute	44.5/ 1.9	47.4/ 3.0
heart rate, max bpm	193.1/ 1.7	190.4/ 3.1
systolic blood pressure, max	217.5/ 1.0	153.8/10.6

Upon arrival in the laboratory, blood was drawn by the application of an intervenous forearm catheter. 40 ml blood were collected immediately, right after the loading, and 20, 40, and 60 minutes later, with the subject lying on a couch. To analyze cortisol, ACTH, vasopressin, prolactin, and human growth hormone (HGH), blood samples were centrifuged, and plasma was frozen immediately. Commercial RIA kits were used for determination of cortisol (DPC), HGH (Sorin Biomedica), prolactin (Serona), and vasopressin (INC). RIA procedure for ACTH measurement is described in detail elsewhere (Bickel et al., 1988). Inter and intra assay variabilities met the standard criteria. Before and after exercising, subjects rated their expectations regarding their performance level and their feelings of strain on a visual analogous scale. At the end of each session subjects filled in one of the following questionnaires: Freiburger Persönlichkeitsinventar (FPI), a common German personality inventory (Fahrenberg et al., 1978), the Streßverarbeitungsfragebogen (SVF, Janke et al., 1986), measuring individual coping styles, and Framingham Activity Survey (FAS, Haynes et al., 1978), in a short version of ten items measuring type-A behavior.

Correlations were calculated between physiological or psychological data and cortisol levels at different points of time. The maximum cortisol secretion reached after loading can be compared to baseline measures at the beginning of the session. However, since novelty enhances cortisol secretion the question arises whether the first measurement upon arrival in the laboratory – where the whole procedure is unknown to the subject – can be considered a "true" baseline. Thus we additionally compared cortisol maxima to the last cortisol level, i.e. the level reached after 60 minutes of resting after loading. On the basis of the correlation matrix we tried to predict individual cortisol responses by multiple stepwise regression analyses. The best combination of physiological and psychological variables should explain individual variance of cortisol reactivity to a considerable degree. Only variables correlated ›0.50 with cortisol scores were used for regression analyses.

Results

The course of the mean cortisol response reflects rather high baseline levels regarding the time of testing (in the afternoon between 15.00 and 17.00 hours) and the expected rise of cortisol just after loading. During the following resting period cortisol levels fell to a minimum at the end of session (see Figure 1).

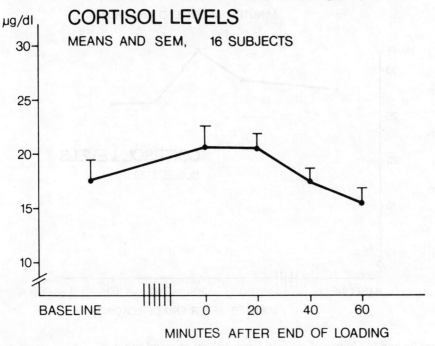

Figure 1. Course of mean of cortisol levles.

A major factor contributing to interindividual differences in cortisol secretion seems to be the relation of the initial baseline measure to maximum and to the last resting measure. Figure 2 depicts the course of cortisol secretion during session 1 in two different subjects. Subject 24 clearly reacts to the stress of the physical load, whereas subject 30 already starts the session with a very high level of cortisol.

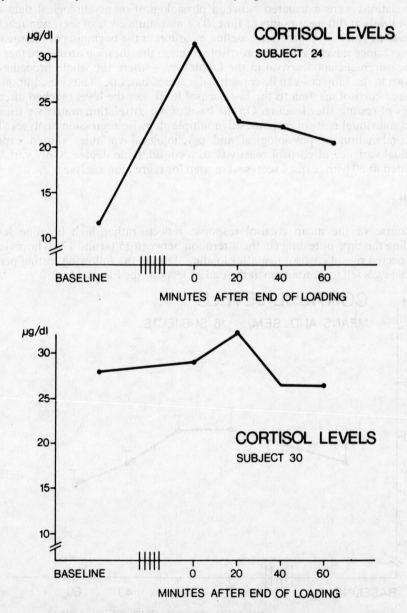

Figure 2a and b. Course of cortisol levels of two selected subjects

Questionnaire data of our sample were within normal range and were mostly normally distributed. Table 2 gives the respective scores.

Table 2. *Questionnaire data*

	mean	SD
Framingham Activity Score	1.40	0.16
Freiburger Persönlichkeitsinventar (stanine scores)		
Nervousness	4.12	1.86
Spontaneous aggressivity	4.50	1.55
Depressivity	4.19	1.64
Irritability	4.31	1.45
Sociability	6.06	2.26
Composedness/self-reliance	4.94	1.95
Reactive aggressivity/dominance	3.81	1.60
Inhibitedness	5.06	2.32
Openness/self-criticism	4.69	1.81
Extraversion	5.75	2.38
Emotional lability	4.56	1.55
Masculinity	5.19	1.80
Streßverarbeitungs-Fragebogen (T-scores)		
Disparagement	49.25	7.31
Diversion from situations	47.94	9.59
Efforts to control situations	54.56	10.47
Efforts to control reactions	49.62	6.21
Positive selfinstructions	53.06	9.33
Need for social support	46.37	6.29
Resignation	46.44	9.42
Self-pity	47.44	8.15
Self-blame	49.69	7.24

On the basis of substantial correlations observed between physiological or psychological parameters on one hand and characteristics of cortisol secretion on the other hand we tried to define the best linear combination of variables to predict cortisol scores. The difference in cortisol secretion between the maximum after loading and the last resting score could be predicted best by a combination of FAS (x_1), nervousness (x_2), and maximum O_2 uptake during loading (x_3) ($R^2 = 0.695$; p < 0.006; $Y = -24.833 + 12.472x_1 + 0.841x_2 + 0.248x_3$): the higher the subject rated on the type-A behavior scale, plus the higher the subject described him/herself as nervous, and the higher the amount of oxygen he/she took during loading, the higher was the amount of cortisol secreted just after loading as compared to resting scores; this combination explains about 70% of variance of cortisol scores.

As described above some subjects showed very high baseline measures of cortisol (see e.g. subject 30, fig. 2). We tried to characterize those subjects who displayed a large difference between baseline scores and the last resting scores. Regression analyses including the respective variables revealed a combination of high resignation measured by SVF, high lactate measures just after the end of loading, and a high maximum breathing frequence during loading as best predictor of high baseline levels of cortisol as compared to resting scores (variance explained: 65%, R^2 = 0.648; p < 0.02). There was a limited number of other variables which had predictive power for the amount of cortisol secretion, but to a lesser degree than those reported above (e.g. maximum diastolic blood pressure, time spent with loading after anaerobic level) as suggested by a stepwise procedure in multiple regression analyses. Regarding the limited sample size more than three predictors would not fit regression analysis.

Discussion

In a standardardized setting, 16 untrained volunteers loaded till exhaustion. Remarkable elevations in blood pressure, heart rate, oxygen uptake, breathing frequence, lactate levels, and hormonal parameters confirm the strain induced by the task. Cortisol levels as well as other hormonal secretion varied considerably between persons, both, regarding the amount of secretion (maximum compared to resting scores) and regarding the time of high cortisol secretion (high anticipatory baseline secretion before loading). In posthoc analyses with our limited sample subjects with high cortisol secretion can be characterized best by high levels of Type A behavior in combination with high nervousness and high oxygen uptake. Persons tending to a high anticipatory secretion of cortisol could be described best by a coping style of resignation, high lactate levels after end of loading, and a high breathing frequence. Anticipation of muscular exercise was reported to elevate cortisol responses by Mason et al. (1973). Figure 1 shows that our sample started with very high cortisol levels regarding time of day which could be interpreted as such an anticipation effect because our subjects were informed that they had to exercise on a bicycle to test their limits.

Psychoendocrine research has widely neglected individual differences in hormonal secretion, although psychoendocrine theories have focussed on the impact of psychological factors modulating hormone secretion from early on (e.g. Mason, 1968; for review see Rose, 1984). Every indicator of activation assessed reflected remarkable variation of the individual response to a given stress situation, as has been demonstrated repeatedly in psychophysiological studies of individual differences in trait, state, or reaction aspects of activation (e.g. Fahrenberg et al., 1983). If hormonal patterns in different stress situations could ever have any predictive value for the development of health and disease, only individual patterns should be taken into account. The apparent contradictory effects of glucocorticoids in maintaining life while suppressing the defense mechanisms of the body at the same time (especially by immune-suppression) have been reconciled, at least in principle, by the hypothesis that the glucocorticoid response to stress prevents an overshoot of the defense mechanisms in response to a challenge (Munck et al., 1984). Our study may be a contribution to elucidate the person x situation interactions, i.e. a combination of personality factors, coping styles, and physiological parameters in the situation, as best predictors for individual hormonal patterns.

Research was supported by DFG, SPP Interozeption und Verhaltenskontrolle

References

Berger, M., Bossert, S., Krieg. J., Dirlich, G., Ettmeier, W., Schreiber, W., and von Zerssen, D. (1987). Interindividual differences in the susceptibility of the cortisol system: An important factor for the degree of hypercortisolism in stress situations? *Biological Psychiatry, 22,* 1327–1339.

Bickel, U., Born, J., Fehm, H. L., Distler, M., and Voigt, K. (1988). The behaviorally active peptide ACTH 4–10, measurement in plasma and pharmacokinetics in man. *European Journal of Clinical Pharmacology, 35,* 371–377.

Fahrenberg, J., Selg, H., and Hampel, R. (1978). Das Freiburger Persönlichkeitsinventar, FPI. (Freiburger Personality Inventory). Göttingen: Hogrefe.

Fahrenberg, J., Walschburger, P., Foerster, F., Myrtek, M., and Müller, W. (1983) An evaluation of trait, state, and reaction aspects of activation processes. *Psychophysiology, 20,* 188–195.

Fehm-Wolfsdorf, G. and Voigt, K. (1989). Physical stress overcomes the dexamethasone suppression of cortisol/ACTH secretion. In H. Weiner, I. Florin, R. Murison, and D. Hellhammer (Eds.), *Frontiers of stress research.* (pp. 372–375). Toronto: Huber.

Haynes, S. G., Levine, S., Scotch, N., Feinleib, M., and Kannel, W. B. (1978). The relationship of psychosocial factors to coronary heart disease in the Framingham study. I. Methods and risk factors. *American Journal of Epidemiology, 107,* 362–383.

Janke, W., Erdmann, G., and Kallus, W. (1985). *Streßverarbeitungsfragebogen, SVF.* (Coping Questionnaire). Göttingen: Hogrefe.

Mason, J. W. (1986). Organisation of the multiple endocrine responses to avoidance in the monkey. *Psychosomatic Medicine, 30,* 774–790.

Mason, J. W., Hartley, L. H., Kotchen, T. A., Mougey, E. H., Ricketts, P. T., and Jones, L. R. G. (1973). Plasma cortisol and norepinephrine responses in anticipation of muscular exercise. *Psychosomatic medicine, 35,* 406–414.

Munck, A., Guyre, P. M., and Holbrook, N. J. (1984). Physiological functions of glucocorticoids in stress and their relation to pharmacological actions. *Endocrine Reviews, 5,* 25–44.

Rose, R. M. (1984). Overview of endocrinology of stress. In G. M. Brown, S. H. Koslow, and S. Reichlin. (Eds.), *Neuroendocrinology and psychiatric disorder.* (pp. 95–122) New York: Raven.

Voigt, K., Ziegler, M., Grünert-Fuchs, M., Bickel, U., and Fehm-Wolfsdorf, G. (1990). Hormonal responses to exhausting physical exercise: the role of predictability and controllability of the situation. *Psychoneuroendocrinology,* in press.

Can Stress Affect Metabolic Disruption in Diabetes Mellitus?

Hans-Joachim Steingrüber, Friedrich W. Kemmer and Rudolf Bisping

The discussion about the effects of psychological stress on poor diabetes control is still controversial. Empirical evidence on endocrine and metabolic regulation suggests that levels of blood glucose, plasma ketone bodies, and free fatty acids may be affected by stress-induced increases of cortisol, catecholamine, glucagon, and growth hormone secretion. Thus, it is reasonable to assume that in diabetic patients these counterregulatory responses may lead to severe metabolic derangements. In fact, some studies report both, the adverse effects of stress and, correspondingly, the favourable effects of relaxation exercises on metabolic control in diabetics (e.g. Hinkle, Conger, & Wolf, 1950; Surwit & Feinglos, 1988). However, critical reviews point out that the majority of relevant investigations suffer from methodological flaws which impede unequivocal conclusions (Lustman, Carney, & Amado, 1981; Barglow, Hatcher, Edidin, & Sloan-Rossiter, 1984; Kemmer, 1988). Points of critique refer to:

1. lack of stressor standardization,
2. no control for order effects,
3. no confirmation that the presumed stressor indeed produces stress,
4. lack of consistent measurements before, during, and after stressor exposure,
5. heterogeneous samples (e.g. pooling Type I and Type II diabetes),
6. poorly-defined therapeutic conditions.

Despite these shortcomings it is interesting to note that most of the findings suggest that blood glucose levels are either unaltered or may even decrease with stress (VandenBergh, Sussman, & Vaughan, 1967; Carter, Gonder-Frederick, Cox, Clarke, & Scott, 1985).

Stress Effects in Type I Diabetics

In an attempt to consider the above-mentioned methodological problems we recently reported an experimental approach designed to examine the effects of acute psychological stress on psychophysiological, hormonal and metabolic variables in patients with Type I diabetes (Kemmer et al., 1986). We compared (a) nine diabetic patients in good metabolic control (injection of usual insulin doses the evening before and on the morning of the study), (b) nine diabetic patients in poor metabolic control (withholding the usual insulin doses on the morning of the study), and (c) nine nondiabetic subjects, all participants being matched for sex, age (variation: 19–36 years), weight, and socioeconomic status. They were exposed to two standardized psychological stressors (mental arithmetic / 45 minutes, public speaking / 15 minutes) and one non-stress situation (reading magazines) on three different days in a systematically permutated order. Before, during, and after exposure to these experimental conditions the following parameters were repeatedly measured: Self-ratings of emotional arousal (eleven-point bipolar scale ranging from "very calm" to "very excited"), heart rate, and blood pressure; free insulin/immunoreactive insulin, plasma levels of epinephrine, norepinephrine, cortisol, glucagon, and growth hormone; blood glucose, ketone bodies, and free fatty acids. Both stress situations caused significant increases of all psychophysiological variables (self-ratings, heart rate, blood pressure) which was associated with increments of plasma catecholamine levels ranging from 50–100 pg/milliliter (epinephrine), and 150–200 pg/milliliter (norepinephrine), respectively (for blood pressure as an example see Figure 1.). The plasma cortisol level increased significantly after public speaking in all groups.

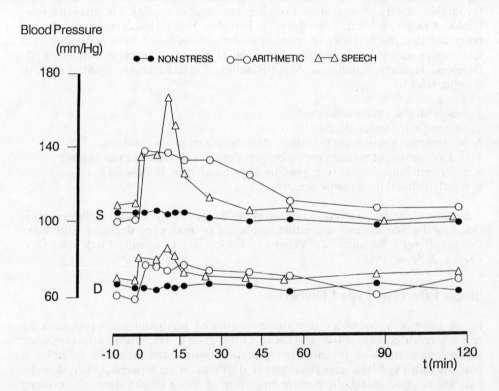

Figure 1. Systolic (S) and diastolic (D) blood pressure in Type I diabetics in good metabolic control before, during and after stress induction (arithmetic: t0-t45; speech: t0-t10 preparing for speech, t10-t15 public speaking)

In contrast, glucagon and growth hormone as well as the metabolic variables remained unaffected by stress. This was true for nondiabetic subjects and for diabetic patients in good and in poor metabolic control.

We concluded that for all subjects arithmetic and public speaking were obviously stressful activities but that the increase of catecholamine and cortisol levels was not sufficient to induce metabolic alterations.

However, taking into account the study design it is not justified to infer from the data that stress in general has no impact on diabetes control. For a definite evaluation further aspects of possible stress effects should be considered first.

Sources of Variance

Type of Stress

In our experiment we examined acute and rather short-lived stress reactions. Regarding the psychophysiological and hormonal alterations they were comparable to those associated with common daily life situations, such as driving motor vehicles or taking examinations (Taggart, Gibbons, & Somerville, 1969; Danner, Endert, Koster, & Dunning, 1981). On the other hand it is uncertain how representative these laboratory conditions are of real life conditions (Dimsdale, 1984): Far more pronounced or exceptional stress situations may occur in real life with marked hormone increments exceeding the threshold for metabolic effects (Cryer, 1980). Moreover, real life stress is often chronic, so that protracted and synergistic action of counterregulatory hormones (especially catecholamines and cortisol) may deteriorate diabetes control. Beside these possible neurohormonal pathways chronic stress can also affect certain behavior patterns which are essential for glucoregulatory control in diabetics: Physical activity, accuracy of diet, glucose monitoring, and insulin application.

Individual Type of Reaction

One of the reasons for contradictory results on stress-related worsening of diabetes control is probably due to the fact that only some patients develop metabolic derangements but others do not. Thus, in the presence of differential reactions group effects may either be weak or not exist because opposite effects will neutralize each other. There is indeed evidence that physiological, psychological, and clinical characteristics could account for metabolic response variation.

Carter et al. (1985) reported that pre-stress blood glucose levels in Type I diabetics predicted blood glucose changes during stress and that direction and degree of blood glucose change turned out to vary between subjects but were stable within subjects. These and other neurohumoral response sets, such as increased sensitivity to stress hormones, may be crucial characteristics of stress reactors. Another approach for discriminating between reactors and non-reactors is the identification of certain personality traits or behavioral patterns. This approach refers not only to a hormonal stress mediation hypothesis but also to behavioral alterations of the diabetic regimen or to psychological coping processes. Thus, Stabler et al. (1987) demonstrated that in childen with Type I diabetes a hyperglycemic response to stress was associated with a Type A behavior pattern. Finally, some data suggest that glucoregulatory responses to relaxation exercises are less consistent in patients with Type I than in Type II diabetes (see Surwit & Feinglos, 1988).

In summary, there is no definite answer to the general question whether stress affects metabolic disruption in patients with diabetes mellitus. Experimental data provide evidence that acute and short-lived stress situations which are typical for daily life do not disturb metabolic control in patients with Type I diabetes. However, systematic investigation is lacking about indications of possible stress effects which are either related to type of stress or to individual type of reaction.

References

Barglow, P., Hatcher, R., Edidin, D. V., & Sloan-Rossiter, D. (1984). Stress and metabolic control in diabetes: psychosomatic evidence and evaluation of methods. *Psychosomatic Medicine, 46*, 127–144.

Carter, W. R., Gonder-Frederick, L. A., Cox, D. J., Clarke, W. L., & Scott, D. (1985). Effect of stress on blood glucose in IDDM. *Diabetes Care, 8*, 411–412.

Cryer, P. E. (1980). Physiology and pathophysiology of the human sympathoadrenal neuroendocrine system. *New England Journal of Medicine, 303*, 436–444.

Danner, S. A., Endert, E., Koster, R. W., & Dunning, A. J. (1981). Biochemical and circulatory parameters during purely mental stress. *Acta Medica Scandinavica, 209*, 305–308.

Dimsdale, J. E. (1984). Generalizing from laboratory studies to field studies of human stress physiology. *Psychosomatic Medicine, 46*, 463–469.

Hinkle, L. E., Conger, G. B., & Wolf, S. (1950). Studies on diabetes mellitus: the relation of stressful life situations to the concentration of ketone bodies in the blood of diabetic and non-diabetic humans. *Journal of Clinical Investigation, 29*, 754–769.

Kemmer, F. W. (1988). Einflüsse von Streßhormonen und psychischen Belastungen auf die diabetische Stoffwechsellage. (Effects of stress hormones and psychological stress on diabetes). München, Wien, Baltimore: Urban und Schwarzenberg.

Kemmer, F. W., Bisping, R., Steingrüber, H. J., Baar, H., Hardtmann, F., Schlaghecke, R., & Berger, M. (1986). Psychological stress and metabolic control in patients with Type I diabetes mellitus. *New England Journal of Medicine, 314*, 1078–1084.

Lustman, P., Carney, R., & Amado, H. (1981). Acute stress and metabolism in diabetes. *Diabetes Care, 4*, 658–659.

Stabler, B., Surwit, R. S., Lane, J. D., Morris, M. A., Litton, J., & Feinglos, M. N. (1987). Type A behavior pattern and blood glucose control in diabetic children. *Psychosomatic Medicine, 49*, 313–316.

Surwit, R. S., & Feinglos, M. N. (1988). Stress and autonomic nervous system in Type II diabetes. *Diabetes Care, 11*, 83–85.

Taggart, P., Gibbons, D., & Somerville, W. (1969). Some effects of motor-car driving on the normal and abnormal heart. *British Medical Journal, 4*, 130–134.

VandenBergh, R. L., Sussman, K. E., & Vaughan, G. D. (1967). effects of combined physical-anticipatory stress on carbohydrate-lipid metabolism in patients with diabetes mellitus. *Psychosomatics, 8*, 16–19.

Section 4

Social Support in Health and Disease

Social Support and Physical Health: An Updated Meta-Analysis

Anja Leppin and Ralf Schwarzer

While several thousand years ago the Apocryphes stated that "a good friend is the best medicine", latter-day empirical science has not quite been able to match this untroubled outlook on the physical benefits of social relations.

Some empirical contributions from the seventies might have given rise to high expectations (Berkman & Syme, 1979; Medalie & Goldbourt, 1976; Nuckolls, Cassel, & Kaplan, 1972). However, while the amount of literature dealing with this issue has steadily increased, sceptical voices have been heard, too.

Thus, Wallston, Whitcher-Alagna, DeVellis, and DeVellis (1983) in their review on social support and health came to quite mixed conclusions. And in a more recent survey Ganster and Victor (1988) have stated: "At this time the literature still has not resolved several fundamental questions of the relationship between social support and health. Perhaps foremost is the ambiguity regarding the impact of social support on physical well-being. Until large-scale prospective studies on a general population sample are conducted, the literature will have to continue to assume that either physical morbidity is unaffected by social support, or that the current research is systematically flawed" (p. 33).

Although the demand for methodologically sound studies to be conducted in the future is very definitely justified, for the time being it might still be necessary and possible to evaluate the evidence that is available on a more systematic basis, for instance on quantitative rather than narrative grounds, i.e. by applying a meta-analysis to the available data.

Also, to find a more reliable answer to the question whether there really is a causal relationship between social integration/ social support and health, it might be helpful to systematically apply explicit criteria to the empirical material. This would mean evaluating the available evidence in terms of standards such as consistency, strength, temporality, and specificity (see Broadhead, Kaplan, James, Wagner, Schoenbach, Grimson, Heyden, Tibblin, & Gehlbach, 1983). While these standards lend themselves to meta-analytic investigation, other important criteria such as coherence or biological plausibility of theoretical models (see Broadhead et al., 1983) have not yet generated a sufficient amount of empirical research, therefore will not be dealt with here. For an extensive overview on theoretical models explaining the support-physical health relationships see Cohen (1988).

Consistency of findings refers to the question of whether the body of results is homogeneous. Have all studies found a negative relationship between social support and illness or were there only a few? And what about the *strength* of these relationships? Have there been large differences or only marginal ones? A first glance at the literature shows that while mainly negative correlations between social support and illness have been reported, positive relationships are no rarity, either.

Temporality also still poses a major problem. Only a minority of all findings is based on longitudinal designs and more often than not these are epidemiological studies dealing with social integration only. A majority of reported findings is therefore wide open for the critical question whether social support has prevented or reduced the incidence of illness or – – vice versa – – illness incidence has disturbed social relationships and thus reduced the quantity of social support.

Another issue is raised by the *specificity* of findings. Does social support always and under all circumstances exert a positive effect on all possible indicators of physical health or are there specific effects? Empirical investigations have been dealing with very different populations, and the widest variety of instruments for measuring social integration or social support have been used while health or illness criteria have been ranging from psychosomatic symptoms to mortality. It seems questionable at best that a variable like social support should have a similarly strong effect in all these cases. But, which precisely are the circumstances that are amenable to social support and which kinds of support or integration are the ones that work best?

Very important, for instance, seems the distinction between social integration in general terms and the more specific functions social integration can provide for the individual. Only these functional aspects will subsequently be referred to as social support, whereas the term "social embeddedness" will be used for both structural and functional aspects. The term social integration generally pertains to the mere existence or the structure of a social network (House & Kahn, 1985; House, Umberson, & Landis, 1988). On an operational level it is indicators like family status, number of friends, numbers of organisations participated in or combined indices that are used most often.

While the availability of a large network certainly provides a potential for helpful and beneficial social interactions, it also offers ample opportunity for social conflict (see, for instance, Argyle & Furnham, 1983). Yet, most often social integration, independent of actual quality of relationships, might be more salutary than social isolation. Social integration might not only entail help in situations of need but also the more general advantages inherent in social relations such as behavior modeling by others and the chance for social role enactment that might be necessary for developing a sense of meaning and coherence in one's life (Thoits, 1985).

And yet, most researchers agree that it is necessary to go beyond existence or lack of social relations and look for what is actually provided or perceived as being present in terms of *beneficial functions*. However, even within this domain of social support, concepts and operationalizations differ widely.

There is a debate, for instance, on whether social support is a unidimensional construct or not. Many researchers have strongly emphasized the necessity to assess various types of support (Barrera, 1981; Cohen & Hoberman, 1983; Cohen & McKay, 1984; Cutrona & Russell, 1989; Dunkel-Schetter, Feinstein, & Call, 1987; House, 1981; Wills, 1985). Some have even argued the case for a 'need-support-specificity-model' claiming that specific types of support are required in specific kinds of situations, for instance material aid in times of economic need (Cohen & Wills, 1985; Wills, 1985). Others, on the contrary, have postulated that only one concept of support, i.e. emotional support (including feelings of belonging and attachment) is essential (Cobb, 1976); Sarason, Levine, Basham, & Sarason, 1983; Sarason, Sarason, & Shearin, 1986; Sarason, Shearin, Pierce, & Sarason, 1987). According to this notion all other 'types' of support such as instrumental or material help derive from this general sense of being loved and cared for. Thus, they are – – at best – – secondary.

Another controversial issue pertains to the relevance and impact of received as compared to perceived support. One prominent approach in recent years has been to consider the general subjective perspective of the recipient not as *one* important criterion, but as *the* essential or even the only one (Sarason et al., 1987; Turner, Frankel, & Levin, 1983). When social support is primarily viewed in emotional terms, i.e. as a general sense of being loved and valued, of being 'safe' within a strong network of others, the concept would come fairly close to reflecting a personality variable rather than referring to actual social interaction (Sarason et al., 1986).

Individual perceptions of resources are definitely highly important when it comes to a person's well-being, for instance in those instances where an event or encounter is evaluated in terms of being stressful and maybe threatening and is weighted against potential coping resources. What, however, would happen if during the actual process of coping with an event the person's beliefs about others' willingness to help are shattered? What if, contrary to all expectations, others do not rally round, do not understand the problem or are reluctant to help? It seems that processes of actual helping behavior are not at all irrelevant to the formation and maintenance of subjective concepts of support, but should contribute to confirm or disconfirm such beliefs.

Received support is the concept that deals with those kinds of beneficial behaviors of others. While it also concerns subjective perceptions of the recipient, these do not pertain to hypothetical situations or general impressions but to behaviors that have been perceived as having actually occured. Consequently this conceptualization of support should be particularly useful when it comes to situations where individuals have to cope with a stressful event.

Social support whether received or perceived can further be assessed in terms of quantitative-descriptive and/or qualitative-evaluative aspects, i.e. one can ask people whether they perceive themselves as potentially supported or have been the recipients of certain benefical actions by others in the past and/or whether they are satisfied with the status quo of their social support.

The relevance of social support within stressful circumstances vs. everyday life is another issue that has given rise to a multitude of differing opinions. Some research has concentrated on direct effects of social support (Barrera, 1986; Thoits, 1985), i.e. effects that come about independent or whether the individual finds him- or herself in a stressful situation or not. Social support, according to this model, would either prevent the event altogether (stress prevention model) or would affect well-being independent of this event (additive model). The buffer model, on the contrary, states that social support plays a role especially under stressful circumstances (Cohen & Wills, 1985). Only when something important is at stake for the individual, the presence or absence of social support makes a difference, i.e. can buffer the deleterious impact of the event by reducing stress appraisal or by giving coping-assistance.

The present meta-analysis is aimed at pursuing the following questions:

Is social support correlated with indicators of physical health and if so, to what degree?

Are these empirical relations different for

a) structural vs. functional aspects or social support/social integration?

b) emotional vs. instrumental aspects of social support?
c) perceived vs. received social support?
d) specific indicators of health and illness?

and in all these cases: is there any difference when stress samples and unselected samples are considered separately?

Method

The Rationale of Meta-Analysis

The aim of meta-analysis is to integrate a multitude of effect sizes, for instances correlations, which are to be found in original empirical studies (Fricke & Treinies, 1985; Hedges & Olkin, 1985). There are a variety of different meta-analytical techniques whose common principle is that they are all trying to integrate the information provided by the original studies on a higher statistical level. The present study is based on the Schmidt-Hunter method (Hunter, Schmidt, & Jackson, 1982). This technique makes use of correlations without being restricted to purely correlational studies. Other statistical values (such as t-, F-, or p-Values) can be transformed into the 'effect size r'. All sample effect sizes are weighted by the corresponding sample size N. The population effect size is, thus, defined as the weighted average of all r's.

The chosen strategy aims at determining a population effect size for a homogeneous data set of effect sizes. This is to be achieved by decomposing the observed variance of effect sizes into variance due to artefacts and variance due to systematic factors (i.e. moderators). Most important for the majority of applications is the determination of this unexplained population variance s^2_{rho} by subtracting the sampling error s^2_e from the observed variance s^2_r.

$$S^2_{rho} = S^2_r - S^2_e$$

The population variance S^2_{rho} is also called the residual variance, and its square root is called residual standard deviation (res_{SD}). An approximation for the sampling error is obtained by

$$S^2_e = ((1-\bar{r}^2_w)^2 {}_* k)/N$$

where $\bar{r}^2_w$ is the squared weighted mean of the effect sizes, k the number of studies, and N the total sample size (Hunter et al., 1982).

It is desirable that all the observed variance s^2_r is made up by the sampling error s^2_e, and that the residual variance s^2_{rho} would become zero. In that case the "percentage of observed variance accounted for by sampling error" would be 100% as an indication of homogeneity. Very often, however, only a small percentage can be explained by artefacts, leaving a state of heterogeneity which requires further searches for moderator variables. A total of 100% is usually very difficult to achieve, so that the rule of thumb by Hunter et al. (1982) is a level of at least 75% of variance explained by artefacts in order to evaluate a data set as being sufficiently homogeneous. The computations have been performed with the meta-analysis programs for personal computers (Schwarzer, 1989).

Database

A systematic literature search was conducted for studies on social support or social integration and health which had appeared between 1976 and early 1988. This search was performed mainly with the help of a computer-based survey done by the Center for Psychological Information and Documentation in Trier (West Germany), a review of the 'Psychological Abstracts' for this period and an additional manual check of 25 relevant scientific journals. Inclusion criteria for articles were a) they had to be written in either German or English, b) they had to be empirical, and c) they had to report correlations or statistics suitable for transformation into effect sizes (such as t, F, p).

Eighty studies were compiled which yielded a total of 110 effect sizes. Samples ranged from n= 17 to n= 6,534 with an overall size of N= 60,936, a mean of $N_M=$ 553 and a median of $N_{Md}=$ 134. The majority of these studies (59) came from North America, 13 from Western Europe, three from Latin America, two from Israel, and three from other countries. Sixty-one of these papers were published as articles in scientific journals, three were book chapters, 16 dissertations, research reports or conference papers. The dates of publication show that the number of studies dealing with that topic has increased rapidly. While only 16 of the studies included here were published between 1976 and 1981, there were 19 within two years 1982/83 alone, 18 in 1984/85 and 27 between 1986 and spring 1988.

The unit of analysis was the subject sample. Some studies were based on more than one independent sample, for instance, in those cases where men and women were dealt with separately. In these cases, each sample was represented by one effect size.

The total amount of 110 samples (=110 correlations) in this meta-analysis was derived from a total of 80 studies. When the authors did not report any correlations, other statistical values were transformed into effect sizes, or the available material was reanalyzed — wherever possible. Many studies dealing with the given topic did not publish any effect sizes but, for instance, risk ratios or exact probabilities. The well-known study by Berkman and Syme (1979), for instance, states that the mortality risk of weakly-integrated persons is about two times higher than that of socially well-integrated men and women. We have estimated an effect size of 'only' r= –0.07 for this risk ratio (a more extensive elaboration on this project can be found in Schwarzer & Leppin, 1989a, pp. 209–213). Such a transformation reveals two things:1) effect sizes are less 'spectacular' than some other statistics, at least in those cases where large samples or extreme groups are involved, and 2) small effect sizes can nevertheless be important, if serious consequences are at stake.

Results

Overall Analysis

All 110 effect sizes were combined to obtain a first estimate to be used later as a yardstick for comparison. These 110 correlations varied from r= –0.43 to r= + ,0.17 The majority of coefficients was located near zero. The population effect size was $\bar{r}_w=$ –0.07. The magnitude of such a correlation might seem small, but is not negligible (see discussion section). As expected the large data set on which this result was based was not homogeneous (38%).

Structural, Functional and Functional-Evaluative Aspects of Social Embeddedness and their Relationship with Illness

The first attempt at specifying the most general result reported above was made in terms of the types of social embeddedness that were dealt with in each study, i.e. structural vs. functional and functional-evaluative support. The present meta-analysis asked which quantitative indicators characterize current research and whether different kinds of social embeddedness are more or less strongly related to health criteria. First, all effect sizes from those studies where network indicators had been used were combined. These were 55 correlation coefficients on the basis of 32, 825 persons. The weighted mean was $\bar{r}_w = -0.07$, indicating a weak relationship between social integration and illness. Well-integrated persons seemed to be somewhat less affected by health problems than persons with few social ties. However, the data set was yet too heterogeneous to classify this finding as reliable. With 42% the homogeneity index was a long way from the required 75% (see Table 1). While there was no noteworthy difference to this finding when social support was under investigation (k = 79; N = 35,257; $\bar{r}_w = -0.08$), the effect size for the evaluative dimension of social support, i.e. satisfaction with support was markedly higher (k= 12; N = 1383; $\bar{r}_w = -0.25$) than for the other two. The large discrepancy between these results makes it even more regrettable that only relatively few studies have dealt with this aspect of support. In any case, none of the results were based on homogeneous data sets (see Table 1).

Table 1. *Structural, functional and functional-evaluative aspects of social embeddedness and their relationship with illness*

Variable	k	N	$\bar{r}_w$	% homogeneity
social integration	55	32,825	−0.07	42
social support	79	35,257	−0.08	26
support satisfaction	12	1,383	−0.25	44

In order to examine the buffer hypothesis, the network and the functional support data set were further divided into stress samples vs. unselected samples (see Table 2).

While for the support data no difference between the two — still heterogeneous — samples became apparent ($\bar{r}_w = -0.09$ and $\bar{r}_w = -0.08$, respectively), in the case of social integration it turned out that the correlation for the stress subsample was slightly higher ($\bar{r}_w = -.10$) than for the unselected one ($\bar{r}_w = -.06$). However, only the stress sample was homogeneous.

Family Integration, Family Support and their Relationship with Illness

As one sample for social integration within different sub-groups and support from different sources, the data set for one type of source, i.e. the large 'family data subset' was looked at in terms of different types of embeddedness and stressed vs. unselected samples (see Table 3).

Table 2. *Structural, functional and functional-evaluative aspects of social embeddedness and their relationship with illness: Stress samples vs. unselected samples.*

Variable	k	N	$\bar{r}_w$	% homogeneity
social integration/ stress sample	17	4,532	–0.10	80
social integration/ unselected sample	35	27,874	–0.06	36
support/ stress sample	31	6,062	–0.09	64
support/ unselected sample	45	28,573	–0.08	18

Table 3. *Family integration, family support and their relationship with illness*

Variable	k	N	$\bar{r}_w$	% homogeneity
social integration	8	5,692	–0.05	100
support	19	2,612	–0.16	44

There was a remarkable difference between social integration and functional support ($\bar{r}_w$ = –0.05 compared to $\bar{r}_w$ = –0.16); however only the former was based on a homogeneous sample. This result might again emphasize the relative importance of subjective indicators of support in contrast to objective-structural measures.

A further breakdown according to stress samples and unselected samples brought about the findings illustrated in Table 4.

Table 4. *Family integration, family support and their relationship with illness: Stress samples vs. unselected samples*

Variable	k	N	$\bar{r}_w$	% homogeneity
stress sample	13	986	–0.15	49
unselected sample	14	7,172	–0.07	34

Although homogeneity could not be achieved in either case, there was another clear indication for a stronger relationship between support and illness within the stress sample ($\bar{r}_w$ = –0.15 as compared to $\bar{r}_w$ = –0.07).

Different Types of Support and their Relationship with Illness: Emotional vs. Instrumental and Advice/Information Support

For the large set of studies which dealt with functional aspects, further specifications were made which have figured prominently in the literature and have been the object of not a few controversies. First, the overall set was divided according to the contents of functions that had been measured, a procedure which yielded three categories: emotional, instrumental and information/advice support (see Table 5).

Table 5. *Emotional vs. instrumental and advice/information support and their relationship with illness.*

Variable	k	N	$\bar{r}_w$	% homogeneity
emotional	34	21,121	–0.05	40
instrumental	15	8,176	–0.17	42
advice/ information	11	1,540	–0.13	41

While none of the data sets came close to the required 75% homogeneity, it is interesting that, contrary to expectations, instrumental and information support seem to be more relevant for physical problems than emotional support ($\bar{r}_w = -0.17$ and $\bar{r}_w = -0.13$ as compared to $\bar{r}_w = -0.05$). However, as long as these results are not reliable, they cannot indicate more than perhaps a trend towards a certain direction.

Different Types of Social Support and their Relationship with Illness: Perceived vs. Received Support

Another comparison, 'perceived vs. received support' yielded the following results (see Table 6):

Table 6. *Perceived and received support and their relationship with illness*

Variable	k	N	$\bar{r}_w$	% homogeneity
perceived	69	34,607	–0.08	25
received	18	1,121	–0.05	50

Obviously in this case the theoretical distinction was not borne out by a differential impact of the two variables on physical illness ($\bar{r}_w = -0.08$ and $\bar{r}_w = -0.05$). Again, however, any conclusion is premature as long as the data sets are heterogeneous. It is obvious, too, that there is a considerable imbalance in the attention that the two concepts have so far found empirically. Sixty nine effect sizes with an N of 34, 607 on "perceived support" were available while there were only 18 effect sizes with an N of 1, 121 for the dimension "received support".

Different Types of Support and their Relationship with Illness: Emotional and Instrumental Support Combined with Received and Perceived Support

Further subdivisions were performed by combining the perceived-received distinction with the emotional-instrumental dimension. The instrumental support data set also included the data on information/advice support. Results are depicted in Table 7.

Table 7. *Emotional and instrumental support combined with received and perceived support and their relationship with illness.*

Variable	k	N	$\bar{r}_w$	% homogeneity
emotional/perceived	27	20,799	−0.04	35
emotional/received	7	342	−0.13	53
instrumental/perceived	15	8,773	−0.18	50
instrumental/received	5	494	−0.03	83

Opposite patterns emerged for the emotional and the instrumental data sets. When emotional support was investigated, the received support subtype was related more strongly to illness($\bar{r}_w$= −0.13) than the perceived one ($\bar{r}_w$ = −0.04). For instrumental support there was an exactly reverse pattern. Perceived support was more closely related to illness ($\bar{r}_w$ = −0.18) than received support ($\bar{r}_w$ = −0.03). However, only the (very small) instrumental/received support subset could match homogeneity standards.

Another interesting possibility for a moderator search was the breakdown according to stress samples vs. unselected samples combined with the various types of support (Table 8).

Table 8. *Emotional and instrumental support and their relationship with illness: Stress samples vs. unselected samples*

Variable	k	N	$\bar{r}_w$	% homogeneity
emotional/stress sample	16	4,245	−0.06	100
emotional/unselected sample	13	16,301	−0.04	23
instrumental/stress sample	10	985	−0.10	74
instrumental unselected sample	10	8,282	−0.18	37

As expected the two stress samples turned out to be more homogeneous (100% and 74% respectively) than the unselected samples (23% and 37%, respectively) and were thus able to meet respective standards. The effect sizes for these two stress samples differed only slightly ($\bar{r}_w$ =−0.06 for emotional, $\bar{r}_w$ = −0.10 for instrumental support), whereas there was a large difference within the unselected group ($\bar{r}_w$ = −0.04 for emotional as compared to $\bar{r}_w$ = −0.18 for instrumental support). Noteworthy is also the discrepancy between the instrumental and emotional subgroups in terms of their differing effect when combined with the two sample types. While emotional support related only weakly to illness within the stress as well as the unselected sample ($\bar{r}_w$= −0.06 and $\bar{r}_w$ =0.04), instrumental support brought about a higher effect size when measured within the unselected than the stress sample ($\bar{r}_w$ =0.18 as compared to $\bar{r}_w$=0.10).

When the perceived-received distinction was aplied to the 'stress vs. unselected samples dimension', it turned out that there was a clear buffer effect for received support while this was not the case for perceived support. Received support yielded an $\bar{r}_w$ = −0.12 for the stress sample as compared to an $\bar{r}_w$ = +0.12 for the unselected sample. Thus the relationship in the unselected sample was even a positive one. For perceived support, on the contrary, effect sizes for both sample types were negative and of a similar magnitude ($\bar{r}_w$ = −0.09 and $\bar{r}_w$ = −0.08).

Table 9. *Perceived and received support and their relationship with illness: Stress samples vs. unselected samples.*

Variable	k	N	$\bar{r}_w$	% homogeneity
perceived/ unselected sample	41	28, 328	−0.08	17
perceived/ stress sample	26	5,781	−0.9	64
received/ stress sample	11	692	−0.12	74
received/ unselected sample	6	385	0.12	100

Relationships Between Social Support/Social Integration and Different Operationalizations of Illness

All findings presented so far have been based on the implicit assumption that health problems should be treated as a unidimensional construct. However, such an approach can be nothing more than a first step. Beyond that it was absolutely essential to have a look at how different indicators of health and illness were affected by social embeddedness. Several subgroups of indicators were formed such as a general health rating, where persons were asked to rate their health on an 'excellent – good – fair – poor' – scale or symptom indices where persons were requested to fill in lists of symptoms such as headache, stomach pains, fever etc. Then there were chronic diseases such as angina pectoris or arthritis. This group was then further split up into one subgroup containing only cardiovascular diseases and another dealing with all other chronic illnesses. Another subcategory was severity of disease, i.e. progress and/or recovery, and, finally, mortality. Table 10 contains the meta-analytic results for each of these categories.

Population effect sizes ranged from $\bar{r}_w$ = −0.03 to $\bar{r}_w$ = −0.13. The more subjective indicators such as general health ratings ($\bar{r}_w$ = −0.10) and symptom indices ($\bar{r}_w$ = −0.11) tended to yield slightly higher effect sizes than more objective criteria like mortality ($\bar{r}_w$ = −0.07) or chronic disease ($\bar{r}_w$ = −0.04). However, it was possible to split up data pertaining exclusively to cardiovascular diseases and contrast them to all other types

Table 10. *Relationships between social support/social integration and different operationalizations of illness.*

Variable	k	N	$\bar{r}_w$	% homogeneity
Health rating	10	10,714	−0.10	43
physical symptoms	45	16,536	−0.11	37
diseases (all)	19	22,787	−0.04	31
diseases (without CHD)	8	3,172	−0.13	100
CHD	12	19,684	−0.03	34
severity of disease	7	1,316	−0.08	83

of chronic disease (which in the majority of cases meant summary indices of chronic diseases). The effect size for cardiovascular diseases was very small (k=12; N=19,684; $\bar{r}_w$=−0.03) and heterogeneous (34%), which was largely due to the impact of two large-scale epidemiological studies on the social integration-coronary artery disease relationship which came up with very small effect sizes. For the subset of all other chronic diseases, on the contrary, a considerably higher population effect size was yielded (k= 8; N= 3,172; $\bar{r}_w$=−0.13) which was based on a totally homogeneous data set. Of the other effect sizes only those for mortality and disease severity could claim reliability.

Discussion

The present meta-analysis reflects the current empirical evidence about the linear statistical relationship between social integration/social support and indicators of physical illness. It has been revealed that the relation between these variables is a negative, if moderate-sized one. Another recent meta-analysis established that social support is much more closely linked to depression than to physical health (Schwarzer & Leppin, 1989a) – a result that does not really come as a surprise considering the conceptual closeness of many definitions of support on one hand, psychological well-being, on the other.

While such moderate and partly small effect sizes might seem somewhat "disappointing" at first sight, a closer look at the practical relevance of these results might change perspectives. If we take, for instance, the population effect size of $\bar{r}_w$=−0.07 found for the relationship between social embeddedness and mortality, this might seem a negligible correlation. Rosenthal's (1984) binomial effect size display, however, demonstrates that such a correlation of −0.07 can be interpreted in a different manner: If there were 100 socially weak embedded people, 53.5% of whom die, another group of 100 socially well embedded persons would loose only 46.5% people during the same time range in comparison. This example may show that correlations can well be of importance where matters of life and death are at stake. This might also be illustrated by looking at relative risk ratios for extreme groups. While Berkman and Syme (1979) in their study reported a relative mortality risk ratio of 2.3 for weak-integrated men as compared to well-integrated men, we estimated an effect size of $\bar{r}_w = -0.07$ on the basis of their published data (Schwarzer & Leppin, 1989a, pp. 209–213, 244ff).

Aboveand beyond that, it has been established that the relationship between social support and physical health is *specific*. Findings differed largely according to concepts and indicators of support/integration and illness used. However, some results lacked sufficient homogeneity to permity definate statements.

Stress was one of the specific factors investigated. Buffer effects of social support on stress experience and consequences are usually tested for by statistical interactions which are hard to recompute by meta-analysis. If a number of studies were to report F-values for exactly the same kind of statistical interactions, e.g. between spouse support, illness symptoms and job stress, it would be possible to estimate an appropriate population effect size. Since this kind of compatibility of data sets was not given within the present data, studies which reported only interaction effects could not be included (e.g., Sarason, Sarason, Potter, & Antoni, 1985; Heitzmann & Kaplan 1984). Buffer effects were instead investigated by separating stressed groups from unselected groups. However, this procedure might underrate true population differences, mostly because the unselected samples contain truly unstressed as well as stressed persons.

Buffer effects were found for family integration and support and particularly for received support, which emphasizes the close linkage between stress situations and actual receipt of support (see below), whereas generally perceived support might be important in everyday life as well as under specifically stressful circumstances. Similarly, specific subtypes of support, i.e. emotional and instrumental support might not be more relevant for stressed than unselected samples. However, what is interesting to note here is that while the correlations for the stress groups were based on homogeneous data sets, those for unselected samples were not. This would indicate that stress might provide a sufficient basis for emotional and instrumental social support to come into effect while in its absence other factors or conditions would have to be present to turn support into an effective weapon against development of disease.

As for relative relevance of social integration as compared to functional aspects (social support), it seems as if support might be more important than mere presence of social relationships (for instance in case of family integration/support or for the physical symptoms subgroup). However, this does not imply that social integration is irrelevant. In stress situations, for instance, availability of social relations and social contacts is obviously more beneficial than lack of those.

Within the domain of social support itself the available data strongly suggest that qualitative aspects are considerably more important than quantitative aspects. Satisfaction with support thus would have a stronger impact than its mere quantity. However, even though the large differences in effect sizes between these different aspects of support are indeed suggestive, the lack of reliability requires further search for moderators in the future. In particular, it is imperative that many more studies include the qualitative aspects in their research designs, instead of relying on quantitative information alone, assuming that more support is always better or always enough.

As for the contents of support perceived and received, it seems that practical kinds of help might be more important here than the more general emotional variety – – a result that might come as some kind of surprise. It is necessary, however, to keep in mind that it is indicators of physical health that are at stake here. Other than psychological comfort and well-being which might be influenced mostly by perceptions of being loved and cared for, physical health might profit relatively more from tangible aid and advice by way of reducing physical strain. However, further specifications clearly indicated that actual help in terms of received support carried little weight compared to perceived instrumental support, while for emotional support this relationship came out the other way round, i.e. the effect size for received emotional support was higher than for perceived emotional support. Such patterns might well be due to further moderating factors which could not be tracked down due to the small number of remaining data sets, but they nevertheless lend some weight to a multidimensional concept of social support (Cohen & Wills, 1985). Especially the tendency of instrumental support to show more "potential" than the emotional variety suggests that it might be premature to conceptualize the latter as the one and only concept of social support (Sarason et al., 1987).

Related to this controversy is the issue of the relevance of perceived as compared to received support. While no general difference could be detected for the relationships between illness and perceived support on one hand, illness and received support on the other, further differentiations in terms of type of support, sample type or type of outcome made it obvious that these two concepts are not simply interchangeable. For instance, it turned out that received support was positively connected with illness within the unselected sample type, whereas this relationship was a negative one within the stress sample. Actually received aid might represent a much more complicated process than the mere hypothetical perception of support. Dunkel-Schetter and Bennett (1988) have made the point that actually received help entail negative side-effects like feelings of obligation, of resentment, of lowered self-esteem which in themselves can decompensate any positive effects help might have had. Above and beyond such side-effects, the whole process during which perceived and received support come into play might be different. First of all, the concept of received support is more strongly tied to stress situations than perception of support. Often, people will offer their help to somebody only after they have noticed that this person has a problem. In this case the problem and/or symptoms due to this problem are causal for the social support coming forward. Thus a mobilization model would explain why physical symptoms might be accompanied by more support – – at least in a cross-sectional perspective which is the most common one taken. Only later should positive effects of social support become apparent and turn the positive correlation with illness into a negative one. Such confoundation problems are emphasized when received support is assessed within unselected samples. Asking for received support within these groups is likely to elicit answers where the receipt of support is confounded with the recent need for aid, i.e. stress experience (see also Barrera, 1986). In a similar vein, Dunkel-Schetter and Bennett (1988) have maintained that until a lot more studies have been conducted investigating the effects of received support within homogeneous samples of people suffering from the same kind of events, conclusions about the impact of theis specific type of support might be premature. The present results, i.e. a negative correlation of $\bar{r}_w = -0.12$ (reliable) for the stress group compared to a positive correlation for the unselected samples of $\bar{r}_w = +0.12$ might add some empirical weight to this argument.

Interpreting the results for different "outcome types" suggests that support integration might be more important for the "weaker", more subjective types of illness indicators such as general health ratings and symptom indices (often meaning psychosomatic symptoms) than for chronic disease, disease severity (i.e. progression or recovery) and mortality. However, there also was an effect size of $\bar{r}_w = -0.12$ for chronic disease when effect sizes for coronary artery disease were excluded. Thus, while it is not particularly surprising that a psychological construct such as social support should be more strongly related to subjective indicators of health than objective ones, more serious conditions such as chronic disease, obviously can be influenced, too. This social support-chronic disease relationship in particular deserves a lot more attention than it has got to date. The very low rate of homogeneity for the overall category as well as for coronary artery disease when compared to other chronic illnesses suggest that a lot more research is needed within this area which would allow for further specification of outcome criteria.

It should also be added that while, for instance, the issue of social integration and mortality might be settled ($\bar{r}_w = -0.07$; 98%), the topic of social support and mortality has not even been tackled yet, as all effect sizes in this meta-analysis for the mortality data were based on measures of social integration only.

There are a number of limitations in this study, some of which pertain to the meta-analytic method, some of which reflect the current empirical status within the field of support research. For instance, it remains unknown whether the compiled 80 studies are representative of research done in this field. Retrieval, publication and reporting bias may all have contributed to an unknown number studies remaining in the "file drawers". While Rosenthal (1984) has developed a method for developing some rough estimate of this bias, this "Fail Safe N-Formula" is not yet applicable to effect sizes r. And yet another meta-analytic deficiency contributes to the problem or representativeness. While methodologically poor studies often can be used in meta-analysis by transforming p-values, cell frequencies or percentage tables to effect sizes r, methodologically sophisticated studies using multiple regressions, structural modeling or log-linear analysis often fail to provide the reader with elementary statistics (such as correlation tables), and, thus, have to be excluded from meta-analytic computations. The same restriction applies for curvilinear relationships.

As has already been pointed out, temporality is a major problem for causal interpretation. As the majority of the studies used were based on cross-sectional designs, the present effect sizes are also affected by this deficiency.

A further shortcoming of this study pertains to the fact that some advanced options available to meta-analysts could not be employed due to limitations inherent in the empirical material. Meta-analytic technique nowadays permits to consider the unreliability of the measures employed, and to compute a population effect size that is not biased by this kind of artefact. However, of the studies on social support and health only a minority reported reliability coefficients, and it did therefore not seem appropriate to provide results for unbiased effect sizes.

Also the currently available empirical material lacks in specificity. Often studies do not separate their samples on the basis of different characteristics, or use very general measures for support or illness. This deficiency make it difficult to break down large samples into smaller, more specific subsamples.

What is therefore needed in the future are controlled longitudinal studies which will not neal with *any* general effect of social support or social integration on *any* kind of health or illness indicator, but very specific research into the effects of different types of support on very *specific* outcome indicators for different people under different circumstances.

Note

This article presents an update of a previous meta-analysis (Schwarzer & Leppin, 1989a, b) that was based on 55 studies and 83 effect sizes only.

References

Argyle, M., and Furnham, A. (1983). Sources of satisfaction and conflict in longterm relationships. *Journal of Marriage and the Family, 45*, 481–493.

Barrera, M. (1981). Social support in the adjustment of pregnant adolescents. In D. Gottlieb (Ed.), *Social support networks* (pp. 69–96). San Francisco, CA: Jossey-Bass.

Barrera, M. (1986). Distinctions between social support concepts, measures, and models. *American Journal of Community Psychology, 14*, 413–445.

Berkman, L. F., and Syme, S. L. (1979). Social networks, host resistance, and mortality: A nine-year follow-up study of Alameda county residents. *American Journal of Epidemiology, 109*, 186–204.

Broadhead, W. E., Kaplan, B. H., James, S. A., Wagner, E. H., Schoenbach, V. J., Grimson, R., Heyden, S., Tibblin, G., and Gehlbach, S. H. (1983). The epidemiologic evidence for a relationship between social support and health. *American Journal of Epidemiology, 117*, 521–537.

Cobb, S. (1976). Social support as a moderator of life stress. *Psychosomatic Medicine, 38*, 300–314.

Cohen, S. (1988). Psychosocial models of the role of social support in the etiology of physical disease. *Health Psychology, 3*, 269–297.

Cohen, S., and Hoberman, H. M. (1983). Positive events and social support as buffers of life change stress. *Journal of Applied Psychology, 13*, 99–125.

Cohen, S., and McKay, G. (1984). Social support, stress, and the buffering hypothesis: A theoretical analysis. In A. Baum, S. E. Taylor, and J. E. Singer (Eds.), *Handbook of psychology and health* (Vol. 4, pp. 253–267). Hillsdale, NJ: Erlbaum.

Cohen, S. M and Wills, T. A. (1985). Stress, social support, and the buffering hypothesis. *Psychological Bulletin, 98*, 310–357.

Cultrona, C. E., and Russell, D. W. (1989). The provisions of social relationships and adaptation of stress. In W. H. Jones and D. Perlman (Eds.), *Perspectives on interpersonal behavior and relationships*. Greenwich, CT: JAI Press.

Dunkel-Schetter, C., and Bennet, T. L. (1989). The availability of social support and its activation in times of stress. In I. G. Sarason, B. R. Sarason, and G. R. Pierce (Eds.), *Social support: An interactional view*. New York: Wiley.

Dunkel-Schetter, C., Feinstein, L., and Call, J. (1987). *A self-report inventory for the measurement of social support.* (Unpublished manuscript). Los Angeles, CA: UCLA, Department of Psychology.

Fricke, R., and Treinies, G. (1985). *Einführung in die Metaanalyse [Introduction to meta-analysis].* Bern, Switzerland: Huber.

Ganster, D. C., and Victor, B. (1988). The impact of social support on mental and physical health. *British Journal of Medical Psychology, 61*, 17–36.

Hedges, L. V., and Olkin, I. (1985). *Statistical methods for meta-analysis.* New York: Academic Press.

Heitzmann, C. A., and Kaplan, R. M. (1984). Interaction between sex and social support in the control of Type II diabetes mellitus. *Journal of Consulting and Clinical Psychology, 52*, 1087–1089.

Holahan, C. J., and Moos, R. H. (1986). Personality, coping, and family resources in stress resistance: A longitudinal analysis. *Journal of Personality and Social Psychology, 51*, 389–395.

House, J. S. (1981). *Work stress and social support.* Reading, MA: Addison-Wesley.

House, J. S., and Kahn, R. L. (1985). Measures and concepts of social support. In S. Cohen and S. L. Syme (Eds.), *Social support and health* (pp. 83–108). New York: Academic Press.

House, J. S., Umberson, D., and Landis, K. R. (1988). Structures and processes of social support. In W. R. Scott and J. Blake (Eds.), *Annual Review of Sociology* (Vol. 14, pp. 293–318). Palo Alto, CA: Annual Review Inc.

Hunter, J. E., Schmidt. F. L., and Jackson, G. B. (1982). *Meta-analysis. Cumulating research findings across studies.* Beverly Hills, CA: Sage.

Leppin, A., and Schwarzer, R. (1989). *The social support-health relationship. Who is better off: Women or men?* Paper presented at the 3rd International Conference on Life-Styles and Health, Utrecht. The Netherlands.

Medalie, J. H., and Goldbourt, U. (1976). Angina pectoris among 10,000 men: 2. Psychosocial and other risk factors as evidenced by a multivariate analysis of a five year incidence study. *The American Journal of Medicine, 60*, 910–921.

Norbeck, J. S., and Tilden, V. P. (1983). Life stress, social support, and emotional disequilibrium in complications of pregnancy: A prospective, multivariate study. *Journal of Health and Social Behavior, 24*, 30–46.

Nuckolls, K. B., Cassel, J., and Kaplan, B. H. (1972). Psychosocial aspects, life crisis and the prognosis of pregnancy. *American Journal of Epidemiology, 95*, 431–441.

Rosenthal, R. (1984). *Meta-analytic procedures for social research.* Beverly Hills, CA: Sage.

Sarason, B. R., Shearin, E. N., Pierce, G. R., and Sarason, I. G. (1987). Interrelations of social support measures: Theoretical and practical implications. *Journal of Personality and Social Psychology, 52*, 813–832.

Sarason, I. G., Levine, H. M., Basham, R. B., and Sarason, B. R. (1983). Assessing social support: The Social Support Questionnaire. *Journal of Personality and Social Psychology, 44*, 127–138.

Sarason, I. G., Sarason, B. R., Potter, E. H., and Antoni, M. H. (1985). Life events, social support, and illness. *Psychosomatic Medicine, 47*, 156–163.

Sarason, I. G., Sarason, B. R., and Shearin, E. N. (1986). Social support as an individual difference variable: Its stability, origins, and relational aspects. *Journal of Personality and Social Psychology, 50*, 845–855.

Schwarzer, R. (1989). *Meta-analysis programs for microcomputers.* Raleigh, NC: National Collegiate Software.

Schwarzer, R., and Leppin, A. (1989a). *Sozialer Rückhalt und Gesundheit: Eine Meta-Analyse [Social support and health: A meta-analysis].* Göttingen: Hogrefe.

Schwarzer, R., and Leppin, A. (1989b). Social support and health: A meta-analysis. *Psychology and Health: An International Journal*, 3, 1–15.

Thoits, P. A. (1985). Social support processes and psychological well-being: Theoretical possibilities. In I. G. Sarason and B. R. Sarason (Eds.), *Social support: Theory, research and applications* (pp. 51–72). Dordrecht, The Netherlands: Martinus Nijhoff.

Turner, R. J. (1981). Social support as a contingency in psychological well-being. *Journal of Health and Social Behavior, 22*, 357–367.

Turner, R. J., Frankel, G., and Levin, D. (1983). Social support: Conceptualization, measurement, and implications for mental health. In J. R. Greenly (Ed.), *Research on community and mental health* (vol. 3. pp. 67–111). Greenwich, CT: JAI Press.

Wallston, B. S., Whitcher-Alagna, S. W., DeVellis, B. M., and DeVellis, R. F. (1983). Social support and physical health. *Health Psychology, 2*, 367–391.

Wills, T. A. (1985). Supportive functions of interpersonal relationships. In S. Cohen and S. L. Syme (Eds.), *Social support and health* (pp. 61–82). New York: Academic Press.

Social Support and Cancer: Main Themes and Problems

Jacques A. M. Winnubst, Adèle L. Couzijn and Wynand J. G. Ros

For most people the diagnosis cancer comes as a blow. The psychological condition that almost immediately occurs is difficult to describe; despair, anxiety, panic and other intense emotions alternate with depression and apathy. The physician informing the patient usually is not very reassuring. A predominantly brief and businesslike attitude (Dunkel-Schetter, 1984). Typically, the physician is very busy and not trained in dealing with feelings of panic. Immediately after the fatal message and quite often for some time thereafter, the patient primarily feels alone. Not only is the doctor at a loss how to react, but also those individuals who are in the immediate environment of the patient are in the same predicament. Is this person doomed to die? What are his/her chances for survival? Will there be a long period of suffering or a quick death? How will the survivors manage? Is it dangerous to touch a cancer patient?

The situation is characterized by fear, ambiguity and insecurity on all sides. Cancer is an illness which immediately disrupts psychological equilibrium and social processes, much more so than most other illnesses. Regaining equilibrium and maintaining social contacts is a difficult task for the cancer patient. In this paper we will elaborate these aspects, by means of the rather recent concept of "social support", a topic given increasing attention in the social sciences. During the last decade research literature on social support has increased exponentially.

It is assumed more and more that social support has a beneficial influence on a number of things such as health, both physical and mental, efficiency, creativity and competence. Social support is thought to protect people against the adverse effects of a crisis. It has been demonstrated in carefully-designed studies – both prospective and longitudinal - that social support has a positive effect on health (see Funch & Marshall, 1983; for a review article, see Wortman & Conway, 1985).

In the last few years in the field of social oncology there have been occasional studies concerning social support and cancer. It has been found that the quality of a person's social network is of importance for the manner in which he or she is able to deal with the disease. The person in question can cope better with shocking news, with the process of illness or recovery as well as with, possibly, approaching death. Approximately 40% of all cancers are cured, but cured patients also encounter problems, namely with reintegrating in the daily routine of living and working.

Social Support: Definition and Sources

First of all it is important to be clear what is to be considered as social support. A frequently used and good definition is the one by Cobb (1976). According to him social support is: "...information leading a person to believe that:

  i. he/she is loved and cared for;
  ii. he/she is esteemed and valued;
  iii. he/she is part of a network of communication and mutual obligation."

Kahn and Antonucci (1980) have especially emphasized the protective aspect of the social network. The metaphor they use is that of a convoy: vulnerable ships are protected by well-armed and fast war ships. This nautical metaphor clearly indicates that a "convoy" in which a person can sail for a long time is of major importance for everyone. The advantage of the above-mentioned definitions is their clarifying character. In much of the former research, definitions were lacking completely or were vague and circular.

Although Cobb (1976) especially mentions mutual obligations as an aspect of social support, it can be observed that most of these definitions are somewhat one-sided. Other authors have placed more emphasis on the mutuality of social support. Shumaker and Brownell (1984) define social support as follows: "Social support is an exchange of resources between at least two people, with the intention, according to the giver or receiver, to enhance the well-being of the receiver."

The question arises what these resources may be. The work of Foa and Foa (1974) is very lucid on this subject. They developed their ideas into a "resource exchange paradigm". They distinguish six categories of resources on the basis of which people can achieve a social exchange: affection, status, information, money, commodities and services. In these six areas people can support or obstruct each other. For instance, information may be given or withheld. The conditions under which these modalities will occur can be studied. The premise in this theory is that people will strive to achieve an optimum in the area of the six sources mentioned, in order to avoid a decrease in well-being. This approach is important in understanding the specific problems of the cancer patient.

Because of the illness, the cancer patient often finds himself in situation of only partial reciprocity: that is to say from a relatively independent position the patient falls into a position of requiring help. One is dependent on a number of others without being able to reciprocate. Therefore it is important, especially with serious illness, to regard the theme of social support from the point of view of differences in power and position and the related problems of reciprocity. We will return to this.

Social Support and Cancer

The obvious starting point for a review of work in this area is the excellent review by Wortman (1984). An important conclusion from studying her work is that the majority of researchers of social support have lost themselves in aspects of the theme which do not touch the crux of the the matter. Much attention has been paid to the structural, quantitative and objectively observable aspects of social networks, to aspects of comprehensiveness and diversity. Besides that, the theme has been studied from a variety of aspects: personality and situational indices, coping styles, main and/or interaction effects. The statistical force of the studies at times makes one long for the descriptive and phenomenological level. The substance of social support, the most relevant aspect is often given too little attention. What characteristics of a social relationship, what attitude, information and emotion causes the cancer patient to actually feel supported. At which substantial aspects should interventions be aimed? Which inequalities in the support system are harmful for the people involved? Wortman (1984) shows us the state of the art in research on cancer and social support and she gives some theoretical notions, but hardly works out the most important inferences. In this article we will connect the most important conclusions with certain theoretical concepts. These concepts are mainly derived from social psychology: Social exchange theory and theoretical notions on affiliation and intimacy and from theories on clinical psychology, namely stress and coping approaches.

Main Themes of Research on Social Support and Cancer

The existing literature on social support and cancer shows the strong and weak points of social support research in general. We will elaborate on those aspects which result from Wortman's work. (Wortman, 1984; Wortman & Conway in press).

Forms of Social Support and the Phase of the Illness

Foa and Foa (1974) and others (e.g. Caplan, 1974; House, 1981) have made it clear that many kinds of social support can be discerned. Simplifying this subdivison to an extent, one can distinguish emotional, informational and material support. Which kind of support is most important depends in part on the phase of the illness. Weisman (1977) distinguishes four main phases in coping with illness (see also: De Haes & Trimbos, 1984; Couzijn, Ros and Winnubst, 1990):

Phase 1. Existential crisis: this phase is characterized by anxious premonitions, diagnosis, panic, acceptance and treatment. After a more or less serious crisis, the patient usually feels active and fights against the disease, is not too affected and feelings of depression alternate with optimism.

Phase 2. Accommodation and mitigation: after treatment the patient has to fight in order to pick up his daily routines. Work and everyday life are resumed but may need to be adjusted. The patient's physical and mental condition go up and down but optimism prevails and problems are treated actively.

Phase 3. Recurrence of the disease: cancer may strike again and this has a severe impact on the patient. Feelings of optimism give way to the fear of not recovering. There is a will to fight and at other times resignation, denial gives way to realism and concern.

Phase 4. Deterioration and death: the patient becomes increasingly dependent upon care by others and becomes passive psychologically as well. Pessimism and depression prevail. The patient starts anticipating death and concern about his relatives starts playing a part.

The psychological phases of Weisman are pertinent to the theme of coping and support: research indicates that the kind of support a patient wants, varies according to the phase. Vachon, Lyall, Rogers, Cochrane and Freeman (1982) concluded that women with breast cancer, in the phase after the amputation, experienced support from group discussions with other women in the same phase. Raphael (1977) concluded from his study of breast cancer patients that material support was related to successful recovery (phase 2), while there was no such relation with other kinds of support. Gordon et al. (1980) found that the patient with a poor prognosis (phase 3 but also phase 1) has less need of information than the patient with a good prognosis. Wortman (1984) points out that the very ill patient, especially in phase 4, has a need for intense relationships directed at emotional support. Dunkel-Schetter and Wortman (1982) and Dunkel-Schetter (1984) concluded from their research that emotional support, more than other types of support, is regarded as essential by cancer patients. More than 90% of the cancer patients in her study referred to emotional support as one of the most appropriate types of support. The study also showed that clear information given by the medical and paramedical staff about disease and treatment is very important in phases 1 and 3. The general picture that emerges is that the medical staff do not live up to the expectations of the patient and his family. In phase 2, in the fight against recurrence, the support systems at home and at work seem of particular importance. In phase 4 those most intimate play a very important part: the spouse, children and close relatives. The role of the doctor in the different phases has been reviewed recently by Couzijn, Ros and Winnubst (1990) who also stress that information is a particularly significant source of support, provided that it is not given in a cool, distant businesslike manner.

Sources of Support and the Dangers of Intimacy

There is a whole series of potential support givers for the cancer patient. These include spouse, family, friends, neighbors, colleagues at work, the general practitioner, medical specialists, nurses, pastoral workers, social workers, psychologists and patient groups. It is important to know who can and who cannot give which kind of support, when, and in which phase of illness or recovery.

Perhaps it is wise to differentiate within the support system between intimates and non-intimates. Hatfield's (1984) approach distinguishes three aspects of intimacy in relations, namely: cognitive, emotional and behavioral. In her view it is characteristic of intimates that they:

i.   are prepared to show their week sides; they provide personal and confidential information to the other and are themselves prepared to listen to confidences of the other (the cognitive dimension);
ii. care deeply about each other. This is shown alternately by love and hate, but never by indifference. Intense, often conflicting emotions are characteristic of an intimate relationship (the emotional dimension);
iii. feel comfortable in close contact with each other and therefore call on each other, touch and caress each other (the behavioral dimension).

Hatfield (1984) also studied the question of why people have so much difficulty in getting close. The causes she gives are based on the fear of people to:

– show their weak points too much;
– lose the other;
– be exposed to anger of the other;
– lose control of their own situation;
– show their own destructive tendencies;
– lose their own individuality to be absorbed by the other.

These theoretical notions on intimacy may help us understand the problems cancer patients and their direct family are confronted with. Cancer is so serious and so much surrounded by taboos (see for the cultural and historical aspects: Sontag, 1977), that the fear of losing intimate contact with the spouse plays a part during a prolonged period of time. Wortman (1984) shows that the tragic part of the situation of the cancer patient lies in the ambivalence in this area since he/she is afraid to repel the other with the illness and at the same time afraid that the other will come too close and gain too much control over the situation. The other is needed more than ever and simultaneously there are worries about being totally in the hands of the other. As she puts it: "Ironically, then, cancer may often undermine one of the strongest potential resources people have in coping with the disease – their social relationships." (p. 2341).

Lowenthal and Haven (1978); consider intimacy as *the* critical variable in research on the relationship between social support and cancer. The proximity of only one person on who one can count completely and who is to be trusted completely, is decisive for the relative well-being of the cancer patient and his capacity to cope with the situation to a degree.

The notions also indicate that the support givers should understand the limitations of their role. Confidentiality is only appreciated with people the cancer patient knows well. For instance, the doctor should on the one hand try to change his businesslike attitude somewhat but on the other should not reduce the psychological distance too much since this will cause the patient to feel threatened. Dunkel-Schetter (1984) concluded from her study that the support a doctor can give lies mainly in the field of medical information. This type of information given by relatives or acquaintances usually does not work well. Van den Borne and Pruyn (1985) showed that other cancer patients are an important source for emotional and informational support. Going through or having gone through the same disease cancer apparently has a strong distance-reducing effect.

Well-Intentioned but Incongruent Help and Power Problems

Older studies on social support give the impression that social support is universally effective and the interest in possible negative aspects has been more recent. Winnubst, Marcelissen and Kleber (1982) concluded that for people with a lot of responsibility at work, adequate social support was related to more rather than fewer complaints of stress. Social support can also give rise to experience that others are meddling and can interfere with the feeling of personal autonomy.

It was shown by Bloom (1981) that the medical specialist was mentioned as the most important source of both social support and stress as well. Peters-Golden (1982) concluded that many patients feel at a loss by the overly helpful attitude of others. Since this can prevent them from doing various small tasks patients feel less competent and this may result in loss of self-esteem. Dunkel-Schetter (1984) paid a lot of attention to so-called non-supportive behavior. She specifically mentions doctors since they give too little information, are cool, distant and do not take enough time. Friends and acquaintances at times try to minimize the problems or give false hopes with such comments as "it might have been worse" or "it will turn out all right". These kinds of inadequate remarks were investigated by Brickman et al. (1982), who concludes that "well-meant remarks" may have as a side-effect so-called victimization or stigmatization. Wortman (1984) also elaborates on the theme of well-meant help and cites a large number of studies. She states that it has been shown that behavior considered supportive by the person who gives help is often not viewed that way by the person receiving it. A lot of this so-called helpful behavior is regarded even as undesirable or annoying. She pleads for research into the convergence and divergence of views on social support and it should be relatively simple to make differences in opinion between those who give or receive social support the subject of research.

However, this observation of Wortman's does not take into account the issue of power to which we referred earlier. Becoming seriously ill signifies not merely physical and mental consequences, but also an attack on the patient's autonomy and position of power. The issue of power can severely complicate the simple establishment of differences in opinions on social support. Quite a bit has been published on aspects of power in the relationship doctor-patient and nurse-patient.

Hatfield, Traupman, Sprecher, Utne and Hay (1984) offer a perspective which enables us to understand the incongruencies in support offered by the spouse. It is interesting that they combine theoretical notions on social exchange theory with ideas derived on intimacy. The authors assume that in intimate relations there is a striving for a fair balance in the division of resources (e.g. Foa and Foa's resources, Foa and Foa, 1974). In a number of propositions they elaborate on the idea that people will continually strive to maximize outcomes. In short these authors reach the conclusion that, in times of stability, couples who consider there relationship based on the principle of just and equal division of resources become more intimate. However, during times of change relationships will tend to get out of balance. When couples are asked before, during and after such crises, it will become clear that they experienced such crises as very distressing. They will strive for a situation of dividing justice as soon as possible... or they will go in the direction of dissolving the relationship." (p.14).

This discussion clearly indicates the stress a relationship may undergo in a crisis involving a serious illness such as cancer. During such a period a major shift occurs in the capacity of a patient to reciprocate help with anything other than affection. At the same time there is an enormous taboo on dissolving a relationship when the spouse is seriously ill. Therefore, in view of the mentioned theory, the question arises as to why many spouses of seriously ill and terminal cancer patients report a number of indeliable and deep personal experiences, despite the lack or reciprocity in a number of areas. Therefore, critics of social exchange theory, as applied to intimate relations, state that intimate relationships are characterized by the lack of exchange principles, especially in times of crisis (e.g. Chadwick-Jones, 1976).

The Capacity to Give or Receive Support

During several decades there has been a literature indicating that cancer patients are characterized by a specific personality structure. Cancer patients were said to exhibit behavior that was in part the opposite of the Type A Behavioral Pattern found in patients with coronary heart disease, whereas the latter was characterized by being in a rush, displaying aggression, and by a very competitive attitude. In contrast, the cancer patient is said to lead a very restrained life, especially as far as showing emotions goes and leading an outwardly calm and uneventful life. This idea has been attacked severely on various grounds as being too simplistic and is supported almost exclusively by retrospective research (see Bouter, Keppel Hesselink, & Winnubst, 1984, for a critical review).

It is strongly doubted that cancer patients have trouble showing their emotions or shaking off what bothers them. When and if this behavior occurs, it can also be explained in terms of the afore-mentioned power perspective. At times patients are so intimidated by the illness and perhaps also by their perception of the dominance of the medical and family support systems, that in certain phases of the illness, they cannot show their emotions adequately. On the other hand, Schmale (1984) points out that lack of social interest on the part of the patient almost completely inhibits the functioning of the support system.

Wortman states that personality and social support are strongly neglected elements in research. In her own research she has shown that traits like empathy and understanding are only minimally correlated to the ability to give support. It is even probable that the most caring and empathic givers of support have a lot of trouble in maintaining interactions with people who suffer intense pain over a prolonged period of time (Coates, Wortman, & Abbey, 1979).

Again we are confronted with apparent paradoxes in the field of support and cancer. Sometimes the cancer patient has trouble in adequately showing his emotions, while research shows that it is precisely emotional support which is the most desired type of support, provided it is attuned to the phase of the illness. And it is this type of support which is the most difficult to give over a prolonged period of time because of symptoms of exhaustion and a lack of reciprocity.

This conclusion focuses attention again on the patients' own skills and coping abilities. While the presence of a social network in itself has positive effects, it is the ability to mobilize the support system which really counts in times of personal crisis. In coping research the ability to mobilize support is one of the significant dimensions of coping scales. Other frequently occuring strategies include handling a problem actively, seeking information, avoidance behavior and palliative behavior (Schreurs, Tellegen, & Van de Willige, 1984). Personality traits closely related to the ability to mobilize support are hardly ever studied systematically. Among those that do get mentioned are "locus of control" and "introversion-extraversion".

Further, the skills perspective is important for determining what skills a person has at his disposal. Wortman considers the work of Heller and Schwindle (in press) as significant. They state a number of aspects that are noteworthy and these include sociability, assertiveness, tolerance of intimacy, low social anxiety, empathy and the ability to handle problems in a relationship. It seems to us that the coping and skills perspectives are closely interwoven, although both are studied too often as separate fields.

Summary and Conclusions

In recent years social research has increased tremendously. In this article we report the attainments of this research in the field of social oncology and have tried to connect them with various theoretical notions. We have done this in order to obtain more insight into the strange ambivalence that cancer patients and those closely related to them experience during the course of the illness. These peculiarities are not yet fully understood.

We did not direct our attention to the methodological shortcomings of social support research. Literature on this is abundant (e.g. Brownell & Shumaker, 1984; Shumaker & Brownell, 1984; Thoits, 1984; Turner, 1984). Among the major criticisms are the many vague and sometimes circular definitions, the lack of agreement on how to measure social support, the interpretation of correlations and, sometimes, causal relations, the lack of a theoretical base and the lack of attention to the negative effects of support. The pedantic discussion as to whether the main effects or the moderator effects of social support are more important is also notorious. However, it should be stated that this is a common critisism during the development of almost any useful concept in the social sciences. The more criticism, the further advanced the concept usually is. Of course this does not free us from the responsibility of doing better research.

It seems to us that the time has come in the field of social support to advance by means of theoretical development. Apparent contradictions become clear with the aid of theoretical notions. We have tried to make a start with this in the specific field of social support and cancer. We have used notions of social exchange theory, theories on intimacy and affiliation, the coping perspective and the skills approach. Van de Borne and Pruyn (1985) have also used insights from attribution theory and social comparison theory in their study of contacts between patients.

Summarizing the theme of social support and cancer we can draw the following conclusions:

1. In the various phases of illness the patient has a need for different types of social support. In some phases the need for emotional support is dominant whereas in others informational support and material support are important, particularly during the period of treatment and reintegration. Emotional support is significant at the time of the first traumatic communication, when a relapse occurs and in the terminal phase;

2. Cancer is a strongly disintegrating disease. While the need for support is strong during various phases of the disease, there are mechanisms that strongly threaten the adequate functioning of the support system. This is caused by power and incongruence problems.

3. There are considerable differences in the way the medical support system and the family support system function. Both are main sources of support. The strength of medical support lies in giving factual information in a warm but not too intrusive manner. The family support system is of special significance in the emotional and intimate sphere and should preferably refrain from providing medical-technical information;

4. The support system has a number of potentially threatening aspects. Thus the distance between people may become too small causing loss of autonomy and feelings of fear, well-meant but totally unwanted support may be given and victimization and stigmatization may occur;

5. There are considerable differences between people in their ability to both mobilize support and to give support. These differences have to do with personality structure, with social skills and with the ability to cope with stress. Providing emotional support during a protracted terminal situation implies a heavy burden on the strength of those involved and can only be maintained if they themselves have a system from which they can derive social support.

This exploration into the developing field of social support and cancer has showed us how important it is to advance further in this area. Providing support to cancer patients is hardly easy because of the various taboos, ambivalence and incongruence mentioned in these pages. It is our hope that future interventions in this field will be based on a number of clear notions derived from both practical experience and scientific research.

References

Bloom, J. R. (1981). Cancer-care providers and the medical care system: facilitators or inhibitors of patient coping responses. In. Elsenier (Ed.), *Coping with cancer* New York: North Holland Press.

Borne, H. W., and Pruyn, J. F. A. van den (1985). *Lotgenotencontact bij kankerpatienten.* Assen/Maastricht: Van Gorcum.

Bouter, L. M., Keppel Hesselink, J. M., and Winnubst, J. A. M. (1984). Stress en kanker. *Maatschappelijke gezondheidszorg, 12*, 3 en 4, 6–11, 26–31.

Brickman, P., Rabinowitz, B. C., Karuza, J., Cohn, E., and Kidder, L. (1982). Models of helping and coping. *American Psychologist, 37*, 368–384.

Brownell, A., and Shumaker, S. A. (1984). Social support: An introduction to a complex phenomenon. *Journal of Social Issues, 40*, 1–10.

Caplan, G. (1974). *Support systems and community mental health.* New York: Behavioral Publications.

Chadwick-Jones, J. K. (1976). *Social exchange theory: Its structure and influence in social psychology.* London: Academic Press.

Coates, D., Wortman, C. B., and Abbey, A. (1979). Reaction to victims. In I. M. Frieze, D. Bar-Tal, and J. S. Caroll (Eds.), *New approaches to social problems* (pp. 21–52). San Francisco: Jossey-Bass.

Cobb, S. (1976). Social support as a moderator of life stress. *Psychosomatic Medicine, 38*, 300–314.

Couzijn, A. L., Ros, W. J. G., and Winnubst, J. A. M. (1990). Cancer. In A.Kaptein, H.M. van der Ploeg, B. Garssen, p.7.G. Schreurs and K. Beunderman (Eds.), *Behavioural medicine: Psychological treatment of sormatic disorders* (pp.231–246) New York: Wiley.

Dunkel-Schetter, C. (1984). Social support and cancer: Findings based on patient interviews and their implications. *Journal of Social Issues, 40*, 77–98.

Dunkel-Schetter, C., and Wortman, C. (1982). The interpersonal dynamics of cancer: Problems in social relationship and their impact on the patient. In H. S. Friedman and M. R. DiMatteo (Eds.), *Interpersonal issues in health care* (pp. 69–100). New York: Academic Press.

Foa, U. G., and Foa, E. B. (1974). *Societal structures of the mind.* Springfield, Ill.: Charles C. Thomas.

Funch, D. P., and Marshall, J. (1983). The role of stress, social support and age in survival from breast cancer. *Journal of Psychosomatic Research, 27*, 77–83.

Gordon, W. A., Freidenbergs, I., Diller, L., Hibbard, M., Wolf, C., Levine, L., Lipkins, R. Ezrachi, O., and Lucido, D. (1980). Efficacy of psychosocial intervention with cancer patients. *Journal of Consulting and Clinical Psychology, 48*, 743–759.

Hatfield, E. (1984). The dangers of intimacy. In E. Hatfield (Ed.), *Communication, intimacy and close relationship.* New York: Academic Press.

Hatfield, E., Traupman, J., Sprecher, S., Utne, L., and Hay, J. (1984). Equity and intimate relations: Recent research. In W. Icker (Ed.), *Compatible and incompatible relationships.* New York: Springer.

Heller, K., and Swindle, R. (in press). Social networks, perceived social support and coping with stress. In R. D. Felner, L. A. Jason, J. Moritsugu, and S. S. Farbes (Eds.), *Prevention psychology: Theory, research and practice in community intervention* (pp. 87–103). New York: Pergamon.

House, J. S. (1981). *Work, stress and social support.* Philippines: Addison Wesley.

Kahn, R., and Antonucci, T. (1980). Convoys over the life course: Attachment, roles and social support: In P. B. Baltes and O. Brim (Eds.), *Life-span development and behavior* (Vol. 3, pp. 253–286). Boston: Lexington Press.

Lowenthal., M. F., and Haven, C. (1986). Interaction and adaptation: Intimacy as a critical variable. *American Sociological Review, 33*, 20–30.

Peters-Golden, M. (1982). Breast cancer: Varied perceptions of social support in the illness experience. *Social Science and Medicine, 16*, 483–491.

Raphael, B. (1977). Preventive intervention with the recently bereaved. *Archives of General Psychiatry, 34*, 1450–1454.

Schmale, A. H. (1984). Response to C. B. Wortman. *Supplement to cancer, 53*, 2360–2362.

Schreurs, P. J. G., Tellegen, B., and Willige, G. van de (1984). Gezondheid, stress en coping: de ontwikkeling van de Utrechtse Coping Lijst. *Gedrag, Tijdschrift voor Psychologie, 12*, 101–117.

Shumaker, S. A., and Brownell, A. (1984). Toward a theory of social support: closing conceptual gaps. *Journal of Social Issues, 40*, 11–36.

Sontag, S. (1977). *Illness as metaphor*. New York: Vintage.

Thoits, P. A. (1984). Coping, social support, and psychological outcomes. The central role of emotion. In P. Shaver (Ed.), *Review of Personality and Social Psychology* (Vol. 5, pp. 219–238). Beverly Hills, CA: Sage.

Turner, R. J. (1983). Direct, indirect and moderating effects of social support on psychological distress and associated conditions. In H. B. Kaplan (Ed.), *Psychosocial stress: Trends in theory and research* (pp. 105–156). New York: Academic Press.

Vachon, M. L. S., lyall, W. A. L., Rogers, J., Chochrane, J., and Freeman, S. J. J. (1982). The effectiveness of psychological support during post-surgical treatment of breast cancer. *International Journal of Psychiatry in Medicine, 11*, 365–372.

Weisman, A. D. (1984). A model for psychosocial phasing in cancer. In R. Moos (Ed.), *Coping with physical illness. 2: New perspectives* (pp. 107–138). New York: Plenum.

Winnubst, J. A. M., Marcelissen, F. H. G., and Kleber, R. J. (1982). Effects of social support in the stressor-strain relationship: a Dutch sample. *Social Science and Medicine, 16*, 475–482.

Wortman, C. B. (1984). Social support and the cancer patient. Conceptual and methodologic issues. *Supplement to Cancer, 53*, 2339–2360.

Wortman, C. B., and Conway, T. (in press). The role of social support in adaptation and recovery from physical illness. In S. Cohen and L. Syme (Eds.), *Social support and health*. New York: Academic Press.

Section 5

Child and Adolescent Health Psychology

Children's Knowledge of Chronic Disease and Implications for Education: A Review

Christine Eiser

Introduction

Some 10% of children suffer from chronic disease (Hobbs & Perrin, 1985) including asthma (2%), epilepsy (1%), cardiac conditions (0.5%), cerebral palsy (0.5%) orthopaedic illnesses (0.5%) and diabetes mellitus (0.1%) (Mattson, 1972). In all these illnesses, there is no magical cure. Rather, children face a life-time of medical care and uncertainty about the future. As a result, it is said that paediatric medicine should have three goals: to treat disease itself; to prevent the disease from interfering with the child's development; and to prevent the disease from adversely affecting the family.

Although chronic diseases vary substantially along a number of dimensions (e.g. severity, chronicity, degree of threat to life, limitations to mobility; Lipowski, 1970), they also share a number of features. In particular, patients and their families must often become responsible for many aspects of daily care. These can include, for example, self-medication, adherence to medical diets, therapeutic exercise or physiotherapy. Since the treatment of childhood chronic disease requires prolonged and close cooperation between doctors, patients, and their families, it is essential that communication be direct and effective. It is generally argued that good doctor-patient communication is associated with improved understanding of the illness and treatment. In turn, this is hoped to increase compliance behaviours and reduce difficult behavioural or emotional reactions. Failure to achieve such rapport jeopardizes the chances of doctor and patient working together to control the disease and may increase the risk of untoward side-effects and long-term complications. It follows that how a diagnosis of chronic disease is made to a child, and updated appropriately, may have far-reaching implications.

While there has been some research concerned with improving how "bad news" is given to parents (Greenberg, Jewett, Gluck, Champion, Leikin, Altieri and Lipnick, 1984; McDonald, Carson, Palmer & Slay, 1982) and documenting how parents react to diagnosis of chronic or potentially fatal disease in their child (Cunningham, Morgan & McGucken, 1984; Myers, 1983), very little is known about how such information is communicated to the child. Partly this can be attributed to the fact that such communications are restricted to parents in many cases, since it is clearly inappropriate to attempt much in the way of explanation to very young children. Partly also hospital rarely have general policies on these matters, but leave decisions to individual consultants and families concerned. The result is that we know very little at a formal level about how explanations of chronic disease are given to children of different ages (Koocher, 1980; Spinetta, 1980).

At a general level, we do know that communication between doctors and paediatric patients is often inadequate. Pantell, Stewart, Dias, Wells and Ross

(1982) video-taped interactions between a doctor, parent and child patient. While doctors made considerable efforts to elicit information from children, they directed almost all information about diagnosis and treatment to the parent. While communication improved with the child's age, doctors consistently addressed more remarks to boys than girls.

To Tell or Not to Tell

Two opposing views to communication with chronically sick children have developed (Share, 1972). This work has focussed almost exclusively on the question of communication and explanations with paediatric oncology patients. The traditional or "protective" approach which was favoured in the 1950s and 1960s advocated that children be shielded from full knowledge of their condition (Bluebond-Langer, 1978; Evans, 1968; Slavin, O' Malley, Koocher & Foster, 1982; Share, 1972). Such knowledge was perceived to be harmful in increasing children's anxieties and fears and subsequently interfering with effective coping (Plank, 1964).

Later research suggested that children were frequently aware of the seriousness of their condition, but also realised that parents and medical staff did not want them to discuss the matter openly. As a result, many children experienced loneliness and isolation (Binger, Ablin, Feuerstein, Kushner, Zoger & Mikkelsen, 1969; Vernick & Karon, 1965; Spinetta, Rigler & Karon, 1973). The lack of openness also meant that some children fantasized about their condition, and consequently became more distressed than if they had been given the real diagnosis (Lindemann, 1981; Perrin & Gerrity, 1984). Recognition of these factors led to a more "open" approach, encouraging parents and physicians to share information about the disease (Novack, Plumer & Smith, 1979). However, very little is known about what, or how, children are given information about serious illness, although Chesler, Paris and Barbarin (1986) found that the decision to inform child oncology patients was based on a number of factors, including the child's age, sibling structure, religious beliefs and parental access to information. Neither has much work been directed at the question of how knowledge of disease relates to subsequent behavioral and emotional adjustment. However, Slavin, O'Malley, Koocher and Foster (1982) argued that adjustment to childhood cancer could be promoted by early and honest explanations. Children who were informed about their condition by the age of 6 years or within 1 year of diagnosis were better adjusted than those informed later or those who learned about the disease by a process of self-education rather than direct information from parents or medical staff.

It remains difficult therefore to advocate that either a "protective" or "open" approach be adopted, until more is understood about how children interpret medical information and the relationship between such information and attitudes and behaviour.

Children's Understanding of Chronic Disease

Despite the fact that little is known formally about how doctors and parents explain chronic illness to children and that many patients are too young or too ill on diagnosis to understand very much about their illness, many researchers have been concerned to assess children's knowledge. This research is usually justified on the grounds that some knowledge is necessary in order that children can assume some responsibility for controlling their own health. Children with asthma, for example, need to be aware of specific environmental or emotional factors that might trigger attacks, and those with diabetes need to understand restrictions on their diet and how to monitor glucose levels and inject insulin. In that diabetes demands a great deal of personal responsibility for self-care, much work has focused on assessing knowledge amongst children with diabetes.

Some of the earliest research was conducted by Etzwiler and his colleagues. Etzwiler (1962) found that 75% of younger children with diabetes (6–7 years) could interpret the results of their urine tests successfully, but difficulties in relating this to their insulin needs were experienced even by the older children (16–17 years). Collier and Etzwiler (1971) reported that children most frequently made errors in relation to recognising symptoms of acidosis, testing for acetones, dietary control and understanding the effects of different types of insulin. Similarly, Garner and Thompson (1974) reported that a lack of knowledge of genetics, inability to calculate dietary intake, and identification of symptoms relating to control were most common, especially for children in the 9–13 year age-range.

These early studies focussed on paper and pencil assessments of children's knowledge, and tended to include a range of questions, some relevant to practical aspects of the disease and others more theoretical (e.g. do you know what causes diabetes?). Some of these more theoretical questions may have little relevance to how conscientiously children perform self-care activities. For this reason, subsequent research shifted in emphasis toward how well children actually performed self-care activities. Garner, Thompson and Partridge (1969) and Garner and Thompson (1974) found that children made gross errors in estimating appropriate-sized servings of food. Lorenz, Christensen & Pichert (1985) demonstrated that children could not select acceptable foods from a canteen menu. Malone, Hellrung, Malphus, Rosenbloom, Grgic and Weber (1976) reported that children lacked accuracy in interpreting urine results; only 41% of children's results corresponded with those made by laboratory technicians.

Similar inaccuracies were reported by Johnson, Pollak, Silverstein, Rosenbloom, Spiller, McCallum and Harkavy (1982). Errors in urine-testing were made by 80% of children; errors in self-injection by 40%. In both cases, children's skill in these practical tasks did not correlate with their scores on a more conventional assessment of diabetes knowledge. While older children were generally more knowledgeable than younger children, girls of all ages were more accurate on the "skills" measures than boys of a similar age.

Work with other groups of chronically sick children has also relied heavily on questionnaire assessment. Martin, Landau and Phelan (1982) reported that young people (aged 21 years) who had suffered from asthma since childhood were ill-informed about various aspects of their illness. They were especially badly informed about the potential dangers of over use of broncho-dilators and did not understand the particular risks to asthmatics associated with smoking. Eiser, Town and Tripp (1988) found that school-aged children knew little about the aetiology of asthma, and were rarely either aware of or prepared to take actions necessary to avoid environmental or emotional triggers likely to precipitate attacks. (For example, children with asthma might report that attacks were precipitated by the family pet, yet take no action to remove the pet from the household.) Children and their mothers did not always agree about what were precipitating factors.

Other work with oncology patients also suggests that children and their parents often differ considerably in their understanding of the disease. Mulhern, Crisco and Camitta (1981) found that children were very much more optimistic about their prognosis than either their mothers or physicians. Levenson, Copeland, Morrow, Pfefferbaum Silverberg (1983) studied 55 cancer patients aged between 11 and 20 years. Again, differences between patients and parents were noted on a number of issues. In particular they tended to disagree over patients' self-help and treatments, the effects of alcohol, tobacco and drugs on the course of the illness and social issues concerned with how the disease was discussed with friends and relatives.

Inadequate knowledge of their disease has also been reported for children with cystic fibrosis. Nolan, Desmond, Herlich and Hardy (1986) found that patients were reasonably informed about treatment protocols, but confused about genetics and implications of the condition for reproductive risk and male sterility.

In summary, then, it is apparent that children with chronic disease can be poorly informed about many aspects of their condition. The finding that they lack information about the cause or physiology of the disease should not be surprising, and has little implication for daily management or general health. Other findings suggesting that children do not understand practical aspects of their treatment are more serious, especially where this results in an inability to handle routine aspects of treatment (Johnson et al, 1982). Among adolescents, there are particular difficulties associated with a lack of understanding of the implications of the disease for sexuality and reproduction on the one hand, and smoking, alcohol and drug-taking on the other.

Interventions with Chronically Sick Children

Increasing Illness-Related Knowledge

Traditionally interventions have focussed on attempts to increase knowledge and understanding of the disease and treatment. This work is based on the assumption that increased understanding is likely to lead to greater compliance with treatment, better "emotional adjustment" and reduced behavioural difficulties (Blos, 1978). In fact, researchers have generally been content to demonstrate increased knowledge following intervention, and the implications for emotional of behavioural adjustment have been left in the balance.

Nevertheless, increases in diabetes-related knowledge have been reported amongst children attending diabetic camp (Schipp, 1963), although more substantial increases occured among older (8+) compared with younger children (Harkavy, Johnson, Silverstein, Spillar, McCallum & Rosenbloom, 1983). While attendence at summer camp did not seem to be associated specifically with increases in knowledge, shifts toward more internal locus of control beliefs were reported by Moffatt and Pless (1983). These authors argued that internal locus of control beliefs have important implications for children's confidence in self-care activities. Also in a summer camp setting, Gilbert, Johnson, Spillar, McCallum, Silverstein and Rosenbloom (1982) demonstrated the effectiveness of a peer-modeling film in teaching self-injection. The film was especially successfull in teaching older (8–9 years) girls compared with same-aged boys or younger children. The results are interpreted in terms of the potential effectiveness of social learning approaches to teaching children practical aspects of self-care and reducing associated anxiety (Bandura, 1977). A programme of increased physical activity and self-treatment was shown to be as efficient as conventional physiotheraphy among children with cystic fibrosis (Blomquist, Freyschuss, Wiman & Strandvik, 1986).

A number of educational packages aimed at helping children manage and reduce the morbidity associated with asthma have also been developed (Creer & Leung, 1981; Scamagas & Rodabaugh, 1981; McNabb, Wilson-Pressano & Jacobs, 1986). However, many programmes have not been evaluated at all, while others have been evaluated ineffectively. Rubin, Leventhal, Sadock, Letovsky, Schottland, Clemente and McCarthy (1986), for example, developed an asthma-specific computer game. While the game itself appears to have considerable merit and ingenuity, the authors compared its effectiveness against routine computer games. It is hardly suprising, therefore, that children who viewed the asthma games showed improved asthma-related knowledge.

A more rigorous evaluation was reported by Lewis, Rachelsefsky, Lewis, de la Suta and Kaplan (1984), who compared two groups of children (aged 8–12 years). A control group received 4½ hours of lecture presentations on asthma and its management. The "experimental" group received five 1-hour sessions on the general theme of *active* control of the disease. Parents and children received separate interventions. Activities involving children were aimed at developing skills to increase personal mastery; parents were encouraged to create a home environment in which children could practice self-care and decision-making. Increases in asthma-related knowledge were reported for both groups, but those in the "experimental" group also showed significant changes in self-reported compliance behaviours and a reduction in emergency treatments and days of hospitalization. This study is exceptional in demonstrating that information in itself is of limited effectiveness. Children need help also in developing a sense of mastery toward the disease and its treatment.

This kind of approach forms the basis of recent school-based programmes designed to reduce tobacco (Botvin, 1983; Flay, 1985), alcohol (Casswell, Brasch, Gilmore & Silva, 1985), and drugs misuse (Eiser & Eiser, 1988). In these contexts, the programmes are reported to have a degree of success, especially in reducing experimentation with legal and illegal substances. Whether or not the programmes improve self-mastery and confidence skills in the long-term is yet to be proven. However, there is evidence that girls are more responsive to these social approaches to education than boys (Eiser & Eiser, 1988). Interventions with chronically sick children need to take greater account of innovations in general health education, and be founded on more rigorous theoretical principles. Research to date has neither taken account of developmental changes in cognitive factors such as learning and memory (cf. Chi & Ceci, 1987) nor of motivational factors affecting learning and emotional responses to illness (Perrin & Gerrity, 1981; Millstein, Adler & Irwin, 1981).

At the same time, very little work has been directed at the questions of how increases in knowledge about disease influence a child's attitude toward disease or effectiveness in self-care activities. As reported earlier, knowledge is not associated with improved self-care among diabetics (Johnson *et* al, 1982). Allen, Affleck, Tennen, McGrade and Ratzan (1984) reported that diabetics with a more sophisticated understanding of the disease were more worried than those with less developed disease-concepts. The authors also argue that education about chronic disease must be integrated within a wider programme aimed also at emotional responses to disease.

Pain-Control

Paediatric cancer patients experience repeated and extremely painful diagnostic procedures. Both parents and children report that Bone Marrow Aspirations (BMAs) are highly traumatic and stressful. In many cases, anticipatory anxiety prior to these procedures can be severe and result in symptoms of nausea, vomiting, skin rashes and insomnia for several days beforehand. During procedures, children can show extremely negative behaviours (including screaming, kicking and resistance) which create difficulties for staff in performing the procedures and anxieties and distress for other patients.

These behaviours were originally described by Katz, Kellerman and Siegel (1980), who reported that younger children reacted in terms of difficult verbal and physical behaviour. While older children showed less overt signs of distress, there was little evidence to suggest that they found the procedure any less distressing. These results were supported by Jay, Ozolins, Elliott and Caldwell (1983). Children less than 7 years old showed stress levels five times higher than older children. While older children showed less behavioural distress, many were highly anxious, and Jay *et* al argued that interventions to reduce stress should therefore include all children, not only those showing overt distress behaviours. They also point to the potential role of parents in helping children who experience painful procedures.

Recent recognition of the degree of distress that medical procedures can create for the child has led to the development and evaluation of a number of intervention procedures. Hypnosis (Hilgard & LeBaron, 1982; Katz, Kellerman & Ellenberg, 1987), puppet therapy (Linn, Beardslee & Patenaude, 1986) and cognitive coping strategies (Worchel, Copeland & Barker, 1987) have all been reported to reduce anxiety and increase a child's feeling of mastery in experiencing BMAs. As childhood pain becomes increasingly acknowledged and understood (Katz, Varni & Jay, 1984), it is likely that this work be extended to include other areas of paediatric medicine, rather than be confined to oncological services.

It is also important to recognise that the noisy and difficult behaviours shown by oncology patients mirror those which are used by all children in responding to stressful situations. Brotman-Band and Weisz (1988) asked healthy children to describe how they coped with everyday stresses, including going to the doctor's for an injection. Six- and seven-year olds were as likely to cope by screaming and kicking as they were to use control strategies such as distraction. The point is that young children do not generally have available a repertoire of primary coping strategies. It may be very stressful for staff when young oncology patients object vociferously to treatment. It should, however, be acknowledged that these responses are normal, rather than indicative of psychopathology.

Discussion

Despite the urgent need to develop appropriate explanations of chronic disease and treatment for children, many interventions are based on altruistic rather than theoretical principals. Others are taken from work with adult populations, with little acknowledgement of differences between adult and child populations in educational needs or abilities to handle information (Drotar, Crawford & Ganofsky, 1984). Many interventions remain reports of clinical case studies and are not evaluated beyond the specific situation in which they were developed.

It is also unfortunate that where interventions are evaluated, basic requirements of experimental design are often not followed. Inadequate programmes are used for comparison purposes, outcome measures are poorly defined, and follow-up is usually of a short-term nature (Roberts & Peterson, 1984).

If interventions are to be improved, researchers need to define both the goals and outcome measures more precisely. Goals of preventive intervention may include 1) mastery of illness-related anxieties, 2) understanding of and adherence to medical regimes, 3) integration of the illness and its treatment with everday life of the family, and 4) integration of the child within home, hospital and school settings (Drotar, Crawford & Ganofsky, 1984). Adequate evaluation of any intervention, regardless of its aim, should not be restricted to global measures of psychological disturbance. Rather, specific measures which are relevant to disease management and coping need to be developed.

At the same time, age appropriate programmes that take account both of children's beliefs about health and illness and their ability to handle medical information need to be developed. It has traditionally been argued that children's beliefs about health and illness develop through a series of stages, paralleling cognitive development in more physical concepts (Bibace & Walsh, 1981). This view implies that children are only able to understand information which is "matched" to their developmental level, and are unable to understand more "mature" explanations (Whitt, Dykstra & Taylor, 1979). This "structuralistic" approach to development has been widely criticised in general psychology (Gelman & Baillargeon, 1983; Carey, 1985; Neisser, 1987). There is now some evidence that children are not necessarily radically different kinds of thinkers compared with adults (Chi, Glaser & Rees, 1982). New research methods which aim to elicit information about what children learn about illness in everday situations (Nelson, 1986) suggest that children may have available more structured and detailed understanding than was originally thought (Eiser, Eiser & Lang, 1989). Interventions with chronically sick children need to be based more firmly within such theoretical approaches which are truly developmental.

References

Allen, D. A., Affleck, G., Tennen, H., McGrade, B. J. and Ratzan, S. (1984). Concerns of children with a chronic illness: a cognitive-developmental study of juvenile diabetes. *Child: care, health and development, 10*, 211–218.

Bandura, A. (1977). *Social Learning Theory*. New Jersey: Prentice-Hall.

Bibace, R and Walsh, M. E. (Eds.). (1981). *Children's conceptions of health, illness and bodily functions*. San Francisco: Jossey-Bass.

Binger, C., Albin, A., Feuerstein, R., Kusher, J., Zoger, S. and Mikkelsen, C. (1969). Childhood leukemia: Emotional impact on patient and family. *New England Journal of Medicine, 280*, 414–418.

Blomguist, M., Freyschuss, U., Wiman, L.-G. and Strandvik, B. (1986). Physical activity and self-treatment in cystic fibrosis. *Archives of Disease in Childhood, 61*, 362–367.

Blos, P (1978). Children think about illness: Their conceptual beliefs. In E. Gellert (Ed.), *Psychosocial aspects of pediatric care* (pp. 1–17). New York: Grune & Stratton.

Bluebond-Langer, M. (1978). *The private world of dying children*. Princeton: Princeton University Press.

Botvin, G. J. (1983). Prevention of adolescent substance abuse through the development of personal and social competence. In Glynn, T. & Lenkereld, C. (Eds.), *Preventing Adolescent Drug Abuse: Intervention Strategies*. DHHS Publication No. (ADM). (pp. 83–128). Washington D.C: U.S. Goverment Printing Office.

Brotman-Band, E. and Weisz, J. R. (1988). How to feel better when it feels bad: Children's perspectives in coping with everyday stress. *Developmental Psychology, 24*, 247–253.

Carey, S. (1985). *Conceptual Change in Childhood*. Massachusetts: MIT.

Casswell, S., Brasch, P., Gilmore, L. and Silvea, P. (1985). Children's attitudes to alcohol and awareness of alcohol-related problems. *British Journal of Addiction*, 191–194.

Chesler, M. A., Paris, J. and Barbarin, O. A. (1986). "Telling" the child with cancer: Parental choices to share information with ill children. *Journal of Pediatric Psychology, 11* 497–516.

Chi, M. T. H. and Ceci, S. J. (1987) Content knowledge: Its role, representation and restructuring in memory development. In H. W. Reese (Ed.), *Advances in Child Development and Behaviour, (Vol.20). (pp.* 91–142). Academic Press, New York.

Chi, M. T. H., Glaser, R. and Rees, E. (1982). Expertise in problem-solving. In R. Sternberg (Ed.), *Advances in the Psychology of Human Intelligence*, Vol. 1. Hillside, N. J.: Lawrence Erlbaum.

Collier, G. and Etzwiler, D. (1971). Comparative study of diabetes knowledge among juvenile diabetics and their parents. *Diabetes, 20*, 51–57.

Creer, T. and Leung, P. (1981). The development and evaluation of a self-management program for children with asthma. In *Self-Management Educational Programs for Childhood Asthma.* Bethesda, MD. National Institute of Allegy and Infectious Disease, Vol. 2, pp. 107–128.

Cunningham, C. C., Morgan, P. A. and McGucken, R. B. (1984). Down's syndrome: Is dissatisfaction with disclosure of diagnosis inevitable? *Developmental Medicine and Child Neurology. 26*, 40–46.

Drotar, D., Crawford, P. and Ganofsky, M. A. (1984). Prevention with chronically ill children. In M. Roberts and L. Peterson (Eds.), *Prevention of problems in childhood.* (pp. 232–265). New York: Wiley.

Eiser, C. and Eiser, J. R. (1988). *Evaluation of "Double Take": A drugs education package*. New York: Springer.

Eiser, C., Eiser, J. R. and Lang, J. (1989). A script analysis of children's reports of medical events. *European Journal of the Psychology of Education, 4*, 377–384.

Eiser, C., Town, C. and Tripp, J. H. (1988). Knowledge and understanding of asthma. *Child: Care, health and development, 14*, 11–24.

Etzwiler, D. (1962). What the juvenile diabetic knows about his disease. *Pediatrics, 29*, 135–141.

Evans, A. (1968). If a child must die. *New England Journal of Medicine, 278*, 138–142.

Flay, B. R. (1985). What we know about the social influences approach to smoking prevention. Review and recommendations. In C. S. Bell and R. Battjes (Eds.), *Prevention research: Deterring drug abuse among children and adolescents.* NIDA Research Monograph 63. A RAUS Review Report.

Garner, A. M. and Thompson, C. W. (1974). Factors in the management of juvenile diabetes. *Pediatric Psychology, 2*, 6–7.

Garner, A. M., Thompson, C. W. and Partridge, J. W. (1969). Who knows best? *Diabetes Bulletin, 45*, 3–4.

Gelman, R. and Baillargeon, R. (1983). Review of some Piagetian concepts. In J. H. Flavell, and E. M. Markman, (Eds.), *Handbook of Child Psychology, Vol. III: Cognitive Development.* New York: Wiley.

Gilbert, B., Johnson, S. B., Spiller, R., McCallum, M., Silverstein, J. and Rosenbloom, A. (1982). The effects of a peer modeling film on children learning learning to self-inject insulin. *Behavior Therapy, 13*, 186–193.

Greenberg, L. W., Jewett, L. S.., Gluck, R. S., Champion, L. A. A., Leikin, S. L., Altieri, M. F. and Lipnick, R. N. (1984) Giving information for a life-threating diagnosis. *American Journal of Diseases of Children, 138*, 649–653.

Harkavy, J., Johnson, S. B., Silverstein, J., Spiller, R., McCallum, M. and Rosenbloom, A (1983). Who learns what at diabetes camp?. *Journal of Pediatric Psychology, 8*, 143–153.

Hilgard, J. R., and LeBaron, S. (1982). Relief of anxiety of pain in children and adolescents with cancer: quantitative measures and clinical observations. *International Journal of Clinical and Experimental Hyposis, 30*, 417–442.

Hobbs, N. and Perrin, J. M. (Eds.) (1985). *Issues in the care of children with chronic illness.* San Francisco: Jossey-Bass.

Jay, S. M., Ozolins, M., Elliott, C. H. and Caldwell, S. (1983). Assessment of children's distress during painful medical procedures. *Health Psychology, 2*, 133–147.

Johnson, S. B., Pollak, T., Silverstein, J. H., Rosenbloom, A. L., Spiller, R., McCallum, M. and Harkavy, J. (1982). Cognitive and behavioral knowledge about insulin dependent diabetes among children and parents. *Pediatrics, 69*, 708–713.

Katz, E. R., Kellerman, J. and Ellenberg, L. (1987). Hypnosis in the reduction of acute pain and distress in children with cancer. *Journal of Pediatric Psychology, 12*, 379–394.

Katz, E. R., Kellerman, J. and Siegal, S. E. (1980). Distress behavior in children with cancer undergoing medical procedures: Developmental considerations. *Journal of Consulting and Clinical Psychology, 48*, 356–365.

Katz, E. R., Varni, J. and Jay, S. M. (1984). Assessment and management of pediatric pain. In M. Hersen and A. S. Bellack (Eds.), *Progress in behavior modification and therapy.* New York: Academic Press.

Koocher, G. P. (1980) Initial consultations with the pediatric cancer patient. In J. Kellerman (Ed.), *Psychological Aspects of Childhood Cancer.* New York: Charles Thomas.

Levenson, P. M., Copeland, D. R., Morrow, J. R., Pfefferbaum, B. and Silverberg, Y. (1983). Disparities in disease-related perceptions of adolescent cancer patients and their parents. *Journal of Pediatric Psychology, 8*, 33–45.

Lewis, E. D., Rachelsefsky, G., Lewis, M. A., de la Sota, A. and Kaplan, M. (1984). A randomized trial of A.C.T. (Asthma Care training) for kids. *Pediatrics, 74*, 478–486.

Lindemann, J. E. (Ed.) (1981). *Psychological and behavioral aspects physical disability.* New York: Plenum Press.

Linn, S., Beardslee, W. and Patenaude, A. F. (1986). Puppet therapy with pediatric bone marrow transplant patients. *Journal of Pediatric Psychology, 11*, 37–46.

Lipowski, Z. J. (1970). Physical illness, the individual and the coping process. *Psychiatry in Medicine, 1*, 91.

Lorenz, R., Christensen, N. and Pichert, J. (1985). Diet-related knowledge, skilled adherence among children with insulin-dependent diabetes mellitus. *Pediatrics, 75*.

Malone, J, Hellrung, I., Malphus, E, Rosenbloom, A. L., Grgic, M. D. and Weber, F. T. (1976). Good diabetic control: A study in mass delusion. *Journal of Pediatrics, 88*, 943–947.

Martin, A. J., Landau L. I. and Phelan, P. D. (1982). Asthma from childhood at age 21: The patient and his disease. *British Medical Journal, 284*, 380–382.

Mattson, A. (1972). Long-term physical illness in childhood: A challenge to psychological adaptation. *Pediatrics, 50*, 801–811.

McDonald, A. C., Carson, K. L., Palmer, D. J. and Slay, T. (1982). Physicians' diagnostic information to parents of handicapped neonates. *Mental Retardation, 20*, 12–14.

McNabb, W. L., Wilson-Pessano, S. R. and Jacobs, A. M. (1986). Critical self-management competencies for children with asthma. *Journal of Pediatric Psychology, 11*, 103–118.

Millstein, S. G., Adler, N. E. and Irwin, C. E. (1981). Conception of illness in young adolescents. *Pediatrics, 68*, 834–839.

Moffatt, M. E. K. and Pless, I. B. (1983) Locus of control in juvenile diabetic campers: Changes during camp, and relationship to camp staff assessments. *Journal of Pediatrics, 103*, 146–150.

Mulhern, R. K., Crisco, J. J. and Camitta, B. M. (1981) Patterns of communication among pediatric patients with leukemia, parents, and physicians: Prognostic disagreements and misunderstandings. *Journal of Pediatricians, 99*, 480–483.

Myers, B. A. (1983). The informing interview. *American Journal of Diseases of Children, 137*, 572–577.

Neisser, U. (1987). *Concepts and Conceptual Development: Ecological and intellectual factors in categorization.* Cambridge: Cambridge University Press.

Nelson, K. (1986). *Event Knowledge: Structure and Function in Development.* New Jersey: Lawrence Erlbaum.

Nolan, T., Desmond, K., Herlich, R. and Hardy, S. (1986). Knowledge of cystic fibrosis in patients and their parents. *Pediatrics, 77*, 229–235.

Novack, D., Plumer, R. and Smith, R. (1979). Changes in physicians' attitudes toward the cancer patient. *Journal of the American Medical Association, 241*, 897–900.

Pantell, R. H., Stewart, T. J., Dias, J. K., Wells, P. and Ross, A. W. (1982). Physician communication with children and parents. *Pediatrics, 70*, 396–402.

Perrin, E. C. and Gerrity, P. S. (1981). There's a demon in your belly: Children's understanding of illness. *Pediatrics, 67*, 841–849.

Perrin, E. C. and Gerrity, P. S. (1984) Development of children with a chronic illness. *Pediatric clinics of North America, 31*, 19–31.

Plank, E. (1964). Death on a children's ward. *Medical Times, 92*, 638–644.

Roberts, M. and Peterson, L. (Eds.). (1984). *Prevention of problems in childhood.* New York: Wiley.

Rubin, D. H., Leventhal, J. M., Sadock, R. T., Letovsky, E., Schottland, P., Clemente, I. and McCarthy, P. (1986). Educational intervention by computer in childhood asthma: A randomized clinical trial testing the use of a new teaching intervention in childhood asthma. *Pediatrics, 77*, 1–10.

Scamagas, P. and Rodabaugh, B. (1981). Development and evaluation of a self-management system for children with asthma. In *Self-management Educational Programs for Childhood Asthma.* Bethesda, MD. National Institute of Allergy and Infectious Disease, Vol. 2, pp. 129–150.

Share, L. (1972). Familt communication in the crisis of child's fatal illness: A literature review and analysis. *Omega, 3*(3), 187–201.

Shipp, J. C. (1963). Florida's first summer camp for diabetic children. *Journal of the Florida Medical Association, 50*, 133.

Slavin, L. A., O'Malley, J. E., Koocher, G. and Foster, D. J. (1982). Communication of the cancer diagnosis to pediatric patients: Impact on long-term adjustment. *American Journal of Psychiatry, 139*(2), 179–183.

Spinetta, J., J. (1980). Disease-related communication: How to tell. In J. Kellerman (Ed.), *Psychological aspects of childhood cancer.* Springfield, Ill: Thomas.

Spinetta, J., Rigler, D. and Karon, M. (1973). Anxiety in the dying child. *Pediatrics, 52*, 841–845.

Vernick, J. and Karon, M. (1965). Who's afraid of death on a leukemia ward? *American Journal of Diseases of Children, 107*, 393–397.

Whitt, J. K., Dykstra, W. and Taylor, C. A. (1979). Children's conceptions of illness and cognitive development. *Clinical Pediatrics, 18*, 327–339.

Worchel, F. F., Copeland, D. R. and Barker, D. G. (1987). Control-related coping strategies in pediatric oncology patients. *Journal of Pediatric Psychology, 12*, 25–38.

Development of Dental Health Beliefs and their Relation to Dental Health Behaviour

Gerry M. Humphris and John Weinman

The study of health beliefs is important in explaining many preventive behaviours, however little research has focused on the development of these beliefs in children particularly with reference to health behaviour. Adler and Stone (1979) suggest that research is sparse on children as health targets. One major difficulty in the study of children's health beliefs and their development is in locating an area of health which is salient to younger people. Thus studies of children's views about cancer or heart disease without experience or knowledge of the illness process may not particularly illuminating or useful. What is more appropriate is for research to concentrate on aspects of health and illness which are meaningful to children and adolescents and there is evidence that dental health meets this criterion. For example, in a recent study by Flaherty (1986) 4–5 year old children were asked their views on what behaviours they considered to be of relevance to their own health. They mentioned toothbrushing after first mentioning eating and visiting the doctor. In another study of young adolescents (mean age: 13 years) the assessment of concerns with respect to 30 topics showed their highest level of concern pertained to dental health followed by friendships and nutrition (Sobal, 1987). Hence there are some reports that aspects of dental health and behaviour are salient for children and adolescents and suggest a possible basis not only for more detailed study of the development of health beliefs but also of explanatory models of preventive health behaviour. Cohen and Jago (1976) advocate the study of dental health in this manner as the mouth, being a relatively closed system, provides the researcher with a unique opportunity to collect easily obtained and fairly objective measures of dental health. The two most common diseases of the mouth (caries and periodontitis) are similar to other chronic physical diseases since they reflect the life style of the individual, have a multifactorial etiology, are largely or wholly preventable and insidious in onset. However dental diseases are unlikely to be life-threating, and in the main, are relatively painless with exception of the acute stages where severe pain may result (Miller, Elwood and Swallow, 1975). In addition there is some evidence that it is possible to assess dental health beliefs and attitudes of children, as demonstrated by the work of Gochman and colleagues (Gochman, 1971; Gochman & Sheiham, 1978).

The present study has three main areas of concern. The first is to investigate the development of dental health beliefs with age. There is already a body of evidence suggesting a strong consistency of health beliefs relating to perceived vulnerability to dental illness across age which tends to hold across samples from the United Kingdom and North America (Gochman, Bagramian & Sheiham, 1972; Gochman & Sheiham 1978) and Australia and New Zealand (Wright, 1982). However these reports are based solely on perceived vulnerability and are cross-sectional. Thus the first aim of this study is to examine, longitudinally, a number of different dental health beliefs in children over a wide age range and from different dental health-care systems to assess consistency as previously shown.

Second, in the investigation of health beliefs it is assumed that beliefs exist in relation to other beliefs. Models have been proposed which suggest a structure of how health beliefs relate to each other, to individual health behaviour and demographic variables, e.g. Health Belief Model (Becker, 1974). There is little developmental data to draw upon here, although one study reported that childrens' perceptions of vulnerability to dental disease does correlate with their intention to visit a dentist (Gochman, 1971). Thus the second aim of this study is to explore the relations between dental health beliefs and to relevant dental health behaviour across age groups.

Third, the implications of a greater understanding of the development of health beliefs and their relation to each other is poorly known with respect to predicting health behaviour. One test of this approach applied to children was the study of a school-based preventive health programme based on tropical fluoride rinsing (Weisenberg, Kegeles & Lund, 1980). Results from this programme demonstrated that children's specific and general health beliefs were not strongly predictive of the behaviour the programme organisers were promoting. The authors of this study remark that confirmation of their predictions using health belief variables was not found although they encourage further study of other dental health behaviours. In addition the Weisenberg et al. study was not a straightforward test of children's health beliefs as predictors of their health behaviour since parental anxieties concerning the use of fluoride may have encouraged parents to exclude their children and bias the child sample. In addition, school and peer pressure was recognised as a possible influence other than the individual's health beliefs. Therefore the third aim of this study was to predict other dental health behaviours prospectively using a variety of health beliefs and attitudes with further samples of children.

Method

A longitudinal study was supported by the Department of Health and Social Security and directed by Professor Naylor of the Department of Preventive Dentistry at Guy's Hospital Dental School. It was conducted with children aged from 6 to 16 years (N=1691) over a three-year period and was originally designed to investigate the influence of dental services upon children and the determinants of their health-related behaviour with respect to dentistry.

Two sample areas were studied. The first was a local authority housing estate (Thamesmead) based on the out-skirts of South-East London with an experimental dental service. The service was planned to provide a strong emphasis on oral hygiene instruction through regular appointments at the dental surgeries where the prophylaxis and the disclosing of dental plaque was conducted. Demonstration of the plaque-removal techniques using the patient's toothbruch and use of encouragement and reinforcement of performance exhibited by the child was routinely provided. Topical fluoride-gel applications were routinely administered at every course of dental treatment. Approximately eighty per cent of children were registered with a dentist at one of the two health-centres with dental surgeries on the estate. The remainder were registered with dentists who were mainly general practioners outside the estate.

The second area, Wandsworth (in the South-west of London) was chosen for comparison purposes. This area was also noted for its large proportion of local authority housing, and characterised by a typical mix of dental services (i.e. general dental practitioners and the Community Dental Service). Approximately eighty per cent of children were registered with general practitioners and the remainder with the Community Dental Service. Therefore the children from the two areas received very different dental services even though the two areas were considered to be very similiar in social characteristics as demonstrated by near identical social profiles from a cluster analysis of London wards using the 1978 Household Survey data (Congdon, 1982).

The sample in the first wave of the longitudinal main study consisted of children of four age groups: 6, 9, 12, 15 years. Sixty-nine per cent of the children were successfully followed-up for a second wave of data collection after three years. The six-year olds from the first wave were omitted because health beliefs were not assessed although their questionnaire replies when they were aged nine years were included in the second-wave data analyses. The fifteen year age group was not followed-up at the second wave data-collection because the majority of the children had left school by that time. This paper will concentrate on the results of the children aged nine years and above.

Table 1: *Sample sizes*

AGE-COHORT	AREA	
	THAMESMEAD	WANDSWORTH
6–9	333	151
	(251)[a]	(107)
9–12	294	164
	(201)	(97)
12–15	245	273
	(184)	(160)
15[b]	131	100

Notes: a) Size of Follow-up sample when child three years older indicated in brackets
b) No Follow-up as children left school over three year period.

Data on child's dental-health knowledge, attitudes, beliefs and behaviour was collected by means of structured interviews and pencil-and-paper questionnaires administered at selected schools involved in the study. All children falling into the pre-specified age ranges defined by the study were included in Thamesmead, and children from schools in the area of Wandsworth were included with similar levels of treatment-need according to yearly-updated local community health inspections. The questionnaires were designed by extensive piloting, pre- and re-testing. All of the attitudinal and belief measures for the children which are quoted were based upon multi-item Likert type 5 point scales, all with Cronbach alpha coefficients calculated for each age group above 0.5 (Ware, 1976). Belief in treatment need, for which the child is simply invited to state how many fillings (restorations) would be required if they were to visit the dentist, indicated test-retest coefficients which were acceptable (i.e. for 9 years age group: $r_s = 0.83$, n=41; 12 years age group: $r_s = 0.66$, n=32).

Dental health behaviour was noted through the self report of the child and inspection of dental clinical records. The child was invited to estimate their frequency of tooth-brushing on five occasions during the day. The correlations between the frequency measures from the pencil-and-paper and interview instruments ranged from 0.57 to 0.75 across age groups. Although frequency of toothbrushing is accepted as only one possible estimate of toothbrushing behaviour (e.g. effectiveness of brushing is also an important variable) the resultant frequency measure was shown to relate significantly in the expected direction to oral hygiene clinical indices, namely: Plaque Index and Gingival Colour Index.

Intention to make a dental visit was tapped through a single 5-category item enquiring of the likelihood that the child would make a dental visit in the near future. The test-retest coefficients for this measure varied according to age (i.e. for 9 years age group: $r_s = 0.19$, n=44; 12 years age group: $r_s = 0.45$, n=35). The low reported coefficients for this variable were dissapointing but may have been due to the six week interval between the two test occasions. The child's estimate of their intention to visit the dentist may have been unduly affected by the passage of this time as the second test occasion would have been closer to any dental visit that potentially could have been planned. The younger age group may have been particularly influenced by this effect.

Each child was asked the duration since they last attended the dentist. The correlations between their replies and dates found in their dental records were as follows: 9 year age group, r=0.42, p<0.001, n=186; 12 year age group, r=0.47, p<0.001, n=109.

Further details of re-test coefficients, confirmatory factor analyses and evidence for validity of derived scales are presented elsewhere (Humphris, 1984).

Results and Discussion

Three sets of results are presented coincident with the three main areas of interest expressed in the introduction. They include first an analysis of the developmental changes in dental health beliefs, attitudes and behaviours in each age group over the two waves of the study. Second to report on how these beliefs and attitudes correlate with each other and dental health behaviour which included toothbrushing and dental visiting. Finally to examine how well the belief and attitudinal factors predicted *prospectively* these dental health behaviours.

Development of Dental Health Beliefs, Attitudes and Behaviour

Multivariate analyses of each wave of data was conducted separately to determine the stability of effects over a three year period. The effects estimated included age, sex and area in which the child resided. All main effects were highly significant for both waves of data (results not displayed for reasons of brevity). Many of the variables for both waves of data showed a strong age-group effect when results of the simple A N O V A' S were inspected. The factors of sex and area of residence appeared significant on only a few variables. Hence only the data across age groups in the form of means are presented in Table 2. It should be noted that the samples in both waves are not independent of each other, so that for example the 9 year old children who replied on the first wave are the same sample who responded on the second wave but of course aged 12 years. A similar position was found with first wave 12 year olds who became 15 years on the second wave. Of course smaller sample sizes in these groups were obtained at the second wave data collection because of natural attrition (e.g. families leaving the area). Change score analysis of these children followed-up over the three year period was conducted and gave similar conclusions to those found on examination of the first and second wave data, hence change scores are not presented here.

Table 2: *Means of belief, attitudinal and behavioural variables across age groups for first and second waves.*

		AGE GROUPS			
		9	12	15	p level
	WAVE				
HEALTH BELIEFS					
Perceived Vulnerability					
	1st	12.8	12.8	11.9	**
	2nd	12.6	12.6	11.6	*
Perceived Seriousness					
	1st	13.5	13.8	14.0	
	2nd	14.6	14.3	13.8	
Benefits of Dental Visit					
	1st	na	7.99	7.66	**
	2nd	na	7.89	7.68	**
Treatment Need					
	1st	0.90	0.62	0.55	
	2nd	0.84	0.56	0.54	
ATTITUDES					
Attitude to the Dentist					
	1st	21.5	21.3	20.5	*
	2nd	21.2	21.4	20.4	**
Dental Anxiety					
	1st	14.6	16.0	15.8	**
	2nd	14.9	15.7	16.4	*
BEHAVIOUR					
Toothbrushing Frequency					
	1st	14.1	14.1	16.0	**
	2nd	13.5	13.6	14.6	**
Intervention to visit dentist					
	1st	3.82	4.18	3.84	*
	2nd	3.85	4.11	3.77	**
Duration					
	1st	4.22	4.76	4.77	
	2nd	4.57	4.46	5.45	**
N	1st	230	240	159	(629)
	2nd	292	218	226	(736)

Notes: na = data not ascertained for 9 year olds
  * = p<0.05; ** = p<0.01

The level of perceived vulnerability (i.e. the expectancy of various dental health problems) was lower with 15 years olds in comparison with younger children, a finding demonstrated in both waves of data. No significant developmental changes were found for their belief in seriousness of dental health problems. Beliefs in the benefits of dental visiting were considered less amongst the elder age group studies. Data was not collected from 9 years olds for this variable for reasons of pressure of space in the questionnaire of this group. Children regarded that they required less dental treatment with age although this was not a reliable effect as reflected in the statistical analysis. The fifteen year olds were less positive about the dentist (semantic differential scale) than their younger counterparts while dental anxiety was appreciably less for the nine year olds.

Very consistent results were obtained for toothbrushing which improved with increasing age even though positive intentions to visit the dentist declined in the oldest age group. Duration since last visit to the dentist (in months) did not produce consistent results on both waves of the study but the data suggest that this tends to increase with age.

The consistency of the effects across age for both waves of data (and regardless of area of residence) provided confirmation that age was indeed associated with many dental health beliefs, attitudes and behaviours. The 15 year olds appear to be less concerned about their teeth and gums, and consider professional dental care to be of less benefit. In contrast, home care practices such as tooth brushing do appear to be more salient in the oldest age group with some evidence for a more limited approach to seeking professional dental services.

Gochman et al. (1972) found older children (14 years and above) to have higher levels of perceived vulnerability than younger children, More recently with further samples of children these results were not confirmed and suggested a complex relationship with age (Gochman & Saucier, 1982). Altman and Revenson (1985) found from a study of 8–14 year olds that there was no difference in perceived vulnerability with age group although the older children were less concerned for their general health, and gave lower self-ratings of health. A reduction in perceived vulnerability to dental health problems with age as found in the present study may be due to the trend of lower caries in UK school children (Allen, Ashley & Naylor, 1983) which is influencing children's health beliefs. In addition the increased tooth brushing frequency found in the oldest age group may also contribute to the child's reduced expectancy of dental problems. The relationship between the home practice behaviour and vulnerability to be examined in the next section may confirm this suggestion.

Relationship of Health Beliefs, Attitudes and Behaviour

The second set of results concentrate on relationships between the health beliefs, attitudinal data and behaviour. First wave results were analysed. There were very few consistent and significant relationships between the health belief variables with exception of how vulnerable they believed they were to dental health problems and the extent that they believed treatment was required. The correlations for all three age groups were significant, i.e. 9 years group: $r = 0.19$, $p < 0.001$; 12 years group: $r = 0.20$, $p < 0.001$; 15 years group: $r = 0.32$, $p < 0.001$, confirming a consistent effect regardless of age. There were no consistent relationships between health beliefs and the attitudes measured. Although older students were sampled, these results are supported by Cummings et al. (1978) who reported that the beliefs of perceived seriousness and vulnerability were substantially although not entirely independent of each other. Beliefs concerning the benefits of health care were uncorrelated with these two other health beliefs, which was supported by the present results.

The relationship of the health beliefs to dental health behaviour produced some interesting results. A high perceived vulnerability to dental problems was related to low toothbrushing frequency and greater intention to visit the dentist. This result supports the previous suggestion that perceived vulnerability among older children may be associated with higher frequency of toothbrushing. Benefits of dental visiting for the two older age groups was positively related to toothbrushing frequency and to some extent with intention to visit the dentist, and negatively with duration since last dental visit.

Dental anxiety relates fairly consistently to toothbrushing frequency, that is the more dentally anxious you are the less you brush your teeth. However, hardly any relationship exists with dental attandance. The correspondence between a child's assessment of their dental anxiety and utilisation is not well documented, however Wright (1980) found no direct relationship between dental anxiety and their estimate of potential dental health behaviour.

Attitude to the dentist is related to tooth brushing frequency so that someone who is positive about dentists will brush more frequently. Only amongst the older age groups is there a suggestion of positive views being associated with more frequent attendance.

Weisenberg et al. (1980) study also found low perceived vulnerability associated with greater involvement in health behaviour in an opposite direction to the traditional Health Belief Model formulation. Further discussion of the relationship of health beliefs and attitudes is continued in the next section concerning prediction of health care practices.

Prediction of Dental Health Behaviour

Toothbrushing

An attempt was made to predict future toothbrushing frequency 3 years prospectively using the children's original attitudes to dental health including whether the child had been shown how to brush their teeth. A number of cross sectional studies have been conducted but none have been prospective (Hodge, Holloway & Bell, 1982). An interesting pattern emerged as shown in an example of a regression from the first wave, 12 year-old age group from Thamesmead (Table 4) and is typical of the result for other groups with respect to age and area of residence.

First, many of the health belief and attitudinal variables were not helpful in predicting who were frequent brushers of their teeth and those who were not. Demonstration to the child how to brush their teeth three years previously was also unimportant in their subsequent toothbrushing frequency. The variables which helped predict toothbrushing three years hence included the initial level of brushing frequency, whether the child has been told to brush their teeth, the sex of the child and the number of sibling they had.

Table 3:   *Pearson correlation coefficients of health beliefs and attitudes related to dental health behaviour of three age groups: 9, 12 and 15 years.*

| | | Behaviour | | |
| | | Home care | Professional care | |
	Age groups	Tooth-Brushing	Intention To visit	Duration Since last Visit
Health beliefs				
1. Perceived	9	−0.11	0.16	
Vulnerability	12	−0.14	0.15	
	15	−0.16	0.17	
2. Perceived	9			
Seriousness	12			
	15			
3. Benefits of	9	na	na	na
Dental	12	0.20		−0.11
Visiting	15	0.16	0.16	−0.17
4. Treatment	9			(0.07)[a]
Need	12			0.17
	15			0.21
Dental attitudes				
5. Dental Anxiety	9	(−0.05)[b]		
	12	−0.11		
	15	−0.18		0.21
6. Attitude	9	0.12		
to Dentist	12	0.11	0.16	
	15	0.16		−0.36

Notes: N by age groups: 9 years = 410   na = data not ascertained
12 years = 460   for this age group
15 years = 205
Correlations displayed if $p < 0.05$, or placed in brackets if two of the three age groups were significant ($a = p < 0.2$; $b = p < 0.25$).

In summary these results show that traditional health attitudes do not help explain future frequency of toothbrushing. Previous workers have suggested that tooth brushing for adolescents is more relevant for them in terms of appearance and general grooming and hygiene (Honkala, Rajola & Rimpela, 1981; Hodge et al., 1982).

To help explain these results it is important to be aware of the characteristic of the behaviour in question, i.e. the number of times that the child brushed their teeth per day. This is likely to be a highly "ingrained" behaviour which is a habit and now not susceptible to traditional change pressures.

Dental Attendance

When the child was asked who decided when they should make a dental visit, the percentage of children replying that they were responsible for seeking professional dental care increased sharply with age such that over a quarter of 15 year olds took responsibility for their own dental check-ups. The majority of

Table 4: *Prediction of toothbrushing frequency in 1981 – a summary multiple regression of the first-wave 12 year olds from Thamesmead*

Variables in Equation	Step	Beta	r	t	p
Dependent variable;					
Brushing frequency (1981)					
Brushing frequency (1978)	1	0.296	0.43	3.56	0.0005
Child told to brush[a]	2	–0.212	–0.26	–2.74	0.007
Sex of child[b]	3	–0.189	–0.29	–2.41	0.017
Number of siblings (log)	4	0.178	0.28	2.22	0.028
(Constant)		11.528		8.62	0.000
Variables not in equation					
Perception of clean mouth[c]				–1.98	0.0502
Child shown how to brush					
Motivation to brush					
Dental anxiety					
Attitude to dentist					
Belief in vulnerability					
Belief in seriousness					
Belief in number of fillings required					
Perception of bleeding from gums					

N=128   R=0.536 R^2=0.29
Notes: a) dichotomous variable, coded: 1 = yes told, 2 = not told. b) coded: 1 = boy, 2 = girl.
c) single 5 category item, coded: 1 = extremely clean, to 5 = not clean at all.

Thamesmead children went to the dentist straight from school often unaccompanied and therefore without parental escort which may increase the likelihood of failure to attend. An analysis of past experiences at the dentist, previous attendance pattern and their attitudes and beliefs concerning dental health may be a fruitful test of the ability of these variables to predict future attendance.

Two cohorts of children aged 9 and 12 years respectively were sampled from the experimental area in the first wave of this survey. Measures of the child's attendance record were collected over the next three years. The sample was split into 3 convenient groups, good attenders (i.e. 3 or more courses of treatment: N=45), poor attenders (1 or 2 courses of treatment: N=103) and the consistent non-attenders (i.e. no visits at all: N=45).

Discriminant analysis was employed to identify the set of independent variables which best discriminated the children into the three attendance groups and whether more than one discriminating function contributed in the classification. Full details of the discriminant analysis are presented elsewhere (Humphris, 1984) as a number of sets of variables were introduced in the analysis. However, for the variables selected a simple summary was described by two functions which may be labelled as Past Experience and Behaviour (Variables numbered 1–5, Table 5) and Health Beliefs and Attitudes (Variables numbered 6–10, Table 5). The two functions enabled a 62% successful prediction of children into the three attendance groups.

As expected the children who attended the dentist more often and failed their appointments less often in the year prior the first wave data collection predicted future attendance in the next three years. However the children who attended for only 1 or 2 courses of treatment (i.e. examination, restorative treatment where necessary, plus a prophylaxis and topical-fluoride application) for the whole 3 year study period were found to be the more anxious, believed they were more susceptible to dental disease and were more negative about the dentist than those who had attended 3 or more courses of treatment *and* those who had never attended in that same period. Hence a non-linear predictive relationship was found.

Table 5: *Means and significance of dental attendance, experience, beliefs and attitudes collected at first-wave data collection by future pattern of dental attendance*

| | Attendance ('78–'81) Course of Treatment | | | | |
	0	1–2	3–6	p	lin
1 Preventive experience	2.31	2.78	2.71	**	**
2 Intention to visit	3.67	4.13	4.18	*	
3 Treatment experience	2.29	2.17	1.87	*	
4 Uncompleted courses of treatment (77–78)	0.40	0.27	0.11	*	
5 Completed courses of treatment (77–78)	0.62	0.95	1.24	***	
6 Regular attendance (self-rated)	0.58	0.60	0.87	**	*
7 Belief in perceived vulnerability	11.47	13.65	11.22	***	***
8 Dental anxiety	15.71	16.48	13.27	**	*
9 Attitude to dentist	21.80	20.62	22.53	**	**
10 Fillings required (log)	0.06	0.09	0.02	*	*
N	45	103	45	df2/190	

Notes: P = p level of anova to test group effect
  lin = p level of test for linearity (significant if non-linear)
  *** = p<0.005
  ** = p<0.01
  * = p<0.05

General Discussion and Implications

The levels of children's dental health beliefs and attitudes varied substantially with age of child in comparison to gender and different systems of health care. These age effects were demonstrated on two occasions, three years apart indicating a notable degree of consistency. A previous report of how health beliefs vary with age produced equivocal findings (Gochman & Saucier, 1982) although Altman and Revenson (1985) found with adolescents that age is not implicated in levels of perceived vulnerability which supports Radius, Dillman, Becker, Rosenstock and Hovrath (1980) and their more general conclusion that health beliefs are largely established by the age of 12 and continue to at least 18 years. The present findings demonstrated a picture of reliable reductions of perceived vulnerability to dental health problems, beliefs in the benefits of dental visiting, attitude towards the dentist, with increased age. The magnitude of the changes may not have been great although they are consistent and suggest, especially when considered with the additional findings of lowered intention to visit the dentist and increased frequency of toothbrushing with age that the older child finds professionally supplied health care less salient. Introduction of novel preventive programmes has proved difficult because of compliance problems of older children (Eckhaus, Silverstein, Fine & Boriskin, 1982) which may support the evidence presented in this study that health service provision by statutory authorities is not attractive to older adolescents.

Many of the health beliefs and attitudes correlated consistently with the health behaviours assessed in this study on inspection of the cross-sectional data. However the direction of the relationships were not always as expected from traditional Health Belief Model predictions. e.g. the high level of perceived vulnerability was associated with a lower (rather than a predicted higher) frequency of toothbrushing. Weisenberg et al. (1980) also indicated a moderate negative relationship of children's perceived vulnerability with compliance with a fluoride mouth-rinsing programme, and a similiar result was found by Kegeles and Lund (1982) who reported children "who brushed more often tended to have lower perceived vulnerability". Janz and Becker (1984) in their review of 13 studies of various preventive health-related behaviours found strong relationships of health beliefs in the direction as expected by the Health Belief Model although their review excluded dental health studies and was restricted to adults. Only 3 of the studies reviewed were prospective. The work with children of Kegeles and Lund (1984) extends the original work of Weisenberg et al. (1980) with further experiments on improving compliance with fluoride rinsing from school and home. These authors present data which has led them to conclude that "health beliefs and the interventions based on them have little relationship to the health habits of adolescents".

The present study has focused not only on cross-sectional relationships between health beliefs and behaviour but also attempted to predict prospectively two dental health behaviours. Very different results were found for each behaviour. Health beliefs were poor predictors of a home care practice (i.e toothbrushing) supporting the above quote of Kegeles and Lund (1984) and the contention of Lund, Kegeles and Weisenberg (1977) that past behaviour is an excellent predictor of future behaviour. For highly repetitive and habitual behaviour, attitudes and beliefs appear to have little relevance. Triandis (1977) has stressed the importance of habits as a mediator in the prediction of behaviour as well as other cognitive variables such as intentions.

Attempts to predict utilisation of professional health care services with health beliefs and attitudes was more successful. Account was also taken of prior behaviour and experience in these analysis. It is interesting that had the analysis relied solely on linear models the influence of the cognitive and affective components would have been overlooked.

It was expected that both previous behaviour and attitudes exhibited at the first wave of data collection would relate to future behaviour in a linear fashion. i.e. better future attendance would be predicted by more favourable attitudes and past attendance pattern. However this picture was only found with regard to previous behaviour and experience of dental procedures and not with respect to the attitude and beliefs held by the child. A more complex and non-linear relationship of attitudes and beliefs to attendance was found for instance the highest level of anxiety and vulnerability was found for poor-attenders rather than for non-attenders as would be expected from traditional formulations. This result may explain previous lack of strong correspondence between health beliefs and behaviour if only linear models are specified in data analyses (Cleary, 1987).

The implications for health promotion are not as straightforward as for instance the proponents of the health belief model may suggest. There is agreement that a generalist approach to modify health beliefs should be targeted at young children well before 12 years of age (Radius et al., 1980) and it has been suggested that interventions should be developed for very young children, i.e. pre-schoolers (Gochman and Saucier, 1982). However attempts to improve appropriate health beliefs such as perceived vulnerability amongst older children and adolescents specifically to increase dental service utilisation are unlikely to be successful without careful appreciation of the relationship of the belief to behaviour. It is not obvious, for example, from the present results which direction to encourage a change in health beliefs with infrequent/poor attenders. Our own work with toothbrushing frequency and that of Kegeles and Lund (1985) with new fluoride-rinse programmes suggests that health beliefs are not helpful in predicting habitual or novel preventive dental health procedures. Dental services utilisation is predicted by a non-linear profile of health beliefs and attitudes. Specification of a series of factors including not only health beliefs but also attitudes, previous experience and behaviour may help to identify target groups for promoting improved dental attendance. Therefore a detailed analysis of the behaviour in question, a sophisticated targeting approach and a study of contingent rewards from the behaviour itself may assist in devising effective preventive efforts.

References

Adler, N. E., and Stone, G. C. (1979). Social science perspective on the health system. In G. C. Stone, F. Cohen and N. E. Adler (Eds.), *Health psychology – a handbook* (pp.79–96). San Francisco: Jossey – Bass.

Allen, C. D., Ashley, F. P., and Naylor, M. N. (1983). Caries experience in 11 year-old school girls between 1962 and 1981: a radiological study. *British Dental Journal, 154*, 167–170.

Altman, D. G., and Revenson, T. A. (1985). Children's understanding of health and illness concepts: a preventive health perspective. *Journal of Primary Prevention, 6*, 53–67.

Becker, M. H. (1974). The health belief model and personal health behaviour. *Health Education Monographs, 2*, 326–473.

Cleary, P. (1987). Why people take precautions against health risks. In N. Weinstein (Ed.), *Taking care: understanding and encouraging self-protection behaviour.* (pp. 119–149). Cambridge: University Press.

Cohen, L. K., and Jago, J. D. (1976). Toward the formulation of sociodental indicators. *International Journal of Health Services, 6*, 681–698.

Congdon, P. (1982). Social and economic characteristics of London wards 1978. *GLC Statistical Series No. 15,* Greater London Council.

Cummings, K. M., Jette, A. M., and Rosenstock,, I. M. (1978). Construct validation of the health belief model. *Health Education Monograph, 6*, 394–405.

Eckhaus, B., Silverstein, S., Fine, J., and Boriskin, J. (1982). Enrolment in and compliance with a community demonstration program of caries prevention for grades Kindergarten through 12. *Journal of Public Health Dentistry, 42*, 142–154.

Flaherty, M. (1986). Preschool children's concepts of health beliefs and potential health behaviour. *Maternal-Child Nursing Journal, 15*, 205–265.

Gochman, D. S. (1971). Some correlates of children's health beliefs and potential health behaviour. *Journal of Health and Social Behaviour, 13*, 285–293.

Gochman, D. S. (1974). Preventive encounters and their psychological correlates. *American Journal of Public Health, 64*, 1096–1098.

Gochman, D. S., Bagramian, R. A., and Sheiham, A. (1972). Cross-national consistency in children's beliefs about vulnerability to health problems. *Health Service Reports, 87*, 282–288.

Gochman, D. S., and Shciham, A. (1978). Cross-national consistency in children's beliefs about vulnerability . *International Journal of Health Education, 21*, 189–193.

Gochman, D. S., and Saucier, J–F. (1982). Perceived vulnerability in children and adolescents. *Health Education Quarterly, 9*, (2&3), 46/142–59/155.

Hodge, H. C., Holloway, P. J., and Bell, C. B. (1982). Factors associated with toothbrushing behaviour in adolescents. *British Dental Journal, 152*, 49–51.

Honkala, E., Rajola, M., and Rimpela, M. (1981). Oral hygiene habits among adolescents in Finland. *Community Dentistry and Oral Epidemiology, 9*, 61–68.

Humphris, G. M. (1984). *Dental attitudes and behaviour in children: a psychological investigation into the dental health behaviour of 6–16 year old school children from two communities receiving different systems of dental care.* Unpublished doctoral thesis. University of London.

Janz, N. K., and Becker, M. H. (1984). The health belief model: a decade later. *Health Education Quarterly, 11*(1), 1–47.

Kegeles, S. S., and Lund, A. K. (1982). Acceptance of a novel preventive dental activity. *Health Education Quarterly, 9*(2&3), 96/192–112/208.

Kegeles, S. S., and Lund, A. K. (1984). Adolescents' acceptance of caries-preventive procedure. In J. D. Matarazzo, S. M. Weiss, J. A. Herd, N. E. Miller and S. M. Weiss. (Eds.), *Behavioral Health: A Handbook of Health Enhancement and Disease Prevention.* (pp. 895–909) New York: Wiley

240 GERRY M HUMPHRIS *ET AL*

Lund, A. K., Kegeles, S. S., and Weisenberg, M. (1977) Motivational techniques for increasing acceptance of preventive health measures. *Medical Care, 15*, 678–692.

Miller, J., Elwood, P. C., and Swallow, J. N. (1975) Dental pain. *British Dental Journal, 139*, 327–328.

Radius, S. M., Dillman, T. E., Becker, M. H., Rosenstock, I. M., and Hovrath, W. J. (1980)., Adolescent perspectives on health and illness. *Adolescence, 15*, 375–383.

Sobal, J. (1987). Health concerns of young adolescents. *Adolescence 22*, 739–750.

Triandis, H. C. (1977). *Interpersonal behaviour*, Monterey, Cal.: Brooks/Cole.

Ware, J. E. (1976). Scales for measuring general health perceptions. *Health Services Research, 11* (4), 396–415.

Weisenberg, M., Kegeles, S. S., and Lund, A. K. (1980). Children's health beliefs and acceptance of a dental preventive activity. *Journal of Health and Behaviour, 21*, 59–74.

Wright, F. A. C. (1980). Relationship of children's anxiety to their potential dental health behaviour. *Community Dentistry and Oral Epidemiology, 8*, 189–194.

Wright, F. A. C. (1982). Children's perceptions of vulnerability to illness and dental disease. *Community Dentistry and Oral Epidemiology, 10*, 29–32.

Family Counseling in Childhood Cancer: Conceptualization and Empirical Results

Meinolf Noeker, Franz Peterman and Udo Bode

Introduction

In the last decades, significant advances in treatment of childhood cancer have led to a considerable increase of survival rates. Instead of the former certainty of an inevitable death the young patient and his family nowadays have to face the uncertainty about the individual prognosis. Childhood cancer has altered from a fatal to a chronic, yet life-threatening illness that entails severe burdens and new chores on the cancer-sick child and the family which they do not feel prepared for.

The suddenness, impact and diversity of the burdens make both the patient and the family members perceive them as a threat. The psychosocial functioning of families confronted with the malignant disease of a child, therefore, usually has been described in terms of stress and coping models (Cohen & Lazarus, 1979; Lazarus & Folkman, 1987). Numerous transactional relationships have been investigated in the complex field of particular illness features, resulting psychosocial stressors, processes of appraisal and coping behaviour, moderating family characteristics and resources, and parameters of psychological adjustment. To date, however, we still lack a consistent theoretical framework to integrate the whole array of interrelating variables (Beutel, 1988; Garmezy, 1985; Wortman, 1984; Taylor, Falke, Shoptaw & Lichtman, 1986). Despite the limited knowledge about coping processes in general and intervention strategies in detail, the necessity of psychosocial support by professionals, however, has become self-evident among physicians and health workers on pediatric oncological wards. As a reaction to these clinical needs and demands, various counseling programs for families with a cancer-sick child have been developed transferring the preliminary findings of health psychology into patient-oriented work (Chesler & Barbarin, 1987; Christ & Adams, 1984; Farrell & Hutter, 1984; Kupst, Tyle, Thomas, Mudd, Richardson & Schulman, 1983; Lansky, 1985; Petermann, Noeker & Bode, 1987; Petermann, Noeker, Bochmann, Bode, Grabisch & Herlan-Criado, 1988). Some conceptualizations concentrate on helping the child and the family to cope with the threat of therapy-failure and death (Adams-Greenly, 1984; Chesler, Paris & Barbarin, 1986; Koocher, 1984, Nitschke, Sexauer, Spencer & Humphrey, 1985). Most of these counseling programs had to combine theoretical stringency with heuristic conceptualizations and pragmatic clinical and ethical considerations.

Psychosocial Adaptation Within The Family

Most authors have analyzed the individual coping process of the cancer-sick child within the context of his ot her family (e.g. Kaplan, Smith & Grobstein, 1972; Calhoun, Selby & Kind, 1976; Lobato, Faust & Spirito, 1988; Varni & Katz, 1988).

241

This is self-evident, since parents and siblings are the main source of emotional, instrumental, informative and evaluative support (House, 1981) for the sick child. Thus, many intervention programs have chosen a family-orientated approach supposing that strengthening the whole family's resources is a powerful way to enhance also the child's coping hehavior (e.g. Farrell & Hutter, 1984; Kupst, Tylke, Thomas, Mudd, Richardson & Schulman, 1983; Petermann, Noeker, Bochmann, Bode, Grabisch & Herlan-Criado, 1988).

A family perspective on childhood cancer has not only been emphasized because parents and siblings share the multiple sorrows of the cancer sick-child, but also because they have to face additional stressors and restrictions of their own. Financial burdens, vocational plans, time-constraints, adaptation to hospital and staff, educational problems, insecure future perspective, occupational limitations, responsibility for treatment decisions, feelings of guilt, self-blame and shame, shifts in family relationships, religious doubts, uncertainty about relapse, existential confrontation with loss and death are some of the major stressors regularly found in parents with a cancer-sick child (Calhoun, Selby & Kind, 1976; Chesler & Barbarin, 1987; Koocher & O'Malley, 1981; Lansky, 1985; Lansky & Cairns, 1979; Levine & Hersh, 1982; Petermann, Noeker & Bode, 1987; Varni & Katz, 1988). Whereas the risk of overstrain can result in marital conflicts (Kansky, Cairns, Haasanein, Wehr & Lowman, 1978; Kaplan, 1982; Schmitt, 1986), mastering the stressors, however, can enhance the family's sense of unity and feelings of personal maturation (Kaplan, Smith, Grobstein & Fischman, 1984; Spinetta & Deasy-Spinetta, 1981). Maladaptive reactons in siblings are more likely to occur if the siblings receive only little information about the illness or run the risk of being neglected on behalf of the ill child (Cairns, 1979; Petermann & Bode, 1986; Sourkes, 1980).

As the discussion about the appropriateness of denial as a coping strategy towards the diagnosis illustrates (Beutel, 1988; Breznitz, 1983), the issue of defining criteria for the adequacy of particular coping behaviors is still unresolved. Nevertheless, various family variables have been found to correlate with certain measures of assumed positive long-term adjustment (cf. Kupst & Schulman, 1988). Most of these variables have become key terms in the conceptualization of counseling programs including the one reported here. They comprise openness in family communication about the illnesss (Fergusson, 1976; Koocher & O'Malley, 1981; Spinetta & Deasy-Spinetta, 1981); emotional support (Futterman & Hoffman, 1973; Kaplan, Grobstein & Smith , 1976; Morrow, Carpenter & Hoagland, 1984), and the quality of the marital relationship (Kaplan, Smith, Grobstein & Fischman, 1973; Sourkes, 1977).

Spinetta, Swarner and Sheposh (1981) related the parents' adjustment to life after their child's death of cancer to the former coping behavior during the course of the illness. Variables that indicated a better adjustment were a consistent philosophy of life, the availability of an ongoing support person and the attitude to give the child the information and the support needed. Referring to clinical counseling the authors draw the conclusion that it is necessary to "strengthen the adaptive capabilities and coping styles specific to each family and to each member of the family... and to give them access to the intrafamilial sources of support they most need to help them in that struggle" (Spinetta, Swarner & Sheposh, 1981, p.261). In one of the few prospective studies in this field, Kupst and Schulman (1988) assessed the long-term coping process of forty-three families with acute leukemia by means of semi-structured interviews, self-ratings and ratings by the staff. The most recent results (medium 6.8 years postdiagnosis) reveal a significant improvement in adjustment over time. Antecedent variables related to coping were coping disposition (fathers), occupational level of fathers, and coping with earlier stages of the illness. Concurrent/consequent correlates of coping were: level of family support, quality of the parents marital relationship, good coping of other family members, lack of other concurrent stresses and open communication within the family.

Social Support and Vulnerability

In the last decade, research on social networks and social support has considerably increased (for a review e.g. Schwarzer & Leppin, 1988). One reason for this interest is the expectation that new prevention and intervention strategies could be found (Cassel, 1976).

The findings seem to indicate that social support both exchanged within the family and received from external sources (neighbors, friends, hospital staff etc.) can exert preventive, buffering and ameliorative effects on psychological well-being in adult cancer patients (e.g. Dunkel-Schetter, 1984; Wortman, 1984; Taylor, Falke, Shoptaw & Lichtman, 1986) and chronically ill children (e.g. Kazak, Reber & Carter, 1988; Perrin & Maclean, 1988).

To date, only a few empirical studies on families with a cancer-sick child have been published. Morrow, Hoagland and Morse (1982) evaluated the perceived sources of support of 107 parents with cancer-sick children. Responding to the question "How helpful and supportive has each source been to you during your child's illness?" they named spouse, other parents and friends, medical staff and relatives. The percentage of parents who contacted counselors was relatively low at that time. The question "What was needed most?" was answered in the following way: counseling or emotional support, clearer communication and medical information, sibling support and financial assistance.

In a subsequent study, Morrow, Carpenter and Hoagland (1984) could identify a positive correlation for the same sample between the perceived quality of support and the parents' psychosocial adjustment to childhood cancer.

Whereas social support acts as a protective factor against stressors imposed by a malignant disease, there are other conditions that create an increased vulnerability and risk for maladjustment towards the stressors (Weisman & Worden, 1977). Miles (1985) found that high concurrent life stresses and a low socioeconomic background correlate with a high risk of developing emotional problems as anxiety, depression, somatization and interpersonal sensitivity in families with a cancer-sick child. In the future, the detection of profiles of vulnerability could accelerate the referral of individuals of families with a high risk of maladjustment to the psychosocial counseling.

Methods

Counseling Program Description

Figure 1 delineates a heuristic model that connects the basic key elements of the coping process in the family with the basic functions of the Family Counseling Program on the background of the literature outlined above.

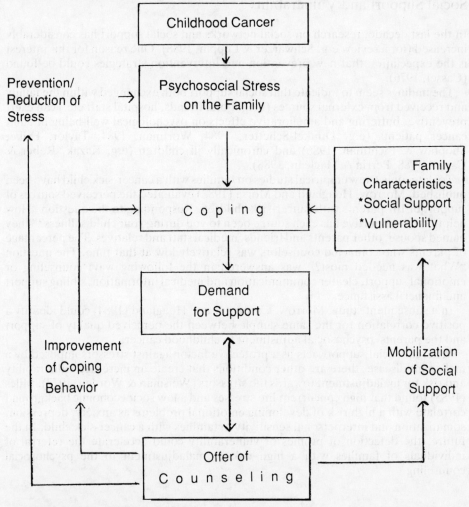

Figure 1. Functions of the Family Counseling Program.

The illness of the child (cancer) puts psychosocial stress on the family members. They make an appraisal of its threatening aspects and of their own capabilities to master it, and exert some kind of spontaneous coping behavior. The coping behavior chosen is moderated by family characteristics, especially by factors of vulnerability and of social support. The coping behavior can lead to a reduction of the psychosocial stress which again alters the subsequent appraisal and coping processes (Lazarus & Folkman, 1987).

If the coping behavior turns out to be ineffective, a demand for support may arise. If this is the case, a counselling offer is indicated.

Along with our conceptualization, the family's demand for support and the clinic's offer of counseling are in a complementary relationship. A basic principle is the orientation of the counseling program to the needs of the child and the family which can vary a lot across all the different sources of stress and the various stages of illness and treatment.

To know the facets of vulnerability in the single family member and in the family unit as a whole can facilitate the recognition to those needs which can be more obvious or hidden.

There are three basic functions by which the counseling program is supposed to influence the key elements of the coping process:

Prevention and Reduction of Stressors. The aim is to minimize the impact of psychosocial stress before it can unfold harmful effects on the psychological well-being of the family. Examples:

– Social work can, in part, prevent financial strains by making available tax reductions or cheaper use of public transport; it can help to find child care for the siblings at home and, thus, preserve the parents' time budget for the hospital visits, for occupational obligations, for social contacts or just for spare time. Arrangement of a rehabilitation after intensive therapy can prevent psychosomatic disturbances, revive family life and communication and enhance physical relaxation.

– To keep the patient integrated among the classmates helps to prevent problems of reentrace in normal school life after the therapy. Individual lessons given on the ward in order to keep up with the lessons of the classmates as far as possible can normalize daily life and affirm the child's self-image. If the counselors visit the class in order to explain and discuss the child's disease, its treatment and the occurence of side-effects (e.g. baldness due to chemotherapy) he/she prevents misconceptions and false phantasies among the classmates (e.g. about an assumed contagiousness of the disease) which otherwise can result in brutal teasing or excluding of the sick child.

Mobilization of Social Support. Unless stressors can be prevented, the aim is to mobilize the intrafamilial and external social support against them. Examples:

– The counselors support an even distribution of the new burdens and chores within the family up to the point that no family member runs the risk of being overstrained (especially the mother) or of being neglected (especially the siblings). This includes to clarify the mutual expectations within the family about which kind of support is desired by whom.

– The counselors prepare the family about the often fearful and ambiguous attitudes and behavior patterns neighbors and friends show when the family returns from her first hospital stay. Instead of social isolation the necessary social support can be experienced.

Improvement of Coping Behavior. Unless the mobilization of social support can hinder a maladjustment the aim is to alter the coping behavior directly. Examples:

– Some parents react to the diagnosis with strong and ongoing feelings of guilt, and they blame themselves of being responsible for the outbreak of the disease. Detailed exploration and gradual restructuring of these cognitions and emotions is also necessary in order to strengthen the parent's compliance with the treatment regimen.

– Educational counseling is often indicated if the parents do not know how to react towards a child that is demanding more from day to day. Parents and counselors search together for a parental behavior that sets limitations to child and, at the same time, shows him or her their unchanged love.

Subjects

The evaluation of the Family Counseling Program is based on a sample of 42 families. All the children were treated at the Children's Hospital at the University of Bonn. The age of the children ranged from two months up to 18 years (Mean age: 8.9 years).

   The exact subtype of childhood cancer in the sample is given according to their general prognosis (see Table 1); lymphoma have the highest, neuroblastoma the lowest survival rates.

Table 1:   Subtype of childhood cancer

Lymphoma	11 cases
Leukemia	22 cases
Osteosarcoma	7 cases
Neuroblastoma	1 case
Other solid Tumors	1 case

Measures

Data were collected by three instruments:
– Detailed protocols of the counseling sessions. The protocols were transformed into descriptive categories. The procedure was adapted to the approach of Mühlfeld (1984).
– A questionnaire. It was designed in order to measure the coping behavior of the family during the intensive therapy in a comprehensive manner. Its items were gathered from three sources: the first 14 items concerning questions of the general development of the child were taken from Petermann and Petermann (1984). 25 items referring to the coping behavior of the family were adopted and partly modified from a previous study on families with leukemic children (Ebeling, 1981). 22 additional items were constructed according to an analysis of literature.

   The questionnaire was completed by the parents about four to six weeks after intensive therapy.
– A five point Likert scale measuring the illness behavior of the child (adopted from Katz, Kellerman and Siegel, 1980). For each child, the scale was completed by his or her parents and by three nurses after the intensive therapy.

Results

Clusteranalysis of the Categories Based on the Counseling Protocols

Twelve categories were deduced representing the contents of the counseling protocols. The category frequencies (in detail see Petermann, Noeker, Bochmann,

Bode, Grabisch & Herlan-Criado, 1988) were the basis of a subsequent hierarchical clusteranalysis (Johnson, 1967). Three clusters were identified.
The clusters are interpreted as:
1. Level of information in the family members (Chi^2 = 32.40)
The cluster represents a close interrelationship of the level of information between father and mother which in turn is connected with the information level of the ill child as well as with that one of the siblings.
2. Coping style of father and mother (Chi^2 = 19.45)
The individual coping styles of father and mother turned out to be closely interrelated.
3. Communication between the parents and the illness behavior of the child (Chi^2 = 16.10)
The mutual parental communication and the child's illness behavior form the third cluster.

Clusteranalysis of the Categories Based on the Questionnaire and on the Likert Scales

Twelve categories based on questioonaire and Likert scales (see Table 2) formed the basis of a second clusteranalysis (Johnson, 1967). For the category frequencies the reader is referred to Petermann, Noeker, Bochmann, Bode, Grabisch and Herlan-Criado (1988).

Table 2. Categories based on questionnaire and Likert scales

cat 0:	Age
cat 1:	Main burden during therapy
cat 2:	Contentment about distribution of burdens
cat 3:	Illness behavior of the child
cat 4:	Communication between the parents
cat 5:	Communication between parents and child
cat 6:	Level of information in the siblings
cat 7a:	Social support given to the parents
cat 7b:	Social support given to the child
cat 8a:	Development of stress symptoms in the parents
cat 8b:	Development of stress symptoms in the child
cat 9:	Reaction of the siblings
cat 10:	Behavioral changes in the child
cat 11:	support by philosophy of life

Four clusters were identified. They were interpreted as:
1. Communication within the family
    (Chi^2 = 12.00; p = 0.01)
The communication between the parents (cat.4) is interrelated with the communication between parents and child (cat. 5).
2. Coping behavior of the siblings
    (Chi^2 = 9.45; p = 0.002)
This cluster connects the level of information of the siblings (cat. 6) and the reaction of the siblings (cat. 9).

3. Behavioral change of the child and parents support by philosophy of life
   (Chi^2 = 6.11; p = 0.013)
This cluster is formed by cat. 10 and cat. 11.
4. Distribution of burdens and contentment about it
   (Chi^2 = 4.67; p = 0.003)
An even distribution of the burdens (cat. 1) is connected with a content about the
way the burdens are shared (cat. 2).

Discussion

The results of the clustering among the categories based on the counseling protocols
are likely to be attributed to the interventions of the counseling program. The first
cluster indicates a close cohesion of the information level of father, mother, ill child
and siblings. The family-orientated approach, the integration of the siblings in the
treatment process and the principle of a "non-protective telling" of diagnosis to all
the family members (Chesler, Paris & Barbarin, 1986) may have contributed to a
"homogenization" of the intrafamilial information level.

Similar reasons may have been responsible for the similarity between the coping
style of father and mother. Counseling stratregies that bring the parental coping
styles into a common line are to encourage the mutual expression of sorrows and
burdens, to clarify expectations, to strengthen the attitude to regard the disease as a
challenge (Petermann & Bode, 1986), and to appeal to a sense of unity and mutual
support. The third cluster underlines the relevance of an open and active
communication between the parents for an appropriate illness behavior of the child.
The basic assumption of the counseling gains new evidence: the necessity to foster
and support the child by providing him or her with the resources of a communicative
and strengthened family gains new evidence.

The results of the clustering among the categories based on the questionnaire and
the Likert scales correspond to those of the counseling protocols. The first cluster
indicates that parents who are able to communicate with each other in a constructive
manner are also able to do so with their child. Intrafamilial communication suffers as
a whole if one member is excluded. The second cluster illustrates that telling the
siblings about the disease and inviting them to see the ill child on the ward prevents
reactions of resentment and feelings of neglect which otherwise can lead to
aggression and somatization. Watching the ill child's treatment and its side-effects
helps the siblings to realize that the child is "really" sick and, therefore, in need of
special parental care.

We could not find a reasonable explanation for the interrelationships represented
in the third cluster, not even after reviewing single-cases.
The fourth cluster strengthens the counselors' task to take care of an even
distribution of the burdens within the family to prevent individual overstrain or
discontentment. We have to keep in mind, however, that the questionnaire data are
subjective data and, thus, represent less the objective distribution of burdens but the
perceived one. Clinically, the impression prevails that the mothers carry the greatest
part of the new duties, responsibilities, restrictions and worries. Nevertheless, they
did not regret their situations as they felt that their ill child suffers so much that
feelings of guilt arise if they would claim priorities for themselves.

Our data indicate that psychosocial counseling is qualified to reduce and prevent stressors imposed on families with childhood cancer, to mobilize social support and to improve illness-related coping behavior.

References

Adams-Greenley, M. (1984). Helping children communicate about serious illness and death. *Journal of Psychosocial Oncology, 2*, 61–72.

Beutel, M. (1988). *Bewältigungsprozesse bei chronischen Krankheiten* [Coping processes in chronic disease]. Weinheim: Edition Medizin.

Breznitz, S. (1983). *The denial of stress*. New York: International Universities press.

Calhoun, L. G., Selby, J., and Kind, H. E. (1976). *Dealing with crisis: A guide to critical life problems*. Englewood Cliffs, N. J.: Prentice Hall.

Cassel, J. (1976). The contribution of the social environment to host resistance. *American Journal of Epidemiology, 104*, 107–123.

Chesler, M. A., and Barbarin, O. A. (1987). *Childhood cancer: Meeting the challenge of stress and support*. New York: Brunner/Mazel.

Chesler, M. A., Paris, J., and Barbarin, O. A. (1986). Telling the child with cancer: Parental choices to share information with ill children *Journal of Pediatric Psychology, 11*, 497–515.

Christ, G., and Adams, M. A. (1984). Therapeutic strategies at psychosocial crisis points in the treatment of childhood cancer.. In A. E. Christ and K. Florenhaft (Eds.), *Childhood cancer: Impact on the family* (pp. 109–128). New York: Plenum.

Cohen, F., and Lazarus, R. (1979). Active coping processes, coping disposition and recovery from surgery. *Psychology reports, 45*, 867–873.

Dunkel-Schetter, C. (1984). Social support and cancer: Findings based on patient interviews and their implications. *Journal of Social Issues, 40*, 77–98.

Ebling, A. (1981). *Untersuchunger zur psychosozialen Problemlage leukämiekranker Kinder und ihrer Familien* [Research on psychosocial problems of children with leukemia and their families]. Unpublished doctoral dissertation, Universtiy of Hamburg.

Farrell. S., and Hutter, J. J. (1984). The family of the adolescent: A time of challenge. In M. G. Eisenberg, K. Sutkin, C. La Faye, and R. A. Jansen (Eds.)., *Chronic illness and disability through life-span. Effects on self and family* (pp. 150–163). New York: Springer.

Fergusson, J. H. (1976). Late psychological effects of a serious illness in childhood. *Nursing Clinics of North America, 11*, 83–93.

Futterman, F. H., and Hoffman, J. (1973). Crisis and adaptation in the families of fatally ill children. In E. J. Anthony and C. Koupernik (Eds.), *The child in his family: The impact of disease and death* (Vol. 2, pp. 127–144). New York: Wiley.

Germezy, N. (1985). Stress resistant children. The search for protective factors. In J. E. Stevenson (Ed.), *Recent research in developmental psychopathology. Journal of child Psychology and Psychiatry* (Book Supplement No. 4, pp. 213–233). Oxford: Pergamon.

House, J. (1981). *Work stress and social support*. Reading: Addision-Wesley.

Johnson, S. (1967). Hierarchical clustering schemes. *Psychometrika, 32*, 241–254.

Kaplan, D. M. (1982). Intervention strategies for families. In J. Cohen, J. W. Cullen, and R. Martin (Eds.), *Psychosocial aspects of cancer*. New York: Raven.

Kaplan, D. M., Grobstein, R., and Smith, A. (1976). Predicting the impact of severe illness in families. *Health and Social Work, 1*, 71–82.

Kaplan, D. M., Smith, A., and Grobstein, R. (1972). *Proceedings of the American Cancer Society's National Conference on Human Values and Cancer*. Atlanta, Georgia.

Kaplan, D. M., Smith, A., Grobstein, R., and Fishman, S. E. (1977). Family mediation of stress. In R. H. Moos (Ed.), *Coping with physical illness* (pp. 81–96). New York: Plenum.

Katz, R. R., Kellerman, J., and Siegel, S. E. (1980). Behavioral distress in children with cancer undergoing medical procedures: Developmental considerations. *Journal of Consulting and Clinical Psychology, 48*, 356–365.

Kazak, A. E., Reber, M., and Carter, A. (1988). Structural and qualitative aspects of social networks in families with young chronicallly ill children. *Journal of Pediatric Psychology, 13*, 171–182.

Koocher, G. P. (1984). Terminal care and survivorship in pediatric chronic illness. *Clinical Psychology Review, 4*, 571–583.

Koocher, G. P., and O'Malley, J. E. (1981). *The damocles syndrome: Psychological consequences of surviving childhood cancer.* New York: McGraw-Hill.

Kupst, M. J., and Schulman, J. L. (1988). Long-term coping pediatric leukemia: a six-year follow-up-study. *Journal of Pediatric Psychology, 13,* 7–22.

Kupst, M. J., Tylke, L., Thomas, L., Mudd, M. E., Richardson, C., and Schulman, J. L. (1983). Strategies of intervention with families of pediatric leukemia patients: a longitudinal perspective. *Social Work in Health Care, 8,* 31–37.

Lansky, S. B. (1985). Management of stressful periods in childhood cancer. *Pediatric Clinics of North America, 32,* 625–632.

Lansky, S. B., and Cairns, N. U. (1979). *The family of the child with cancer.* New York: American Cancer Society.

Lansky, S. B., Cairns, N. U., Haasanein, R., Wehr, J., and Lowman, T. (1978). Childhood cancer: Parental discord and divorce. *Pediatrics, 65,* 184–190.

Lazarus, R. S., and Folkman, S. (1987). Transactional theory and research on emotions and coping. *European Journal of Personality, 1,* 141–170.

Levine, A. S., and Hersh, S. P. (1982). The psychosocial concomitants of cancer in young patients. In A. S. Levine (Ed.), *Cancer in the young* . New York: Masson.

Lobato, D., Faust, D., and Spirito, A. (1988). Examining the effects of chronic disease and disability on children's sibling relationship. *Journal of Pediatric Psychology, 13,* 389–407.

Miles, M. S. (1985). Emotional symptoms and physical health in bereaved parents. *Nursing Research, 34,* 76–78.

Morrow, G. R., Carpenter, P. J., and Hoagland, A. C. (1984). The role of social support in parental adjustment to pediatric cancer. *Journal of Pediatric Psychology, 9,* 317–330.

Morrow, G. R., Hoagland, A. C., and Morse, I. P. (1982). Sources of support perceived by parents of children with cancer: Implications for counseling. *Patient Counseling & Health Education, 4,* 36–40.

Nitschke, R., Sexauer, C. L., Spencer, B., and Humphrey, G. B. (1985). Psychische Betreuung chronisch erkankter Kinder mit progressivem Krankheitsverlauf [Psychological care of chronically ill children with progressive course of illness]. *Monatsschrift für Kinderheilkunde, 133,* 374–378.

Perrin, J. M., and MacLean, W. E. (1988). Children with chronic illness. *The Pediatric Clinics of North America, 35,* 1325–1337.

Petermann, F., and Bode, U. (1986). Five coping styles in families of children with cancer. *Pediatric Hemotology and Oncology, 3,* 299–309.

Petermann, F., Noeker, M., and Bode, U. (1987). *Psychologie chronischer Krankheiten im Kindes- und Jugendalter* [Psychology of chronic diseases in childhood and adolescence]. München: Psychologie Verlags Union.

Petermann, F., Noeker, M., Bochmann, F., Bode, U., Grabisch, B., and Herlan-Criado, H. (1988). *Beratung von Familien mit krebskranken Kindern: Konzeption und emprische Ergebnisse* [Counseling families of children with cancer: Concepts and results]. Frankfurt: Peter Lang.

Petermann, F., and Petermann, U. (1984). *Training mit aggressiven Kindern* [Training of aggressive children] (2nd ed.). München: Psychologie Verlags Union.

Schmitt, G. (1986). Die Lebenssituation des krebskranken Kindes [The state of children with cancer]. In K. H Wiedl (Ed.), *Rehabilitationspsychologie* (54–67). Stuttgart: Kohlhammer.

Schwarzer, R., and Leppin, A. (1988). Social support: The many faces of helpful social interactions. *International Journal of Educational Research, 2,* 333–345.

Sourkes, B. M. (1977). Facilitating family coping with childhood cancer. *Journal of Pediatric Psychology, 2,* 65–67.

Sourkes, B. M. (1980b). Siblings of the pediatric cancer patient. In J. Kellerman (Ed.), *Psychosocial aspects of childhood cancer.* Springerfield: Thomas.

Spinetta, J. J. (1981). Adjustment and adaptation in children with cancer. In J. J. Spinetta and P. Deasy-Spinetta (Eds.), *Living with childhood cancer.* St Louis: Mosby.

Spinetta, J. J., and Deasy-Spinetta, P. (Eds.). (1981). *Living with childhood cancer*. St. Louis: Mosby.

Spinetta, J. J., Warner, J. A., and Sheposh, J. P. (1981). Effective parental coping following the death of a child from cancer. *Journal of Pediatric Psychology, 6*, 251–263.

Taylor, S. E., Falke, R. L., Shoptaw, S. J., and Lichtman, R. R. (1986). Social support, support groups, and the cancer patients. *Journal of Consulting and Clinical Psychology, 54*, 608–615.

Varni, J. W., and Kratz, E. R. (1988). Psychological aspects of childhood cancer: A review of research. *Journal of Psychosocial Oncology, 5*, 93–119.

Weisman, A. D., and Worden, J. W. (1977). *Coping and vulnerability in cancer patients. Project Omega*. Boston: privately printed.

Wortman, C. B. (1984). Social support and the cancer patient. *Cancer, 53*, 2339–2360.

Children's Concepts of Symptoms, Causality, and the Course of Physical Illness

Lothar R. Schmidt and Irmgard Weishaupt

Concepts of Disease

Research about children's concepts of diseases and of health problems is important for several reasons: As *basic* research it might contribute to the description of the interaction between disease concepts and developmental periods as well as to the description of children's models of illness.

On the other hand, this research has many *applications*, such as providing

- a better understanding of how coping processes of ill children are influenced by different information and medical or psychological treatments and helping to prepare the child accordingly;
- better counseling for families and medical personnel, leading to improvement of the interactional processes between the child, the family, and the medical system;
- a better understanding of attitudes and prejudices toward children with severe diseases and handicaps.

Interesting reviews about the development of children's concepts of diseases have been provided by Eiser (1985), Varni (1983) and Karoly, Steffen and O'Grady (1982). A review and critique of the cognitive-developmental literature has been provided by Burbach and Peterson (1986).

Bibace and Walsh (1979, 1980) have theoretically out-lined and empirically examined the development of children's concepts of illness in the light of Piaget's and Werner's theories of development. They found very important theoretical and practical relationships between the level of sophistication of illness concepts and the age of the children. However, they did not always specify the diseases and did not differentiate the causality of different disease concepts. Furthermore, they have not discussed different attributes of illnesses (cf. Leventhal & Nerenz, 1985), since they have mainly focussed on aspects of illness explanations. Other critical aspects are discussed by Burbach and Peterson (1986).

Method and Results

In the following *descriptive* study about children's concepts of diseases, we analyzed three specific health problems and their attributes, namely symptomatology, causality and course, and primarily their treatment. In order to select the three illnesses, we excluded all health problems preschoolers did not know well enough in exploratory interviews and we looked for some heterogeneity in the nature of the problems. We chose *cold, measles* and *injuries* and applied semi-structured interviews containing the three illness attributes mentioned above.

255

The 40 subjects were preschoolers with a mean age of roughly 5 years and elementary school children with a mean age of roughly 9 years. In a screening test all school children and three preschoolers ($N = 20$) had reached the Piagetian *concrete operational* period. The remaining 20 Ss were in the *preoperational* period.

The data were analyzed both qualitatively and quantitatively. We developed a content analytical category system which allowed the answers to be ranked according to the level of cognitive development (Weishaupt & Schmidt, in preparation). Besides "No understanding" there were three categories for symptomatology and four for the more complex aspects of causality and treatment (Table 1). Examples of the categories are given in Table 2.

Table 1. *Content analysis: categories*

Categories	Symptomatology	Causality/ Treatment
no understanding	0	0
confabulation	1	1
concrete, unspecific/ associated phenomena	2	2
concrete, specific phenomena, some explanation	3	3
generalized, sophisticated explanation		4

Only a few results of the *qualitative* analysis can be reported here. First, we should consider the cognitive level of the children's illness concepts in the two developmental groups. In many instances, especially if the illnesses have concrete attributes, the level of the preschoolers' answers was surprisingly good.

Figure 1 shows that the *symptomatology* of *colds* is well understood even by children in the preoperational period.

The first category (see also Tables 1 and 2) of all the *histograms* contains answers at the very low level between no understanding and partly wrong verbalisations (scores 0–1.5), the second category describes concrete associated phenomena (score 2), the third category includes answers with at least some concrete specific phenomena and some correct explanations (score 2.5) and the fourth category stands for the answers of a higher, concrete operational level with more sophisticated explanations (scores 3 and 4). Thus the bars in the right half contain the answers at the higher levels of illness concepts.

The *causality* of colds (Figure 1), however, differentiates the two groups more than could be expected on the basis of the results of other studies (cf. Bibace & Walsh, 1979, 1980). The result for the *treatment* of colds is quite surprising; the graphs demonstrate a very high level of information for children in both groups.

Cold is an "easy" disease in terms of concreteness and it may be observed rather frequently in the family and in the child's own experience; thus it might not be representative for children's concepts of diseases in general. This explanation is strengthened by the results regarding *measles* (Figure 2). About half of the children in the preoperational period do not know enough about the symptomatology of

Table 2. *Examples of the categories for "cold"*

Symptoms	
Confabulation (1)	the teeth are loose; one has cancer and might die
Concrete, associated phenomena (2)	one cannot sleep, one must stay in bed; one cannot go to school
Concrete specific phenomena (3)	cough, catarrh, fever, headache, earache
Causality	
confabulation (1)	it comes from the trees, from the sky, from the acid in the mouth
Concrete, associated phenomena (2)	if one stays outdoors too much when it is cold
Concrete specific phenomena (3)	when it is infectious, the ill child is breathing ill air
Highest level (4)	germs
Treatment	
Confabulation (1)	it needs surgery of the mouth
Concrete, associated phenomena (2)	eat healthy stuff
Concrete specific phenomena (3)	cough drops, nose spray
Highest level (4)	process of healing, including battle against germs, blood flow

measles, and the causal explanations are weak for all but three children. As one would expect it, the concepts of treatment of measles are also rather unsophisticated.

Let us now turn briefly to *injuries* (Figure 3). The symptoms which define injuries are known to all children, in most cases at the highest level (only seven children in the preoperational period were in category "3"), and the concepts of treatment are also well developed.

The knowledge of concepts of *causality* is greatly dependent upon whether the child's focus is on *bleeding* or on *pain*. The causality of bleeding shows some variance, whereas with regard to pain, only one child reached a satisfactory level of explanation.

For quantitative analyses we dichotomized the answers according to their level. We grouped children into two groups: (a) those with no answer at a level higher than 2; (b) those with at least one answer at level 3 together with answers at level 2 or higher, but not at level 1. We compared the two groups in a 2x2 table using chi-quare. Using a significance level of $p < 0.01$, a number of significant differences between the two groups were found and these are shown in Table 3.

More important than the number of significant differences between the two groups was the variance of the concepts in some categories. The greatest differences between the two groups or the most marked developmental effects were found for *measles* with regard to all attributes, and for *causality* with regard to all diseases except for pain. Symptomatology and treatment are more similar in the two groups.

Additionally, the answers were analyzed without considering the highest level a child reached. We therefore calculated the percentage of correct answers by dividing

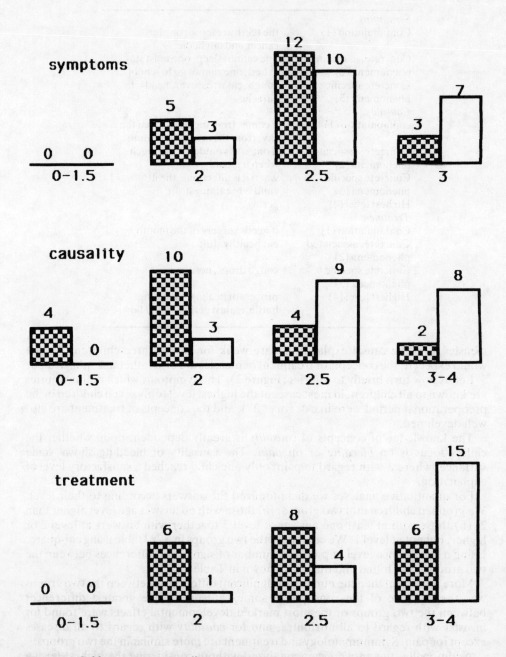

Figure 1. *Cold:* symptoms, causality, treatment
  – children in the preoperational period: checkered bars
  – children in the concrete operational period: white bars

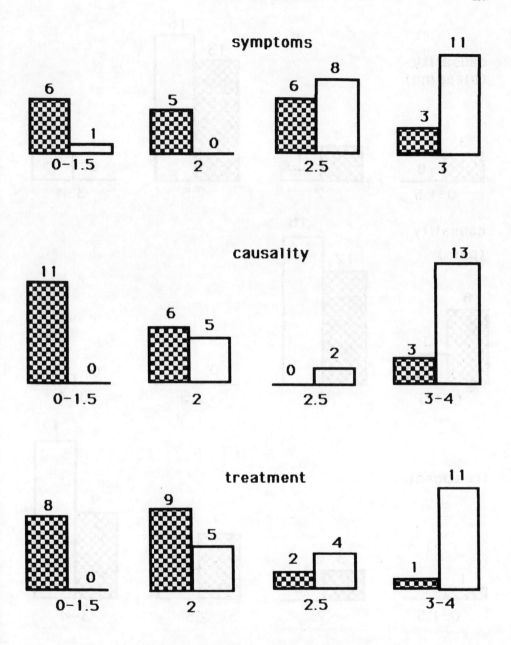

Figure 2. *Measles:* symptoms, causality, treatment
- children in the preoperational period: checkered bars
- children in the concrete operational period: white bars

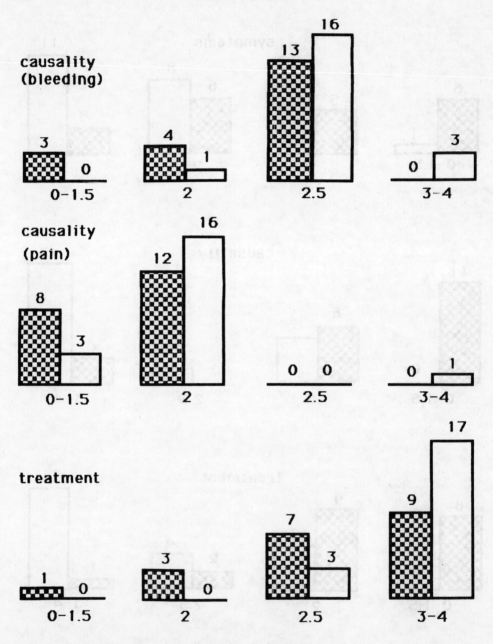

Figure 3. *Injuries:* causality (bleeding and pain), treatment
"Symptoms" are omitted because all children in the concrete operational period and 13 children in the preoperational period were in category "4"; the rest in category "3"
– children in the preoperational period: checkered bars
– children in the concrete operational period: white bars

Table 3. *Significant differences (+) between the children in the preoperational and the concrete operational period (p<0.01)*

Disease attributes	Significance
cold	
symptoms	
causality	+
treatment	
measles	
symptoms	+
causality	+
treatment	+
injuries	
symptoms	
causality (bleeding)	+
(pain)	
treatment	

Table 4. *Percentage of correct answers of the children in the preoperational (po) and the concrete operational (co) period*

Disease attributes	cold		measles		injuries	
	po	co	po	co	po	co
symptoms	62	82	62	86	86	100
causality	35	63	37	88	36	79
treatment	52	75	28	52	66	90

the number of correct answers by the number of all answers. Table 4 provides the main information about the two groups.

In the preoperational group roughly 50% of all answers were correct. With 35% correct responses, the comprehension of causality is the least developed attribute of the three diseases in study. The children in the concrete operational period with a mean age of nine years achieved 80% correct answers altogether.

Discussion and Future Research

This study is intended to be just one more stone in a large mosaic; more studies on this topic are planned with further groups of healthy and sick children and adults. In these studies some of the critical aspects of methodology by Burbach and Peterson (1986) should be regarded.

Our results show that illness concepts were influenced not only by cognitive development but also by the specific characteristics or attributes of diseases, especially their concreteness. Children's answers in the preoperational period were rather unspecific and pertained to action. They focused on concrete, external characteristics of diseases. However, if the diseases have concrete aspects in symptomatology and treatment, than these children were able to answer in a more sophisticated way.

Our results emphasize the need to tailor the research differentially to specific diseases and their attributes. Therefore, general conclusions about the illness concepts of children at a certain age or developmental period are not possible. This is important when considering the provision of information and the preparation for children who are ill or about to undergo treatment or investigations.

Obviously, even children in the preoperational period are able to understand illnesses which contain concrete aspects. In these cases one should provide the children with concrete, detailed information. Also it might be misleading to generalize from recommendations such as that by Potter and Roberts (1984, p. 22) who maintained that: "... it seems that preoperational children benefit most from a global nonspecific explanation while concrete operational children are more apt to comprehend detailed information." Their studies were concerned with childrens' concepts of diabetes and epilepsy and may not therefore relate to all other diseases.

One has to find a balance between explanations which are not too simple, too limited by the child's supposed developmental period and those which are far beyond the cognitive abilities of the child. Some of Bibace and Walsh's suggestions about information seem to be based too much on children's shortcomings and might lead to an attitude that young children be informed mainly with regard to the equipment or the personnel.

On the other hand, the kind and amount of information children have about diseases and medical procedures might be subject to great *cross cultural differences* (cross cultural comparison studies are planned in cooperation with the colleagues Roger Bibace and Mary Walsh). American films about the preparation of children for surgery or bone marrow aspirations show that American professionals verbalize much more and at a much higher level than Germans.

The high level of information about the treatment of the three diseases raises some hope about the effect of children's information on compliance, insofar as compliance does not depend too much on motivational and emotional variables. Parents themselves need to be well informed and should know more about how to inform their children. Often the information parents give their children seems to be too simple or too external, like wearing warm clothes, going to the physician or the hospital.

The results of this and other studies need to be discussed in the light of their implications for illness *models* and models of health-related behavior, like the Health Belief Model. Jordan and O'Grady (1982, p. 72) summarize: "For the most part, the strategies suggested by the Health Belief Model affect parent-initiated health behaviors through modification of parents' health beliefs. Child health care may be improved through direct modification of children's health beliefs... as well." In order to accomplish such changes they suggest an integration of the public health approach with the developmental approach.

The aspect of *personal control* seems to be especially important, both in general and specifically with regard to compliance. In contrast to other studies *magic beliefs*, attributions of guilt or of amoral misbehaviors as causes of illness were extremely rare in our investigation. This might be due to the selection of common health problems and/or to the interviewer (second author) who was, apart from interviewing using a Piagetian approach, rather precise and concentrated on the topics of the interview. She did not intentionally encourage magical or other irrational statements. On the other hand, she did not inhibit them, either.

Usually, the evaluation of children's illness concepts is based on the knowledge of the science of medicine. It might be very interesting to compare this with the knowledge of average adults and adults as patients (cf. Linden, 1985; Bibace & Walsh, 1989) and to study adult illness concepts more thoroughly. Without doubt, most adults have a lot of difficulties explaining the phenomena of pain or asymptomatic illnesses like hypertension, as Leventhal and his coworkers have shown (Leventhal & Nerenz, 1985).

Generally, it seems that adults and even the field of medicine prefer simple models. Sometimes these are described as the medical model which is particularly applicable to infectious disease with one major or "real" cause, a clear course and few relations to the personality and other conditions of the person who gets sick.

References

Bibace, R., and Walsh, M. E. (1979). Developmental stages in children's conceptions of illness. In G. Stone, F. Cohen, and N. Adler (Eds.), *Health psychology: A Handbook* (pp. 285–301). San Francisco: Jossey-Bass.

Bibace, R., and Walsh, M. E. (1980). Development of children's concepts of illness. *Pediatrics, 66*, 912–917.

Bibace, R., and Walsh, M. E. (1989). The patient as a person: Eliciting personal meaning of illness. In preparation.

Burbach, D. J., and Peterson, L. (1986). Children's concepts of physical illness: A review and critique of the cognitive-developmental literature. *Health Psychology, 5*, 307–325.

Eiser, C. (1985). *The psychology of childhood illness*. New York: Springer.

Jordon, M. K., and Grady, D. J. (1982). Children's health beliefs and concepts: Implications for child health care. In P. Karoly, J. J. Steffen, and D. J. O' Grady (Eds.), *Child health psychology* (pp. 58–76). New York: Pergamon.

Karoly, P., Steffen, J. J., and O'Grady, D. J. (Eds.). (1982). *Child health psychology*. New York: Pergamon.

Leventhal, H., and Nerenz, D. R. (1985). The assessment of illness cognition. In P. Karoly (Ed.). *Measurement strategies in health psychology* (pp. 517–554). New York: Wiley.

Linden, M. (1985). Krankheitskonzepte von Patienten [Concepts of illness of patients]. *Psychiatrische Praxis, 12*, 8–12.

Potter, P. C., and Roberts, M. C. (1984). Children's perceptions of chronic illness: The roles of disease symptoms, cognitive development, and information. *Journal of Pediatric Psychology, 9*, 13–27.

Varni, J. W. (1983). *Clinical behavioral pediatrics*. New York: Pergamon.

Weishaupt, I., and Schmidt, L. R. (in preparation). *Kindliche Konzepte von Krankheit* [Illness concepts of children].

Health Related Behaviour and Coping with Illness in Adolescence: A Cross-Cultural Perspective

Inge Seiffge-Krenke

Introduction

The coping skills of young people in dealing with age-specific problems have so far been considerably underestimated. In this paper, studies in health related behaviour and coping with illness are summarized. Starting with a review of the author's own research, involving over 3000 12- to 20- year-olds from various cultures, the problems typical of this developmental phase and the way of coping with these normative demands are presented.

Stress and Coping in Adolescence: Normative Demands and Critical Life Events

Adolescence is a developmental period in which the individual is confronted not only with a dramatic change in bodily contours but at the same time with a series of complex and interrelated developmental tasks which have to be mastered. Of special relevance for the health care of adolescents is their way of coping with these normative demands (see for a summary Seiffge-Krenke, 1986a).

Usually, small homogeneous groups of adolescents who have experienced extremely stressful, non-normative events such as kidnapping, rape or severe illness like cancer, are analysed (see e.g. more recently Compas, 1987a, 1987b; Wagner, Compas & Howell, 1988). Earlier studies in particular thus tended to start from a clinical perspective. Samples where highly selective and the operational definition of coping was heavily dominated by defense aspects. Because of this bias, the coping skills of young people in dealing with problems typical of their age-group, such as detachment from parents, hetrosexual relationships, building up an occupational identity etc. have been largely neglected.

At present, a shift of emphasis can be observed which is probably due to recent developments in the theory of adolescence: The continuity aspect is being more heavily stressed and the activity of the individual is being reasserted. The adolescent is regarded increasingly as the "producer of his own development" (Lerner & Busch-Rossnagel, 1981), who masters the transition to adulthood by continually tackling and coping with relevant developmental tasks (Coleman, 1974).

Ways of Coping with Age-Related Problems

Research with non-clinical groups has revealed that their responses to developmental tasks in such areas as peer group, school or future can be described in

267

terms of three main coping modes (Seiffge-Krenke, 1984a): (a) *active coping*, involving activities such as information-seeking or taking advice; (b) *internal coping*, emphasizing the adolescent's appraisal of the situation and internal reflection on possible solutions; and (c) *withdrawal*, which may be regarded as dysfunctional in the sense that no immediate solution is reached; this dimension includes intrapsychic defenses such as denial, regression and withdrawal.

In a study of 2000 West German adolescents aged 12 to 19 years, young subjects presented themselves as competent copers, well able to deal with problems arising in developmental areas such as school, parents, peers, opposite sex etc. Functional coping modes dominated, dysfunctional coping being employed very rarely and only for certain types of problems. This latter mode occurred particularly often with self-related problems (e.g. "discontented with oneself"), where about a third of responses involved withdrawal (Seiffge-Krenke, 1989). The general ratio of functional to dysfunctional coping was highly stable over time (Seiffge-Krenke, 1984a) and cross-culturally comparable (Seiffge-Krenke & Shulman, 1989).

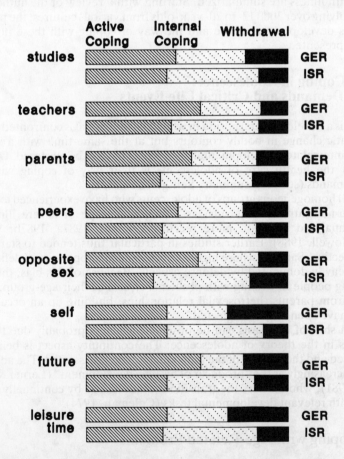

Figure 1: Differences in three coping styles measured by the Coping-Questionnaire (Seiffge-Krenke, 1990) between German (n = 353) and Israeli (n = 187) Adolescents

The tendency to apply dysfunctional coping across all situations was generally low and similar for both German and Israeli samples (21% and 16% respectively see Figure 1). Recent research in a Scandinavian sample found a corresponding percentage here, too. In general, the use of internal forms of coping ("I analyse the problem and work out possible solutions") and the willingness to compromise increase with age. There are striking sex differences in the use of social resources: As they grow older girls seek advice, help, comfort or symathy from others more often than boys, regardless of the nature of the problems (see Figure 2).

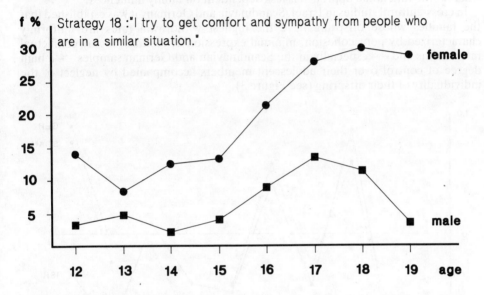

Figure 2: Sex differences in use of social resources by 479 male and 549 female adolescents

Girls discuss their problems with others more often and try to clarify their difficulties by talking them over openly. Male and female adolescents differ further in their appraisal of the same normative demand. Girls assess the same events (bad marks at school, quarrel with the family etc.) as being four times more threatening than do boys of the same age (Seiffge-Krenke, 1988).

Coping Behaviour of Disturbed Adolescents

Turning from "normal" adolescents to the clinical groups, which comprised some 10–20% of the original sample, a different picture emerges.

Among drug abusers and adolescents with interpersonal problems or depression, defense mechanisms are far more prominent. At the same time, their use of both active and internal coping does not differ significantly from that of nonclinical subjects; in these respects their approach is as functional as that of their nonclinical peers. It is thus typical of all adolescents with high problem intensity to have simultaneously high scores in both coping and defending (Seiffge-Krenke, 1984b). Perhaps this behaviour pattern should be regarded as a preventive strategy that has the effect of protecting the adolescent against physical symptoms or more serious neurotic or antisocial developments. Being in treatment reduced a disturbed adolescent's withdrawal score to a level comparable with that of the nonclinical control group.

This was confirmed by a further investigation analysing the relationship between personality type and coping behaviour (Seiffge-Krenke, Lipp & Brath, 1989). 15- to 19-year-old adolescents were grouped by cluster analysis on the basis of their scores on a personality questionnaire. The groups of adolescents with different personality structures differed neither with respect to active coping and support-seeking nor in their internal reflection on possible solutions, but systematic discrepancies were found in their withdrawal scores. This situationally invariant withdrawal tendency is strongly influenced by family climate (Shulman, Seiffge-Krenke & Samet, 1987), whereas the functional approach is less dependent on family influences.

In cross-cultural studies in Israel, Scandinavia and Germany it was established that the families whose offspring have the highest withdrawal rates are uniformly characterized by poor cohesion, minimal expression of feelings, highly conflictual interactions and – – especially in the Scandinavian and German samples – – a high degree of control over their adolescent members accompanied by neglect of the individuality of their offspring (see Figure 3).

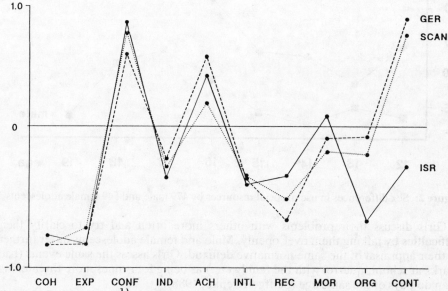

Figure 3: Family climate[1])and Coping behavior (un)structured conflict oriented families

Coping with Illness

In the spontaneous statements of the nonclinical subjects the issues "health" and "illness" do not arise as problem areas even though, or perhaps because, adolescents are so very preoccupied with their physical development and the fact that at this age "everyone wants to be normal". At the same time, it should not be forgotten that currently at least 3% of all families, at least in West Germany, are caring for a chronically ill adolescent (Angermeyer & Wolff, 1980), whilst comparable surveys in America and Britain place this figure at between 7 and 10% (Rutter, Tizard & Whitmore, 1970; Mattson, 1972). If visual, hearing and speech defects as well as learning and behaviour disorders are included, it has been estimated that 30% of all children under 18 are suffering from one or more long-term disorder (Stewart, 1967). According to Antonovsky (1981), individuals tend to become more vulnerable during periods of biological, social and psychological transition. A 14-year-old adolescent will clearly be affected in quite a different way by a critical life event such as major illness than a young adult of 24, who has already solved most of the developmental tasks still confronting the 14-year-old.

Empirical studies about coping with illness in adolescence have shown that the mastery of relevant developmental tasks is impeded or delayed by illness.

Hauser et al. (1983) found specific arrests in ego development among diabetic adolescents. As medical treatment frequently interferes with school and leisure activities, ill adolescents are socially more isolated (Weitzman, 1984), and start dating later than others (Sinnema, 1986).

Ill adolescents are less likely to have a driver's licence (Orr, Wellers, White & Pless, 1984) whether due to the illness itself or to parental refusal.

Future plans become unpredictable (Becker, 1979) and career plans are reported less frequently (Orr et al., 1984). There is some evidence that the spectrum of potential occupations tends to favour the medical professions (Fröhlich, 1986).

Twice as many ill adolescents never partake in joint family activities (Orr et al., 1984). Role expectations and assignments tend to shift within the family (Becker, 1979), the ill adolescent becoming the unwilling object of attention, the focus of family anxiety. The normal process of detachment from parents becomes very difficult (Hauser, 1980).

Developmental Dynamic of Health-Related Behaviour

Not only is the mastery of age-related developmental tasks delayed, impeded or prevented altogether by illness, but additional problems arising in connection with the specific developmental dynamics of this age group may furthermore have serious consequences for the adolescent's diagnosis, treatment and compliance:

Daydreaming, Fantasy and Illness Conceptions

Surgical interventions and physiologically disruptive or intrusive diagnostic procedures are most acutely experienced as menacing invasions during the adolescent years, when patterns of self- perception and body image are undergoing natural changes. Analysing adolescents' behaviour in hospital, Becker (1979) found that these young patients' imaginations were often very highly activated, particularly under conditions of physical immobilization. Daydreaming and fantasy production are normally increased during this developmental period (Giambra, 1974) and clearly become further stimulated by illness conditions. Furthermore, even where cognitive development is generally mature, certain basic misconceptions may persist. Thus, even young diabetics who had been well informed as to the nature of their disease continued to have certain cognitive visions of their pancreas being "riddled with holes" or "split in half", or believed that they had especially large stomachs, since they had to eat more frequently than other children (Kaufman & Hersher, 1971). Adolescent conceptions of illness differ from those of children. They are in general reasonably correct, but some erroneous beliefs may still persist, a fact which is closely associated with the general tendency amongst adolescents to fantasize (Zeltzer & Lebaron, 1986). It is important that health professionals be aware of the fact that adolescent beliefs and assumptions regarding the nature of health and illness have important implications for health care.

Transient Egocentricity

Intense daydreaming and fantasizing are closely related to egocentric behaviour in early adolescence. At this stage adolescents are preoccupied with the restructuring of identity – – an undertaking described by Havighurst (1972) and Erikson (1968) as the primary developmental task confronting them during this period. Earlier self-definitions are losing their relevance in the face of the rapid physical and social changes taking place; they must be re-modelled according to the perceived characteristics of important others, especially parents and peers (Seiffge-Krenke & Olbrich, 1982). Elkind (1967) and Elkind and Bowen (1977) describe two major manifestations of this transient egocentricity: The imaginary audience (the feeling that one is being constantly observed and judged by others) and the personal fable (experience of uniqueness: "Nobody understands me; my thoughts and feelings are exceptional"). At about the age of 13, when this sort of egocentricity is at its peak, adolescents are intensely concerned about the integrity of their body image and extremely sensitive to the prospect of physical disruption or distortion.

At the same time, this preoccupation with the self can easily give rise to misjudgements about real dangers. It is the personal fable phenomenon ("such things cannot happen to me") that is held partly responsible for the high incidence of accidents and teenage pregnancies. In our research we have found a systematic tendency amongst healthy adolescents, especially the younger groups, to underestimate the likelihood that they may themselves fall ill. The possibility that they may have an accident also continues to be misjudged even among the older age groups.

Change in Disclosure Partner

At nearly the same time, a shift in disclosure partner, usually from parents to peers, can be observed (Rivenbark, 1971; Youniss, 1980). As early as 12 years of age adolescents are already beginning to differentiate between private and public information and are no longer so willing to talk to anyone about intimate, private things (Laufer & Wolfe, 1974). In their self-presentations they now distinguish between an inner "true self" and an outer "facade". Their readiness to accept their parents as disclosure partners is clearly waning, as very personal thoughts and feelings are more and more reserved for peers.

As recent results show (Seiffge-Krenke, 1987), West German adolescents talk more frankly with their mothers than with their fathers. As they grow older, however, the preference for both parents dwindles as friends become more important. This change of preferred disclosure partner and the process of selecting which information is considered suitable for which target person is generally regarded as an indicator of social maturity (Chelune & Waring, 1984). However, it inevitably also gives rise to certain problems related to the health status of adolescents.

Firstly, it makes it more difficult to assess symptoms since diagnostic uncertainty is highest in this age group. In a German sample 20% of disturbed adolescents are diagnosed as having disorders of an unspecified nature (Seiffge-Krenke, 1986b). In an American study Weiner and Del Gaudio (1976) found that this diagnosis was applied to 36% of adolescent patients, as compared with 5% of adults. Where definite diagnoses are reached, they often prove unreliable. This partly has to do with the fact that developmental changes not only cause disturbances but can also bring about spontaneous remissions and the solution of old conflicts.

Secondly, the shift in disclosure partner is probably responsible for the fact that offers of professional help are rarely taken up by adolescents.

Detachment From Parents

Comparing adolescents with high and low problem intensity, young people are often caught up in a dilemma between the strong desire to give voice to their worries and an equally strong inhibition preventing them from doing just that (Seiffge-Krenke, 1984b). This can partly be explained in terms of the age-related change in disclosure partner and self-presentation, but there are also some indications that difficult relations with their families are at least partly responsible for this highly ambivalent attitude towards the offers made by health professionals (Seiffge-Krenke, 1989b). In general, any attachment to an adult in a developmental phase where detachment from parents is a central developmental issue may well cause problems.

It is therefore not surprising that ill adolescents who are dependent on the assistance of others over longer periods of time often develop close, highly aggressive attachments to the caring adult, usually the mother (Lepontois, 1975). Relieving and sustaining as the family network may be for the ill adolescent, their parents' unlimited care and concern is nevertheless an enormous problem for them, since their naturally accelerated drive towards detachment is thereby retarded, postponed or even blocked altogether. Since adequate schooling is often no longer possible and social contacts with other adolescents are restricted, adolescents suffering from severe illnesses inevitably find themselves in a situation that is deficient in many respects.

Diagnosis and management of a disease represents a prolonged crisis for parents as well (Burton, 1975; Eiser, 1985), demanding adaptation to a whole series of different stressors, so that one not surprisingly finds depression, marital discord, school and work troubles, as well as additional health problems in the families of chronically ill adolescents (Petermann, Noeker & Bode, 1987). The most frequent parental coping mode, overprotectiveness, interferes with the primary developmental task of gaining independence. The result is that the adolescent's attainment of adult responsibilities, detachment from the family and achievement of an adult status are delayed. Studies investigating coping with illness and family climate in adolescence show that the family coping strategies that contribute most to successful adjustment include normalisation (maximal integration of the chronically ill child into the mainstream of society) and the establishment of a wider social support system through which the burden of the illness can effectively be shared out (Holladay, 1984). It is interesting to observe that in such families, overprotectiveness actually decreases during the course of the illness, whilst in less adapted families dependency and control tend rather to increase.

Conformity with Peer Norms and Risk-Taking Behaviour

The results just reported show that social support not only has a stress-buffering function but can also have its price. The same holds true for peer relations. Especially for the 14- to- 18-year-olds conformity with peer norms is crucial.

At this point it is necessary to take into account the political and economic context of health behaviour: Whilst for adults it has been shown that knowledge about risk factors affecting morbidity and mortality has, during the past 20 years, resulted in a positive modification in life style, the percentage of teenagers involved in nicotine, alcohol or drug abuse, as well as dangerous driving, has increased over the same period (Jessor, 1986). The fact that health practice and preventive health behaviour during this phase of development deviates from overall population trends can be traced back to an age-related difference in the manner in which such risk-taking behaviour is perceived and evaluated. For the young people in question risk-taking is an integral part of the life-style of their peer group and excessive risk-taking is seen as a demonstration of adult status. This also explains why smoking and drug abuse is especially widespread amongst growing girls and, in West Germany, is at present on the increase in country areas, where young people enjoy a lower social status than their city-bred peers. In our own studies, drug abuse is actually not very common and is used as a coping strategy only in very special problem situations e.g. with the opposite sex.

Turning to the results of prospective longitudinal studies such as those made by Kandel (1986) or Jessor (1986), it is apparent that much of the age-appropriate risk-taking behaviour fades out towards the end of adolescence and that a persistently unhealthy life-style can be predicted by the personality dimension "conventionality – unconventionality".

For ill adolescents, conformity to peer norms becomes a very pressing problem. They are generally considered "deviant" (Silber, 1983) and may find friendship only through the common bond of illness (Wolfish & McLean, 1974). If they are able to remain in the healthy peer group, the peer norms become a permanent temptation to noncompliance. The rapid change in peer-group status which a severe illness usually entails is extremely disturbing to young people, adding a further problem to the threat of the illness itself and the associated physical handicap. Male adolescents appear to be especially hard hit by any impairment to their strength and physical prowess (Hofmann & Becker, 1973), whilst female adolescents suffer more from changes affecting their outward appearance (Weinberg, 1968).

Conclusions

The results so far show that in coping with problems in developmental fields such as school, parents, opposite sex etc., adolescents by and large employ functional strategies, which means that they do in fact manage to tackle and successfully master the problem in hand. Only about 15–20% of reactions are dysfunctional, in the sense of substituting a classical defense mechanism like withdrawal, denial etc. for an immediate solution to the problem. This ratio of functional to dysfunctional coping, as well as age and sex differences in the use of various coping strategies, was found to apply fairly uniformly across cultures. In clinical subjects it appeared that coping and defending scores were evenly balanced, which can partly be interpreted as a preventive strategy on the part of troubled adolescents. Defense mechanisms were applied fairly indiscriminately across situations and their use proved to be strongly influenced by family climate.

Considering the extent to which their mastery of developmental tasks is impeded and the detrimental conditions discouraging their normal drive towards detachment from adult caregivers, the overall adaptation of chronically ill adolescents is quite remarkable. The majority of them, far from being the helpless victims of a progressive illness, apparently make good use of active and internal coping strategies, of comparative optimizing (Petermann & Bode, 1986; Rose, 1984), and are capable to adaptively applying the mechanism of denial for dealing with an uncertain future (Mattson, 1972) or as a defense against stressful situations which are unalterable. These young people are faced with the difficult task of discovering how to develop a new set of intrapsychic devices and coping mechanisms for dealing with their illness, while at the same time trying to remain an accepted member of their peer group. Severe maladjustment or self-destructive behaviour occurs in only a small percentage of ill adolescents. Thus, only 10–20% of cases of juvenile diabetes belong to the group of "brittle diabetics" (Ahmed & Ahmed, 1985). This unexpectedly positive picture is consistent for different types of illness.

On the other hand, there is an increasing incidence of psycho-social maladjustment with a higher risk of becoming mentallly ill than healthy adolescents . These ill young people thus prove to be basically competent copers, like their healthy fellows, but at the price of their mental health in other respects. In classifying emotional and psychosocial maladjustment in adolescence, the pronounced "adolescent pattern" is striking (Becker, 1979): (a) one group is characterized by anxiety, inactivity, depression, lack of outside interests and a marked dependency on the family; (b) the second group is excessively independent, may engage in prohibited and risk-taking activities and display strong denial of real dangers and fears.

This splitting between passive dependency and rebellious, independent behaviour represents two equally attractive pulls in normal development, but can become self-destructive when severe illness exacerbates the age-related vulnerability typical of this period.

Health professionals must realize that illness conditions stand in complete opposition to the major developmental forces of adolescence, and that it is important to allow adolescents to make their own decisions about their illness as far as possible in order to gain a sense of mastery and control. This may include tolerating less than optimal therapy in order to prevent severe psychosocial maladjustment, accepting a certain degree of noncompliance with the therapeutic regime and understanding the young patients' counselling aversion without taking it personally. The ultimate aim must be to optimalize the adolescent's physical health without impairing his or her mental development in the process.

References

Ahmed, P. I., and Ahmed, N. (1985). *Coping with juvenile diabetes*. Springfield, IL: Charles C. Thomas.

Angermeyer, M., and Wolff, G. (1980). Chronisch kranke Kinder und Jugendliche in der Familie. [Chronically sick children and adolescents in the family]. *Fortschritte der Medizin, 41*, 1575–1578.

Antonovsky, A. (1981). *Health, stress, and coping*. San Francisco: Jossey-Bass.

Becker, R. D. (1979). Adolescents in the hospital. *Israel Annals of Psychiatry & Related Disciplines, 17*, 328–352.

Burton, L. (1975). *The family life of sick children*. London: Routledge and Kegan Paul.

Chelune, C. J., and Waring, E. M. (1984). Nature and assessment of intimacy. In P. McReynolds (Ed.), *Advances in psychological assessment* (Vol. 6). San Francisco: Jossey-Bass.

Coleman, J. S. (1974). *Relationships in adolescence*. London: Routledge and Kegan Paul.

Compas, B. E. (1987a). Stress and life events during childhood and adolescence. *Clinical Psychology Review, 7*, 275–302.

Compas, B. E. (1987b). Coping with stress during childhood and adolescence. *Psychological Bulletin, 101*, 393–403.

Eiser, C. (1985). *The psychology of childhood illness*. New York: Springer.

Elkind, D. (1967). Egocentrism in adolescence. *Child Development, 38*, 1025–1034.

Elkind, D., and Bowen, R. (1977). Imaginary audience behavior in children and adolescents. *Developmental Psychology, 15*, 38–44.

Erikson, E. H. (1968). *Identity, youth and crisis*. New York: Norton.

Fröhlich, F. (1986). *Die seelische Verarbeitung lebensbedrohlicher Krankheit im Jugendalter. Grundprobleme und Möglichkeiten einer stützenden Therapie*. [Coping with life-threatening diseases in adolescence]. Basel: Schwade.

Giambra, L. (1974). Daydreaming across the life-span. Late adolescence to senior citizen. *International Journal of Aging and Human Development, 5*, 115–140.

Hauser, S. T. (1980). Familial contexts of ego-development and self-image integration in diabetic adolescents: Longitudinal studies. In B. Hamburg, L. Lipsett, G. Inoff, and A. L. Drash (Eds.), *Behavioral and psychosocial issues in diabetes: Proceedings of the National Conference* (pp. 65–85). Washington, DC: Government Printing Office.

Hauser, S. T., Jacobson, A. M., Noam, G., and Powers, S. (1983). Ego-development and self-image complexity in early adolescence. Personality studies of psychiatric and diabetic patients. *Archives of General Psychiatry, 40*, 325–332.

Havighurst, R. J. (1972). *Developmental tasks and education* (3rd ed.). New York: McKey.

Hofmann, A. D., and Becker, R. D. (1973). Psychotherapeutic approaches to the physically ill adolescent. *International Journal of Child Psychotherapy, 2*, 492–511.

Holladay, B. (1984). Challenges of rearing a chronically ill child. Caring and coping. *Nursing Clinics of North America, 19*, 361–368.

Jessor, R. (1986). Adolescent problem drinking: Psychosocial aspects and development outcomes. In R. K, Silbereisen, K. Eyferth, and G. Rudinger (Eds.), *Development as action in context* (pp. 241–264). New York: Springer.

Kandel, D. P. (1986). Processes of peer influences in adolescence. In R. K. Silbereisen, K. Eyferth, and G. Rudinger (Eds.), *Development as action in context* (pp. 203–228). New York: Springer.

Kaufman, R. V., and Hersher, B. (1971). Body image changes in teenage diabetics. *Pediatrics, 48*, 123–128.

Laufer, R., and Wolfe, M. (1974). The concept of privacy in childhood and adolescence. In D. H. Larson (Ed.), *Man-environment interactions. Proceedings of EDRA* (pp. 29–45). Washington, DC: Environmental Design Research Association.

Lepontois, J. (1975). Adolescents with sickle-cell anemia deal with life and death. *Social Work in Health Care, 1*, 71–80.

Lerner, R. M., and Busch-Rossnagel, N. A. (Eds.). (1981). *Individuals as producers of their own development: A longitudinal perspective*. New York: Academic Press.

Mattson, A. (1972). Long-term physically illness in childhood: A challenge to psychosocial adaption. *Pediatrics, 50*, 801–811.

Orr, D. P., Wellers, S. C., Whie, B., and Pless, I. B. (1984). Psychosocial implication of chronic illness in adolescence. *Journal of Pediatrics, 104*, 152–157.

Petermann, F., and Bode, U. (1986). Five coping styles in families of children with cancer. *Paediatric Haematology and Oncology, 3*, 299–309.

Petermann, F., Noeker, M., and Bode, U. (1987). *Psychologie chronischer Krankheiten im Kindes und Jugendalter* [Psychology of chronic diseases in childhood and adolescence]. Weinheim: Psychologie Verlagsunion.

Rivenbark, W. H. (1971). Self-disclosure among adolescents. *Psychological Reports, 28*, 35–42.

Rose, M. H. (1984). The concepts of coping and vulnerability as applied to children with chronic conditions. *Issues in Comprehensive Pediatric Nursing, 7*, 177–186.

Sanok, R. J. (1975). *Egocentric conceptualizations among adolescents and adults*. Unpublished manuscript.

Seiffge-Krenke, I. (1984a). *Problembewältigung im Jugendalter*. [Coping in adolescence]. Unpublished habilitation. University of Gießen.

Seiffge-Krenke, I. (1984b). Problembewältigung bei besonders belasteten Judgendlichen. [Coping of adolescents at risk]. In E. Olrich, and E. Todt (Eds.), *Probleme des Jugendalters. Neuere Sichtweisen* (pp. 353–386). Berlin: Springer.

Seiffge-Krenke, I. (1986a). Problembewältigung im Judgendalter, [Coping in adolescence]. *Zeitschrift für Entwicklungspsychologie und Pädagogische Psychologie, 18*, 122–152.

Seiffge-Krenke, I. (1986b). *Psychoanalytische Therapie Jugendlicher*. [Psychoanalytic therapy of adolescents]. Stuttgart: Kohlhammer.

Seiffge-Krenke, I. (1987). Psychische Konstruktionen bei Jugendlichen: Der imaginäre Gefährte. [Psychological constructions of adolescents: The imaginainary companion].*Zeitschrift für Entwicklungspsychologie und Pädagogische Psychologie, 19*, 14–31.

Seiffge-Krenke, I. (1988). Kognitive Kontrolle als bedeutsame Dimension bei der Bewältigung von Alltagsereignissen. [Coping with daily events]. *Zeitschrift für Pädagogische Psychologie, 2*, 37–49.

Seiffge-Krenke, I. (1989). Developmental processes in self-concept and coping behavior. In S. Jackson, and H. Bosma (Eds.), *Self-concept and coping in adolescence*. New York: Springer.

Seiffge-Krenke, J. (1990). Bewältigung alltäglicher Problemsituationen: Ein Coping-Fragebogen für Jugendliche. [Coping with everday problems: A coping questionnaire]. Zeitschrift für Differentielle und Diagnostische Psychologie, 10, 201–220.

Seiffge-Krenke, I., and Olbrich, E. (1982). Psychosoziale Entwicklung im Jugendalter. [Psychosocial problems in adolescence]. In W. Wieczerkowski, and H. zur Oeveste (Eds.), *Lehrbuch der Entwicklungspsychologie* (Vol. 2, pp. 99–144). Düsseldorf: Schwann.

Seiffge-Krenke, I., and Shulman, S. (1989). Coping style in adolescence: A cross-cultural study. *Journal of Cross Cultural Psychology*, (in press).

Seiffge-Krenke, I., Lipp, O., and Brath, K. (1989). Persönlichkeitsstruktur und Bewältigungsverhalten bei Jungendlichen. [Personality and coping of adolescents]. *Zeitschrift für Klinische Psychologie, 18*, 1–18.

Shulman, S., Seiffge-Krenke, I., and Samet, N. (1987). Adolescent coping style as a function of perceived family climate. *Journal of Adolescent Research, 2*, 367–381.

Silber, T. (1983). Chronic illness in adolescents: A sociological perspective. *Adolescence, 18*, 675–677.

Sinnema, G. (1986). The development of independence in chronically ill adolescents. *International Journal of Adolescent Medicine and Health, 2*, 1–14.

Stewart, W. (1967). The unmet needs of children. *Pediatrics, 39*, 157–160.

Wanger. B. M., Compas, B. E., and Howell, D. C. (1988). Daily and mojor life events: A test of an integrative model of psychosocial stress. *American Journal of Community Psychology,* *16,* 189–205.

Weinberg, S. (1968). Seminars in nursing care of the adolescent. *Nursing Outlook, 16,* 18–23.

Weiner, I. B., and Del Gaudio, A. C. (1976). Psychopathology in adolescence: An epidemiological study. *Archives of General Psychiatry, 33,* 187–193.

Weitzmann, M. (1984). School and peer relations. *Pediatric Clinics of North America, 31,* 59–69.

Youniss, J. (1980). *Parents and peers in social development.* Chicago: University of Chicago Press.

Zeltzer, L., and Lebaron, S. (1986). Fantasy in children and adolescents with chronic illness. *Journal of Developmental and Behavioral Pediatrics, 7,* 195–198.

Section 6

Behavioural Factors in Coronary and Cardiovascular Disease

Cardiovascular Reactivity: Physiological or Psychological

Ray H. Rosenman

Psychophysiologic theory has long hypothesized that individuals with increased cardiovascular responses to external stimuli are predisposed to develop hypertension, and that the repetitive and summated occurence of such heightened responses in their natural environment play a pathogenetic role in the development of essential hypertension and possibly also of coronary atherosclerosis (Clarkson, Manuck & Kaplan, 1986; Herd, 1986; Manuck & Krantz, 1986; Schneiderman, 1983). However, a massive literature developed over many decades of research (Mathews, Weiss, Detre et al., 1986; Steptoe, Ruddel & Neus, 1985) has failed to document this still widely held belief (Krantz & Manuck, 1984; Julius, Weder & Hinderliter, 1986).

The concept that cardiovasuclar reactivity may be pathogenetic does not appear to consider the fact that resting and reactive blood pressures are under a dual system of regulation. There are different anatomic central areas and pathways that regulate basal and reactive blood pressures and, to a significant degree, these are independently controlled (Reis & LeDoux, 1987).

Heart rate and blood pressure are commonly measured in the laboratory setting during exposure of subjects to a wide variety of external stimuli that include cognitive mental tasks, static and dynamic physical taks, cold, stressful interviews, reaction time tasks, competitive tasks and diverse other psychomotor situations. The responses are taken to reflect an individual's cardiovascular "stress reactivity" (Krantz & Manuck, 1984; Steptoe et al., 1985). It is believed that individual patterns of laboratory reponses are generalizable to the natural environment and that increased "cardiovascular reactivity" would predict increased magnitude of responses and variability of the blood pressure in the milieu.

Blood pressure responses to laboratory stressors involve a complex interaction between the heart and peripheral vasculature, carefully mediated through the central nervous system via the sympathetic nervous system (SNS) and locally by factors that are responsible for auto-regulation at the arteriolar level (Esler, Jennings, Korner et al., 1988; Schrager & Ellestad, 1983). The control of peripheral sympathetic nerve transmission is thus extrordinarily complex (Esler et al., 1988; Francis, 1988). The stimuli that are commonly used to elicit responses in laboratory testing variably affect heart rate and systolic and diastolic blood pressures since they have different predominant effects on alpha- and beta-adrenoreceptor activity, hence also on circulating and urinary catecholamines (Ward, Mefford, Parker et al., 1988). Heightened blood pressure responses during laboratory testing may be due to increased central SNS outflow. However, they may also result from increased peripheral release or decreased uptake of norepinephrine during neural stimulation or from increased peripheral adrenoreceptor responsiveness or density. It was appropriately emphasized by Krantz and Manuck (1984) that there is sometimes a naive tendency to regard laboratory assessments "as if it comprised a single physiologic response dimension – which fails to recognize the fact that apparently

283

similar blood pressure responses to stressors reflect distinctly cardiovascular dynamics" and that "the simple notion of a singular 'hot' versus 'cold' cardiovascular reactor may be oversimplified." In fact, search of the literature cited in recent reviews (Eliot, 1988; Elbert, Langosch, Steptoe & Vaitl, 1988) fails to uncover any follow-up data that might confirm a role of cardiovascular reactivity in the pathogenesis of either hypertension or ischemic heart disease (IHD). Moreover, there is a notable lack of scientifically documented, follow-up findings to support the belief (Eliot, 1988) that it is important to evaluate patients by use of special methodology to measure possible "hot reactivity".

Different investigators may find different results for the same laboratory stress tests. This may stem partly from varied methodologic problems that include lack of standardization for test procedures (Kranz & Manuck, 1984; Steptoe et al., 1985). Moreover, reactivity studies often pay inadequate attention to the fact that cardiovascular responses are influenced by age and sex (Frankenhaeuser, 1988), and race (Fredrikson, 1986), psychosocial influences (Frankenhaeuser, 1988; Fredrikson, 1986a), state and trait psychological and emotional dimensions and responses to test procedures (Sullivan, Schoentgen, DeQuattro et al., 1981), active versus passive coping with tasks (Obrist, Langer, Light & Koepke, 1983), cognitive task appraisal (Lazarus), heart rate responses (Light, Koepke, Obrist & Willis, 1983), variable catecholamine responses to different stressors (Dimsdale, Hartley, Ruskin et al., 1984; Ward et al., 1988;), variable duration of effects of discontinued medications that cause up- and down-regulation of adrenergic and muscarinic receptors (Ruddell, 1985), family history of hypertension (Rose, 1986; Havlik & Feinleib, 1982), lean body mass and other relevant anthropometric variables, body position during testing (Jorde & Williams, 1986), sleep and fatigue, duration of abstinence from alcohol, nicotine, caffeine, chocolate and commonly used short-term drugs, relevant dietary backgrounds and habitual and recent dietary intake of several electrolytes, physical conditioning (Harrison, 1985), circadian rhythm (Francioso, Johnson & Tobian, 1980) and blood volume (Falkner, Gaddo & Angelakos, 1981; Falkner & Light, 1986; Light et al., 1983). It is unfortunate that too many studies have given little attention to most of these potentially counfounding influences (Rosenman, 1987).

Despite the complexity of the many endogenous factors that differentially regulate heart rate and systolic and diastolic blood pressures and the multiple exogenous factors that can influence cardiovasular responses to behavioral challenges, there is some replicability of individual patters over time (Krantz & Manuck, 1984). This is greater in younger subjects, in whom cardiovascular responses tend to generalize across laboratory test procedures that require qualitatively different behavioral responses (Mathews, Rakaczy, Stoney & Manuck, 1987). However, such findings strongly suggest that individual patterns of cardiovascular responses in the laboratory are due to anthropometric factors that are genetically determined (Carmelli, Chesney, Ward & Rosenman, 1985; Rose, 1961), rather than to behavioral differences of cognitive perception of the tasks, and thus fail to support the concept of "stress reactivity".

The etiology of essential hypertension is multifactoral and one contributing factor may be SNS overactivity since the hyperkinetic state of borderline hypertensives is neurogenically mediated (Julius et al., 1986). Borderline hypertensives and offspring of hypertensive parents are at increased risk for development of sustained hypertension. They tend to exhibit exaggerated cardiovascular reactivity in laboratory tests (Eliasson, Hjemdahl & Kahan, 1983; Falkner & Kushner, 1981; Light & Obrist, 1980; Nestler, 1969). However, this only occurs in response to cognitive stressors (Falkner, Onesti & Angelakos, 1979; Julius, Weder & Egan, 1983; Julius et al., 1986) and not during responses to such other stimuli as dynamic exercise (Julis & Conway, 1968; Lund-Johansen, 1967; Sannerstedt, 1966), isometric exercise (Sannerstedt & Julius, 1972), cold pressor testing (Eliasson et al., 1983 Thomas & Duszynski, 1982; Eich & Jacobsen, 1967) and orthostatic stress (Eliasson et al., 1983; Sannderstedt, Julias & Conway, 1970). Moreover, higher prevalence of hypertension in black compared to white subjects is not associated with consistent racial differences in reactivity (Myers, Morell, Shapiro at al., 1985).

Subjects at increased genetic risk for hypertension thus do not exhibit generalized autonomic dysregulation (Julius et al., 1986, Julius, 1988) since their exaggerated reactivity is limited to behavioral tasks (Falkner et al., 1979). However, even these responses to mental stressors vary widely from high to low (Julius & Ellis, 1974) and, when heightened, are of small magnitude (Julius et al., 1983; Weder & Julius, 1985) and may in part be due to salt-loading (Falkner et al., 1981; Falkner & Light , 1986).

If cardiovascular reactivity is pathogenetically or even predictively linked to hypertension it would be expected that young borderline hypertensives would exhibit exaggerated blood pressure responses and variability in their natural environment. However, ambulatory monitoring during usual daily activities has failed to document expected findings. Physical and mental activities are determinants of blood pressure changes during usual life routine (Clark, Denby, Pregidon et al., 1987; James, Yee, Harshfield et al., 1986) and the observed changes are reproducible (Fitzgerald, O'Malley & O'Brien, 1984; Weber & Drayer, 1986) provided that such activities are of generally similar nature (Harshfield, Pickering, Yee & Marion, 1985; Pickering, Harshfield & Kleinart, 1984). Julius and Schork (1971) early found that blood pressure variability in borderline hypertensives is no greater that that which occurs in normotensives. Spontaneous blood pressure flucuations of considerable magnitude occur in the natural environment in most individuals but are no greater in hypertensives than in normotensives (Harshfield et al., 1985; Horan, Kennedy & Padget, 1981; Julius et al., 1983; Julius & Johnson, 1984; Kannel, Sorlie & Gordon, 1980; Mancia & Ferrar, 1983; Messerli & Glade, 1982; v.Eiff, Gogolin, Jacobs & Neus, 1985; Weder & Julius, 1985;). Moreover, although blood pressure variability in the natural environment shows some correlation with resting levels (Kannel et al. 1980), subjects with higher reactivity in the laboratory setting show only small increases of systolic pressure in the natural environment, compared to individuals with low stress responses (v.Eiff et al., 1985). High reactors in laboratory stress tests also do not exhibit increased blood pressure variability in daily life routines (Harshfield et al., 1985) and any increased variability "accounted for" by laboratory stress responses is not only very small (Floras, Hassan, Jones & Sleight, 1987) but is not related to SNS activity (Clement, Mussche, Vanhouette & Pannier, 1979). Cardiovascular reactivity in the laboratory setting thus does not predict either blood pressure variability in the natural environment or blood pressure changes that occur from one day to another daily activity (Harshfield et al., 1985).

It can be seen that, despite widespread belief to the contrary, laboratory stress reactivity does not predict blood pressure changes that occur in routine daily life. There is thus little support for the expectation that hyperreactors in the laboratory would exhibit increased variability in their natural environment or that hypertension

can be pathogenetically related to a summation of exaggerated pressor responses
that occur over time. Moreover, there is little evidence that pressor responses and
blood pressure variability that are behaviorally-induced play a contributing role in
the pathogenesis of hypertension (Julius, 1988). The specificity of exaggerated
cardiovascular responses in borderline hypertensives to mental stressors may be
found in a subset of hypertensives but is improperly interpreted to mean that
behaviorally-induced blood pressure reactivity is the mechanism by which
hypertension develops (Julius et al., 1986). It is therefore emphasized that little
support can be found for use of laboratory stress testing to delineate either the
pathogenesis of hypertension (Julius, 1988) or the evaluation of hypertensive
subjects (Harshfield et al., 1985).

The increased risk for hypertension that is associated with exaggerated
cardiovascular reactivity in borderline hypertensives (Falkner & Kushner, 1981;
Lund-Johansen, 1984) is not very great and the substantial majority do not progress
to substained hypertension (Julius et al., 1983). Moreover, there are no population-
based studies which have found hyperreactors to be more likely to develop
hypertension with passage of time (Weber & Julius, 1985). A large number of
subjects with mild-to-moderatly elevated blood pressures during screening in the
Australian Trial (1980) were later found to be normotensive without therapy and
regression toward the mean can account for some of the findings in borderline
hypertensives (Eich & Cuddy, 1966; Weiss & Safar, 1978). There remains some
question about the potential ability of cold pressor testing to predict hypertension
(Krantz, Menkes, Lundberg et al., 1988), but the evidence is weak, if any (Eich &
Jacobsen, 1967; Harlan, Osborne & Graybiel, 1964; Julius et al., 1986; Thomas &
Duszynski, 1982). Moreover, neither the response to cold pressor testing nor
cognitive stressors predict blood pressure responses to antihypersive therapy.

Established hypertensives may exhibit increased cardiovascular reactivity to
dynamic exercise, compared to normotensives, but have a normal response to static
exercise (Conway, Julius & Amery, 1968), tilt (Sannerstedt et al., 1970) and blood
volume expansion (Julius & Pascual, 1971). Thus, older hypertensives may exhibit
increased response to tasks that require active coping, but the differences from
normotensives are quantitative rather than qualitative and are specific for the
cardiovascular system, without evidence of generalized SNS activation (Fredrikson,
1986a). Another relevant finding is that enhanced reactivity shows contrasting
differences for systolic and diastolic blood pressure, depending on whether subjects
have borderline or established hypertension (Julius et al., 1986; Fredrikson, 1986a).

Higher noradrenergic responses are often exhibited by Type A compared to Type
B males during competitive, cognitive challenges in the laboratory setting
(Friedman, Byers, Diamant & Rosenman, 1975) as well as in the natural
environment (Friedman, St. George, Byers & Rosenmann, 1960). A large number
of studies have measured cardiovascular reactivity in Type A and B subjects (Glass
& Contrada, 1984; Houston, 1983; Krantz & Manuck, 1984; Manuck & Krantz,
1986; Mathews, 1982; Rosenman & Chesney, 1982). In general, during exposure to
a wide variety of stressors in the laboratory setting, differences in catecholamine and
cardiovascular responses have often been found in Type A and B subjects (Krantz &
Manuck, 1984). The largest Type A-B differences tend to occur during tasks that are
associated with more rapid pace, greater task difficulty or when subjects are
challenged to perform more difficult tasks in a competitive manner under time
pressure (Rosenman, 1987; Ward et al., 1988). However, the pattern and the lack of

consistency of these differences in many studies (Krantz & Manuck, 1984) strongly suggest that Type A and B individuals do not have any intrinsic differences of reactivity but only that Type A's tend to have heightened perception of relevant stressors that are found to be challenging, in turn associated with a more active coping style that increases SNS responses (Light, 1981). However, despite their tendency to exhibit increased SNS responses to perceived relevant challenges in both the laboratory setting and natural environment, neither Type A's in general nor those with exaggerated cardiovascular reactivity exhibit either higher levels of resting blood pressure or increased prevalence of essential hypertension (Rosenman, 1987). This finding prevails despite the tendency of Type A's to exhibit higher anger/hostility dimensions (Rosenman, 1985; 1987) which are believed to be related to higher levels of blood pressure (Cottington, Matthews, Talbott & Kuller, 1986; Diamond, 1982; Julius, Schneider & Egan, 1985; Kahn, Medalie, Neufeld et al., 1972; McClelland, 1979; Rosenman, 1985; Schneider, Egan, Johnson et al., 1986), heightened cardiovascular reactivity (Goldstein, 1981) and increased variability of the blood pressure during ambulatory monitoring in the natural environment (Harshfield et al., 1985).

Anxiety is often believed to be causally related to hypertension and to be associated with increased cardiovascular reactivity. However, it is doubtful that there is validity for either belief. In fact, subjects with generalized anxiety disorders have a very low prevalence of hypertension (Devereux, Brown, Lutas et al., 1982; Rosenman, 1990). Moreover, a large number of studies have failed to find that cardiovascular reactivity is increased in subjects who exhibit anxiety or have long-standing anxiety disorders (Glass, Lake, Contrada, et al., 1983; Grunhaus, Gloger, Birmacher et al., 1983; Hodges, 1968; Holden & Barlow, 1986; Holroyd, Westbrook, Wolf & Badhorn, 1978; Kelly, Mitchell-Heggs & Sherman, 1971; Klorman, Wiensenfield & Austin, 1975; Knight & Borden, 1979; Mantysaari, Antila & Peltonen, 1988; Nesse, Cameron, Curtis et al., 1984; Orlebeke & van Doornen, 1977; Roth, Teich, Taylor et al., 1986; Smith, Houston & Zurawski, 1984; Steptoe, Melville & Ross, 1984; Sullivan et al., 1981; Taylor, Sheikh, Agras et al., 1986; Turner, Beidel & Larkin, 1986; Wing, 1964; Woods, Charney, McPherson et al., 1987).

The dual regulation of basal and reactive blood pressures (Reis & LeDoux, 1987) probably explains why antihypertensive medications that affect the central regulation involved in basal blood pressure levels do not affect the central regulation of blood pressure lability or variability or the responses to environmental stressors. A large number of studies have measured cardiovascular reactivity in the laboratory setting to a wide variety of physical and mental stressors given in hypertensive subjects before and after short- and long-term therapy with sodium restriction and antihypertensive medications that operate through different central and peripheral mechanisms. Blood pressure variability in the natural environment also has been well studied with ambulatory monitoring in treated hypertensives, often in close temporal proximity to laboratory testing. In studies of the effects of a wide variety of antihypertensive medications that effectively normalized resting blood pressure levels, there has not been observed any associated change or reduction of cardiovascular reactivity. Moreover, antihypertensive therapy has not been found to diminish ambulatory blood pressure variability in the natural environment of treated subjects (Clement, Bogaert & Pannier, 1977; Dimsdale et al. 1984; Eliasson, Kahan, Hylander & Hjemdahl, 1986; Floras, Phil, Hassan et al., 1986; Francois, Cahen,

Gravejat & Estrade, 1984;Gascon, de Ros, Reig et al., 1988; Kaiser, Hylander, Eliasson & Kaiser, 1985; McAllister, 1979; Reuben, Gale & Blake, 1979; Trap-Jensen, Carlsen, Hartling et al., 1982; Velasco, Romerto, Bertoncini et al., 1976; Virtanen, Janne & Frick, 1982; Weder & Julius, 1985; Weder, Takiyyuiddin, Sekkarie et al., 1987). These and many other studies have consistently found that effective antihypertensive therapy has neither reduced spontaneous fluctuations of blood pressure occuring in the 24 hour cycle or ambulatory blood pressure variablility in natural environments nor diminished laboratory measures of cardiovascular reactivity to mental stress, emotionally stressful situations, static and dynamic exercise, isometric handgrip, cold pressor, Valsalvia maneuver or other stressors. These findings are of increased significance considering that the medications have differeing effects on heart rate, systolic and diastolic blood pressures, blood volume, release and plasma level of catecholamines, reflex SNS stimulation and balance of alpha- and beta-adrenergic tone, and that they lower basal blood pressures by a wide variety of different central and peripheral mechanisms.

It is also important to note that there is little evidence to document a belief that stress reactivity is a predictor of cardiovascular morbidity in hypertensives (Pickering & Devereux, 1987; Wood, Sheps, Elveback & Shrirger, 1986). Nor does variability of the blood pressure appear to be a predictor of structural cardiovascular damage in either hypertensives (Sokolow, Werdeger, Kain & Hinman, 1966) or normotensives (Krantz, Schaeffer, Davia et al., 1981).

It has become clear that blood pressure regulation in hypertension is normal and that cardiovasular reactivity cannot explain either the development of hypertension or the shifting hemodynamic pattern that occurs in the transition from borderline to established hypertension (Julius, 1988). The concept of cardiovascular reactivity may require a change (Rosenman & Ward, 1988) in favour of viewing it as engendered by physiological rather than psychological factors. Stress responses should probably be considered to be homeostatically appropriate rather than as "reactive" and possible pathogenetic.

References

Report by the Management Committee. (1980). Australian therapeutic trial in mild hypertension. *Lancet, 1*, 1261–1269.

Carmelli, D., Chesney, M. A., Ward, M. M., and Rosenman, R. H. (1985). Twin similarity in cardiovascular stress response. *Health Psychology, 4*, 413–423.

Clark, L. A., Denby, L., Pregibon, D., Harshfield, G. A., Pickering, T. G., Blank, S., and Laragh, J. H. (1987). A quantitative analysis of the effects of activity and time of day on the diurnal variations of blood pressure. *Journal of Chronic Disease, 40(7)*, 671–681.

Clarkson, T. B., Manuck, S. B., and Kaplan, J. R. (1986). Potential role of cardiovascular reactivity in atherogenesis. In K. A. Matthews, S. M. Weiss, T. Detre, T. M. Dembroski, B. Falkner, S. B. Manuck, and R. B. Williams (Eds.), *Handbook of stress, reactivity and cardiovascular disease* (pp. 35–47). New York: Wiley.

Clement, D. L., Boegaert, M. G., and Pannier, R. (1977). Effect of beta-adrenergic blockade pressure variation in patients with moderate hypertension. *European Journal of Clinical Pharmacology, 7(11)*, 325–327.

Clement, D. L., Mussche, M. M., Vanhouette, G., and Pannier, R. (1979). Is blood pressure variablility related to activity of the sympathetic system? *Clinical Science, 57*, 217s–219s.

Conway, J., Julius, S., and Amery, A. (1968). Effect of blood pressure level on the hemodynamic response to exercise. *Hypertension, 16*, 79–85.

Cottington, E. M., Matthews, K. A., Talbott, E., and Kuller, L. H. (1986). Occupational stress, suppressed anger, and hypertension. *Psychosomatic Medicine, 48*, 249–257.

Devereux, R. B., Brown, W. T., Lutas, E. M., Kramer-Fox, R., and Laragh, J. H. (1982). Association of mitral valve prolapse with low body-weight and low blood pressure. *Lancet, 2*, 792–795.

Diamond, E. L. (1982). The role of anger and hostility in essential hypertension and coronary heart disease. *Psychological Bulletin, 92*, 410–433.

Dimsdale, J. E., Hartley, L. H., Ruskin, J., Greenblatt, D. J., and LaBrie, R. (1984). Effect of beta-blockade on plasma catecholamine levels during psychological and exercise stress, *American Journal of Cardiology, 54*, 182–185.

Eich, R. H., and Cuddy, R. P. (1966). Hemodynamics in labile hypertension. A follow-up study. *Circulation, 34*, 299–307.

Eich, R. H., and Jacobsen, E. D. (1967). Vascular reactivity in medical students followed for 10 years. *Journal of Chronic Disease, 20*, 583–592.

Eiff, A. W. von, Gogolin, E., Jacobs, U., and Neus, H. (1985). Heart rate activity under mental stress as a predictor of blood pressure development in children. *Journal of Hypertension, 3*, Suppl. 4, 589–591.

Elbert, T., Langosch, W., Steptoe, A., and Vaitl, D. (Eds.). (1988). *Behavioural medicine in cardiovascular disorders*. Avon: Wiley.

Eliasson, K., Hjemdahl, P., and Kahan, T. (1983). Circulatory and sympathoadrenal responses to stress in borderline and established hypertension. *Journal of Hypertension, 1*, 131–139.

Eliasson, K., Kahan, T., Hylander, B., and Hjemdahl, P. (1986). Reactivity to mental stress and cold provocation during long-term treatment with metroprolol, propranolol or hydrochlorothiazide, *Hypertension, 4*, Suppl. 6, 263s–265s.

Eliot, R. (1988). The dynamics of hypertension – an overview: Present practices, new possibilities, and new approaches. *American Heart Journal, 116*, 583–589.

Esler, J., Jennings, G., Korner, P., Willett, I., Dudley, F., Hasking, G., Anderson, W., and Lamberg, G. (1988). Assessment of human sympathetic nervous system activity from measurements of norepinephrine turnover. *Hypertension, 11*, 3–20.

Falkner, B., Gaddo, O., and Angelakos, E. (1981). Effect of salt-loading on the cardiovascular response to stress in adolescents. *Hypertension, 3*, II–195–II–199.

Falkner, B., and Kushner, H. (1981). Cardiovascular characteristics in adolescents who develop essential hypertension. *Hypertension, 3*, 521–527.

Falkner, B., and Light, K. C. (1986). The interactive effects of stress and dietary sodium on cardiovascular reactivity. In K. A. Matthews, S. M. Weiss, T. Detre, T. M. Dembroski, B. Falkner, S. B. Manuck, and R. B. Williams (Eds.), *Handbook of stress, reactivity, and cardiovascular disease* (pp. 329–341). New York: Wiley.

Falkner, B., Onesti, G., and Angelakos, E. T. (1979). Cardiovascular responses to mental stress in normal adolescents with hypertensive parents. *Hypertension, 1*, 23–30.

Fitzgerald, D. J., O'Malley, K., and O'Brien, E. T. (1984). Reproducibility of ambulatory blood pressure recordings. In M. A. Weber and J. I. M. Drayer (Eds.), *Ambulatory blood pressure monitoring* (pp. 71–74). New York: Springer.

Floras, J. S., Hassan, M. O., Jones, J. V., and Sleight, P. (1987). Pressor responses to laboratory stresses and daytime blood pressure variability. *Hypertension, 5*, 715–719.

Floras, J. S., Phil, D., Hassan, M. O., Jones, J. V., and Sleight, P. (1986). Cardioselective and nonselective beta-adrenoceptor blocking drugs in hypertension: A comparison of their effect on blood pressure during mental and physical activity. *Hypertension, 4*, Suppl. 6, 263s–265s.

Francioso, J. A., Johnson, S. M., and Tobian, L. J. (1980). Exercise performance in mildly hypertensive patients. *Chest, 78*, 231–237.

Francis, G. S. (1988). Modulation of peripheral sympathetic nerve transmission. *Journal of American College of Cardiology, 12*, 250–254.

Froncois, R, Cahen, R., Gravejat, M. F. and Estrade, M. (1984). Do beta blockers prevent responses to mental stress and physical exercise? *European Heart Journal, 5*, 348–353.

Frankenhauser, M. (1988). Stress and reactivity patterns at different stages of the life cycle. In P. Pancheri and L. Zichella (Eds.), *Biorhythms and stress in the physiopathology of reproduction* (pp. 31–40). New York: Hemisphere.

Fredrikson, M. (1986a). Behavioral aspects of cardiovascular reactivity in essential hypertension. In T. H. Schmidt, T. M. Dembroski, and G. Blumchen (Eds.), *Biological and psychological factors in cardiovascular disease* (pp. 418–446). New York: Springer.

Fredrikson, M. (1986b). Racial differences in cardiovascular reactivity to mental stress in essential hypertension. *Hypertension, 4*, 325–331.

Friedman, M., Byers, S. O., Diamant, J., and Rosenman, R. H. (1975). Plasma catecholamine response of coronary-prone subjects (Type A) to a specific challenge. *Metabolism, 4*, 205–210.

Friedman, M., St. George, S., Byers, S. O., and Rosenman, R. H. (1960). Excretion of catecholamines, 17-ketosteroids, 17-hydroxindole in men exhibiting a particular behavior pattern (A) associated with high incidence of clinical coronary artery disease. *Journal of Clinical Investigation, 39*, 756–764.

Gascon, J. V. G., de Ros, O., Reig, J., Ferrer, J., Martinez, H. M., Siscar, P. B., and Floras, J. S. (1988). Exercise stress test in young hypertensive patients. response to vasodilators (prazosin) vs. beta-blocker (atenolol) agents. *Clinical Cardiology, 11*, 24–34.

Glass, D. C., and Contrada, R. J. (1984). Type A behavior and catecholamines: A critical review. In M. G. Ziegler and C. R. Lake (Eds), *Norepinephrine: Clinical aspects* (pp. 348–367). Baltimore: Williams & Wilkins.

Glass, D. C., Lake, C. R., Contrada, R. J., Kehoe, K., and Erlanger, L. R. (1983). Stability of individual differences in physiological responses to stress. *Health Psychology, 2*, 317–341.

Goldstein, I. B. (1981). Assessment of hypertension. In C. K. Prokop and L. A. Bradley (Eds), *Medical Psychology : Contributions to Behavioral Medicine* (pp. 38–56). New York: Academic Press.

Grunhaus, L., Glober, S., Birmacher, B., Palmer, C., and Ben-David, M. (1983). Prolactin response to the cold pressor test in patients with panic attacks. *Psychiatry Research, 8*, 171–177.

Harlan, W. R., Osborne, R. K., and Graybiel, A. (1964). Prognostic value of the cold pressor test and the basal blood pressure. *American Journal of Cardiology, 13*, 683–687.

Harrison, D. C. (1985). Beta blockers and exercise: physiologic and biochemical definitions and new concepts. *American Journal of Cardiology, 55*, 29D–33D.

Harshfield, G. A., Pickering, T. G., Yee, L. S., and Marion, R. M. (1985) Does blood pressure predict reactivity under natural conditions? *Psychophysiology, 22*, 594.

Havlik, R. J., and Feinleib, M. (1982). Epidemiology and genetics of hypertension. *Hypertension, 4*, Part II, 121–127.

Herd, J. A. (1986). Neuroendocrine mechanisms in coronary heart disease. In K. A. Matthews, S. M. Weiss, T. Detre, T. M. Dembroski, B. Falkner, S. B. Manuck, and R. B. Williams (Eds.), *Handbook of stress, reactivity, and cardiovascular disease* (pp. 49–70). New York: Wiley.

Hodges, W. F. (1986). Effects of ego threat and threat of pain on state anxiety. *Journal of Personality and Social Psychology, 8*, 364–372.

Holden, A. E., and Barlow, D. H. (1986). Heart rate and heart rate variability recorded in vivo in agoraphobics and nonphobics. *Behavior Therapy, 17*, 26–42.

Holyroyd, K. A., Westbrook, T., Wolf, M., and Badhorn, E. (1978). Performance, cognition, and physiological responding in test anxiety. *Journal of Abnormal Psychology, 87*, 442–451.

Horan, M., Kennedy, H., and Padget, N. (1981). Do borderline hypertensive patients have labile blood pressure? *Annals of Internal Medicine , 94*, 466–468.

Houston, B. K. (1983). Psychophysiological responsivity and the Type A behavior pattern. *Journal of Research in Personality, 17*, 22–39.

James, G. D., Yee, L. S., Harshfield, H. A., Blank, S. G., and Pickering, T. G. (1986). The influence of happiness, anger and anxiety on the blood pressure of borderline hypertensives. *Psychosomatic Medicine, 48*, 502–508.

Jorde, L. B., and Williams, R. B. (1986). Innovative blood pressure measurments yield information not reflected by sitting measurements. *Hypertension, 87*, 252–257.

Julius, S. (1988). The blood pressure seeking properties of the central nervous system. *Hypertension, 6*, 177–185.

Julius, S., and Conway, J. (1986). Hemodynamic studies in patients with borderline blood pressure elevation. *Circulation, 38*, 282–288.

Julius, S., and Ellis, C. N. (1974). Home blood pressure determination: value in borderline ("labile") hypertension. *Journal of American Medical Association, 229*, 663–666.

Julius, S., and Johnson, E. H. (1984). Stress, autonomic hyperactivity and essential hypertension: an enigma. *Journal of Hypertension, 3*, Suppl. 4, 511s–517s.

Julius, S., and Pascual, A. V. (1971). Relationship between cardiac output and peripheral resistance in borderline hypertension. *Circulation, 43*, 382–390.

Julius, S., and Schork, M. A. (1971). Borderline hypertension: a critical review. *Journal of Chronic Disease, 23*, 723–754.

Julius, S., Schneider, R., and Egan, B. (1985). Suppressed anger in hypertension: Facts and problems. In M. A. Chesney and R. H. Rosenman (Eds.), *Anger and hostility in cardiovascular and behavioral disorders* (pp. 127–139). New York: Hemisphere.

Julius, S., Weder, A. B., and Egan, B. M. (1983). Pathophysiology of early hypertension: implication for epidemiologic research. In F. Gross and T. Strassers (Eds.), *Mild hypertension: recent advances* (pp. 219–236). New York: Raven Press.

Julius, S., Weder, A. B., and Hinderliter, A. L. (1986). Does behaviorally induced blood pressure variability lead to hypertension? In K. A. Matthews, S. M. Weiss, T. Detre, T. M. Dembroski, B. Falkner, S. B. Manuck, and R. B. Williams (Eds.), *Handbook of stress, reactivity, and cardiovascular disease* (pp. 71–82). New York: Wiley.

Kahn, H. A., Medalie, J. H., Neufeld, H. N., Riss, E., and Goldbourt, V. (1972). The incidence of hypertension and associated factors: The Israeli ischemic heart disease study. *American Heart Journal, 84*, 171–182.

Kaiser, P., Hylander, B., Eliasson, K., and Kaiser, L. (1985). Effect of beat-1 selective and nonselective beta-blockade on blood pressure relative to physcial performance in men with systemic hypertension. *American Journal of Cardiology, 55*, 79D–84D.

Kannel, W., Sorlie, P., and Gordon, T. (1980). Labile hypertension: A faulty concept: The Framingham Study. *Circulation, 61*, 1183–1187.

Kelly, D., Mitchell-Heggs, N., and Sherman, D (1971). Anxiety and the effects of sodium lactate assessed clinically and physiologically. *British Journal of Psychiatry, 119*, 129–141.

Klorman, R., Wiesenfeld, A. R., and Austin, M. L. (1975). Autonomic responses to affective visual stimuli. *Psychophysiology, 12*, 553–560.

Knight, M. L., and Borden, R. J. (1979). Autonomic and affective reactions of high and low socially-anxious individuals awaiting public performance. *Psychophysiology, 16*, 209–213.

Krantz, D. S., and Manuck, S. B. (1984). Acute psychophysiologic reactivity and risk of cardiovascular disease: A review and methodology critique. *Psychological Bulletin, 96*, 435–464.

Krantz, D. S., Menkes, M. S., Lundberg, U., Matthews, K. A., Mead, L. A., Liang, K. Y. Thomas, C. B., and Pearson, T. A. (1988). Cardiovascular reactivity to the cold pressor and prediction of subsequent hypertension. (Abstract). *Psychosomatic Medicine, 50*, 192–193.

Krantz, D. S., Schaeffer, M. A., Davia, J. E., Demonski, T. M., MacDougall, J. M., and Shaffer, R. T. (1981). Extent of coronary atherosclerosis, Type A behavior and cardiovascular response to social interaction. *Psychophysiology, 18*, 654–664.

Lazarus, R. S. (1988). Psychological stress and coping in adaptation and illness. *International Journal of Medicine, 5*, 321–333.

Light, K. C. (1981). Cardiovascular responses to effortful active coping: Implications for the role of stress in hypertension development. *Psychology, 18*, 216–225.

Light, K. C., Koepke, J. P, Obrist, P. A., and Willis, P. W. (1983)). Psychological stress induces soidum and fluid retention in men at high risk for hypertension. *Science, 220*, 429–431.

Light K. C. and Obrist, P. A. (1980). Cardiovascular reactivity to behavioral stress in young males with and without marginallly elevated casual systolic pressures. Comparison of clinic, home, and laboratory measurements. *Hypertension, 2*, 802–808.

Lund-Johansen, P. (1967). Hemodynamics in early essential hypertension. *Acta Medica Scandinavica, 482*, 1–105.

Lund-Johnsen, P. (:1984). Hemodynamic concepts in essential hypertension. *Triangle, 23*, 13–23.

Mancia, G., and Ferrar, A. (1983). Blood pressure and heart rate variabilities in normotensive and hypertension human beings. *Circulation Research, 53*, 96–104.

Mantysaari, M. J., Antila, K. J., and Peltonen, T. E. (1988). Blood pressure reactivity in patients with neurocirculatory asthenia. *American Journal of Hypertension, 1*, 132–139.

Manuck, S. B., and Krantz, D.S. (1986). Psychophysiologic reactivity in coronary heart disease and essential hypertension. In K. A. Mathews, S. M. Weiss, T. Detre, T. M. Dembroski, B. Falkner, B. S. Manuck, and R. B. Williams (Eds.), *Handbook of stress, reactivity, and cardiovascular disease* (pp. 11–34). New York: Wiley.

Matthews, K. A., Rabaczky, C. J., Stoney, C. M., and Manuck, S. B. (1987). Are cardiovascular responses to behavioral stressors a stable individual difference variable in childhood? *Psychophysiology, 24*, 464–473.

Matthews, K. A., Weiss, S. M., Detre, T, Dembroski, T. M., Falkner, B., Manuck, B. S., and Williams, R. B. (Eds.). (1986). *Handbook of stress, reactivity, and cardiovascular disease*. New York: Wiley.

Matthews, K. (1982). Psychological perspectives on the Type A behavior pattern. *Psychological Bulletin, 91*, 293–323.

McAllister, B. B. (1979). Effect of adrenergic receptor blockage on the responses to isometric handgrip: studies in normal and hypertensive subjects. *Journal of Cardiovascular Pharmacology, 1*, 253–263.

McClelland, D. C. (1979). Inhibited power motivation and high blood pressure. *Journal of Abnormal Psychology, 88*, 182–190.

Messerli, F., and Glade, L. (1982). Diurnal variation of cardiac rhythm, arterial pressure, and urinary catecholamines in borderline and established essential hypertension. *American Heart Journal, 104*, 109–114.

Myers, H. F., Morell, M. A., Shapiro, D., Goldstein, J., Armstrong, M., and Drew, C. R. (1985). Biobehavioral stress reactivity in black and white normotensives. *Psychophysiology, 22*, 605–606.

Nesse, R. M., Cameron, O. G., Curtis, G. C., McGann, D. S., and Huber-Smith, M. J. (1984). Adrenergic function in patients with panic anxiety. *Archives of General Psychiatry, 41*, 771–776.

Nestel, P. J. (1969). Blood pressure and catecholamine excretion after mental stress in labile hypertension. *Lancet, 1*, 692–694.

Obrist, P. A., Langer, A. W., Grignolo, A., Light, K. C., Hastrup, L. McCubbin, J. A., Koepke, J. P., and Pollack, M. H. (1983). Behavioral-cardiac interactions in hypertension. In D. S. Krantz, A. Baum, and J. E. Singer (Eds.), *Handbook of Psychology and Health* (pp. 199–231). Hillsdale: Erlbaum.

Orlebeke, J. F., and Van Doornen, L. J. P. (1977). Preception (UCR dimonution) in normal and neurotic subjects. *Biological Psychology, 5*, 15–22.

Pickering, T. G., Harshfield, G. A., and Kleinert, H. D. (1984). Comparison of blood pressure during normal daily activities, sleep and exercise in normal and hypertensive subjects. *Journal of American Medical Association, 147*, 922–926.

Pickering, T. G., and Devereux, R. B. (1987). Ambulatory monitoring of blood pressure as a predictor of cardiovascular risk. *American Heart Journal, 114*, 925–928.

Reis, D. J., and LeDoux, J. E. (1987). Some central neural mechanisms governing resting and behaviorally coupled control of blood pressure. *Circulation, 76*, Suppl., 1–9.

Reuben, S. R., Gale, E. V., and Blake, P. (1979). The effects of alpha- and beta-adrenergic receptor blockers on the pressure responses to isometric exercise in hypertensive patients. *British Journal of Clinical Pharmacology, 8*, 365–368.

Rose, R. J. (1986). Familial influences on cardiovascular reactivity to stress. In K. A. Matthews, S. M. Weiss, T. Detre, T. M. Dembroski, B. Falkner, B. S. Manuck, and R. B.Williams (Eds.), *Handbook of stress, reactivity, and cardiovascular disease* (pp. 260–272). New York: Wiley.

Rosenman, R. H. (1985). Health consequences of anger and implications for treatment. In M. A. Chesney and R. H. Rosenman (Eds.), *Anger and hostility in cardiovascular and behavioral disorders* (pp. 103–127). New York: Hemisphere.

Rosenman, R. H. (1987). Type A behavior and hypertension. In S. Julius and D. R. Bassett (Eds), *Handbook of hypertension: Behavioral factors in hypertension* (pp. 141–149). Amsterdam: Elsevier.

Rosenman, R. H. (1990). Pathogenesis of the relationship of anxiety to mitral valve prolapse. In D. G. Byrne and R. H. Rosenman (Eds.), *Anxiety and the heart*. Washington, D. C: Hemisphere.

Rosenman, R. H., and Chesney, M. A. (1982). Stress, Type A behavior, and coronary disease. In L. Goldberger and S. Breznitz (Eds.), *Handbook of stress* (pp. 547–566). New York: Macmillan.

Rosenman, R. H. and Ward, M. W (1988). The changing concept of cardiovascular reactivity. *Stress Medicine, 4*, 241–251.

Roth, W. T., Teich, M. J., Taylor, C. B., Sachitamo, J. A., Gallen, C. C., Kopell, M. L., McClenahan, K. L., Agras, S., and Pfefferbaum, A. (1986). Autonomic characteristics of agoraphobia with panic attacks. *Biological Psychiatry, 21*, 1133–1154.

Rüddel, H. (1985). The effects of antihypertensive medication and its withdrawal on psychophysiological examinations. In A. Steptoe, H. Rüddel, and H. Neus (Eds.), *Clinical and methodiological issues in cardiovascular psychophysiology* (pp. 127–130). Heidelberg: Springer.

Sannerstedt, R. (1966). Hemodynamic response to exercise in patients with arterial hypertension. *Acta Medica Scandinavica, 458*, Suppl., 1–83.

Sannerstedt, R., Julius, S., and Conway, J. (1970). Hemodynamic response to tilt with beta-adrenergic blockade in young patients with borderline hypertension. *Circulation, 42*, 1057–1064.

Sannerstedt R., and Julius, S. (1972). Systemic hemodynamics in borderline arterial hypertension. response to static exercise before and under the influence of propranolol. *Cardiovascular Research, 6*, 398–403.

Schiffer, F., Hartley, L. H., Schuman, C. L., and Abelman, W. H. (1976). The quiz electrocardiogram. A new diagnostic and research technique for evaluating the relation between emotional stress and ischemic heart disease. *American Journal of Cardiology, 37*, 41–47.

Schneider, R. H., Egan, B. B., Johnson, E. H., Drobny, H., and Julius, S. (1986). Anger and anxiety in borderline hypertension. *Psychosomatic Medicine, 48*, 242–249.

Schneiderman, N. (1983). Behavior, autonomic function and animal models of cardiovascular psychology. In T. M. Dembroski, T. H. Schmidt, and G. Blumchen (Eds.), *Biobehavioral bases of coronary disease* (pp. 304–364). Basel: Karger.

Schrager, B. R., and Ellestad, M. (1983). The importance of blood pressure measurement during exercise testing. *Cardiovascular Reviews & Reports, 4*, 381–386.

Smith, T. W. Houston, B. K., and Zurawski, R. M. (1984). Irrational beliefs and the arousal of emotional distress. *Journal of Counseling Psychology, 31*, 190–201.

Sokolow, M., Werdegar, D., Kain, H. K., and Hinman, A. T. (1966). Relationship between level of blood pressure measured casually and by portable recorders and severity of complications in essential hypertension. *Circulation, 34*, 297–298.

Steptoe, A., Melville, D., and Ross, A. (1984). Behavioral response demands, cardiovascular reactivity, and essential hypertension. *Psychosomatic Medicine, 46*, 33–48.

Steptoe, A., Rüddel, H., and Neus, H. (Eds.). (1985). *Clinical and methodoligical issues in cardiovascular psychophysiology*. Heidelberg: Springer.

Sullivan, P., Schoentgen, S., DeQuattro, V., Procci, W., Levine, D., Van der Meulen, J., Bornheimer, J. (1981). Anxiety, anger and neurogenic tone at rest and in stress in patients with primary hypertension. *Hypertension, 3*, Suppl. II, 119–123.

Taylor, C. B., Sheikh, J., Agras, W. S., Roth, W. T., Margraf, J., Ehlers, D., Maddock, R. J., and Grossard, D. (1986). Ambulatory heart rate changes in patients with panic attacks. *American Journal of Psychiatry, 143*, 478–482.

Thomas, C. B., and Duszynski, K. R. (1982). Blood pressure levels in young adulthood as predictors of hypertension and the fate of the cold pressor test. *John Hopkins Medical Journal, 151*, 93–100.

Trap-Jensen, J., Carlsen, J. E., Hartling, O. J., Svendsen, T. L., Tango, M., and Christensen, N. J. (1982). B-adrenoceptor blockade and psychic stress in man. A comparison of the acute effects of labetalol, metoprolol, pindolol, and propranolol on plasma levels of adrenaline and noradrenaline. *British Journal of Clinical Pharmacology, 13*, 391s–395s.

Turner, S. M., Beidel, D. C., and Larkin, K. T. (1986). Situational determinants of social anxiety in clinic and non-clinical samples: Physiological and cognitive correlates. *Journal of Consulting and Clinical Psychology, 54*, 523–527.

Velasco, M., Romerto, E., Bertoncini, H., Urbina-Quitana, A., Guevara, J., and Hernandez-Pieretti, O. (1976). Effect of propranolol on sympathetic nervous activity in hydrallazine-treated hypertensive patients. *British Journal of Clinical Pharmacology, 6*, 217–220.

Virtanen, K., Janne, J., and Frick, M. H. (1982). Response of blood pressure and plasma norepinephrine to propranolol, metroprolol and clonidine during isometric and dynamic exercise in hypertensive patients. *European Journal of Clinical Pharmacology, 21*, 275–279.

Ward, M. M., Mefford, I. N., Parker, S. D., Chesney, M. A., Taylor, C. B., Keegan, D. L., and Barchas, J. D. (1988). Epinephrine and norepinephrine responses in continuously collected human plasma to a series of stressors. *Psychosomatic Medicine, 45*, 471–487.

Weber, M. A., and Drayer, J. I. M. (1986). Role of blood pressure monitoring in the diagnosis of hypertension. *Journal of Hypertension, 4*, S325–S327.

Weber, A. B., and Julius, S. (1985). Behavior, blood pressure variability and hypertension. *Psychosomatic Medicine, 47*, 406–414.

Weber, A. B., Takiyyuiddin, M., Sekkarie, M. A., Schork, N. J., and Julius, S. (1987). *Lack of control of cardiovascular reactivity during antihypertensive therapy with clonidine and atenolol.* Presented at Conference on Catapres-TTS, Tucson, AZ, May 28–31, 1987.

Weiss, Y. A., and Safar, M. E. (1978). Repeat hemodynamic determinations in borderline hypertension. *American Journal of Medicine, 64*, 382–388.

Wing, L. (1964). Physiological effects of performing a difficult task in patients with anxiety states. *Journal of Psychosomatic Research, 76*, 283–294.

Wood, D. I., Sheps, S. G., Elveback, L. R., and Schirger, A. (1986). Cold pressor test as a predictor of hypertension. *Hypertension, 6*, 301–306.

Woods, S. W., Charney, D. S., McPherson, C. A., Gradman, R. J., and Grossard, D. (1987). Situational panic attacks. *Archives of General Psychiatry, 44*, 365–375.

Approach-Avoidance and Illness Behavior in Coronary Heart Patients

Stan Maes and Eline Bruggemans

Introduction

The recent literature with respect to coping with the stresses of illness refers to two basic modes of coping: approach and avoidance (Roth & Cohen, 1986; Suls & Fletcher, 1985). These concepts are not new since they have been used under different labels for more than 25 years to describe coping in different groups of patients. Some of the terms used are, for example, sensitization-repression (Byrne, 1961), vigilant focussing-minimization (Lipowsky, 1970), non-denial-denial (Croog et al., 1971; Gentry et al., 1972; Stern et al., 1976), vigilance-avoidance (Cohen & Lazarus, 1973), monitoring-blunting (Miller, 1980), attention-rejection (Mullen & Suls, 1982), and monitoring-distraction (Leventhal et al., 1984). The approach dimension refers to a tendency to approach, focus upon, or even maximize the significance of the stressful event. The avoidance dimension, on the other hand, refers to a tendency to avoid, ignore, deny, or minimize the significance of the threat.

Mullen and Suls (1982) and Suls and Fletcher (1985) reported the results of a series of meta-analyses to document the relative effectiveness of approach and avoidance strategies in coping with stressful events. They divided studies into those with short-term and those with long-term outcomes. In general, avoidance strategies were associated with more positive adaptation in the short-term, while approach strategies were associated with more long-term positive outcomes. This conclusion is consistent with Lazarus' (1983) point of view, and may suggest that shortly after confrontation with a stressor avoidance strategies are more efficient than approach strategies, since an individual needs time to adapt to (or accept) the stressor before he can mobilize available resources in order to adequately cope in a more confrontive, problem-focussed way.

Where approach and avoidance seem to be useful concepts to describe adjustment to stressful events (including the stresses of illness) in general, one could ask whether they are relevant for patients with coronary heart disease. While there are virtually no studies on the effectiveness of the approach strategy, there are several studies in the literature which relate the avoidance strategy to illness behavior in coronary patients. Croog et al. (1971) were among the first to study the effects of denial in male coronary patients. The most relevant association between denial and illness behavior in this study was the tendency for deniers to resist medical advice related to work, rest and smoking one month after myocardial infarction. In addition, deniers reported fewer symptoms than non-deniers. A follow-up study, one year later, suggests that for many of the initial deniers this strategy became a long-term mode of coping. Gentry et al. (1972) investigated the role of denial as a determinant of anxiety and perceived health status in a Coronary Care Unit (CCU). Results indicated that patients with myocardial infarction who deny their illness experience less anxiety than non-denying patients, but have a less realistic perceived health status. Levenson et al. (1984) found that unstable angina patients in the CCU who were identified as deniers became medically stabilized twice as quickly as non-deniers. Levine et al. (1987) investigated the relationship between denial and recovery in coronary patients. They found that strong deniers spent fewer days in the CCU and had fewer signs of cardiac dysfunction during their hospitalization compared to weak deniers. In contrast, in the year following discharge, strong deniers were less compliant with medical recommendations and were rehospitalized more often than weak deniers.

To some extent these studies are in line with the results of the meta-analyses of Mullen and Suls (1982) and Suls and Fletcher (1985), and with the widely-accepted clinical opinion that denial can be regarded as an adaptive coping strategy during the first days following acute myocardial infarction, but is less adaptive at later stages of the illness (Soloff, 1978). Although this conclusion seems to apply in general, two remarks must be made. First, the results may depend largely on the types of outcome behavior studied, as at least one study demonstrates that denial may have beneficial effects on return to work (Stern et al., 1976). Second, other studies by Stern et al. (1977); Dimsdale and Hackett (1982); and Shaw et al. (1985) did not find any significant relationship between denial and medical outcome in coronary patients after hospital discharge.

The fact that not all evidence points in the same direction may be due to the different ways in which approach and avoidance were measured in the existing studies (Shaw et al., 1985; Levine et al., 1987). A major remark with regard to the existing measures is related to the fact that the avoidance strategy received the most attention: most measures differentiate deniers or repressors from non-deniers or non-repressors. The best-known example is the Hackett and Cassem (H-C) Denial Scale (Hackett & Cassem, 1974), a quantitative rating-scale which has been used in several studies carried out with coronary patients (e.g. Stern et al., 1977; Dimsdale & Hackett, 1982; Levenson et al., 1984). Similar assessment procedures have been used in two recent studies in coronary patients. Shaw et al. (1985) used a modification of the H-C Denial Scale and the H-C Denial Scale was the starting point for the development of the Levine Denial of Illness Scale (Levine et al., 1987). Another way to identify repressors is by means of the procedure introduced by Weinberger et al. (1979). This combines low and high anxiety as measured by the Taylor Manifest Anxiety Scale with low and high defensiveness as measured by the Marlowe Crowne Social Desirability Scale. Repressors are considered to score low on anxiety and high on defensiveness, while non-repressors are those who score low on defensiveness and low or high on anxiety (Van Heck, 1981). However, it seems impossible to characterize all the patients involved in a specific study in terms of repressors or non-repressors by means of this procedure, as was illustrated in an unpublished study by Chatrou and Maes (1984).

In conclusion, virtually all studies carried out with coronary patients focus on the avoidance strategy, thus neglecting the possible effects of approach. There are, however, studies outside the domain of coronary heart disease in which both coping aspects were measured. The most commonly-used measure to assess both approach and avoidance is the Byrne Repression-Sensitization Scale (Byrne, 1961). Although the idea is sound, this scale has received severe criticism because of its uni-dimensionality and because it correlates 0.80 or higher with anxiety scales (Van Heck, 1981; Shaw et al. 1985). As a consequence, the scale must be considered an anxiety measure rather than a valid coping measure. A more recent attempt to differentiate between approach and avoidance is the Miller Behavioural Style Scale (MBSS) (Miller, 1987). This scale measures monitoring and blunting by means of reaction statements related to four hypothetical stress-evoking scenes and has been used by Miller and associates in several studies (Miller & Mangan, 1983; Miller & Brody, 1985; Miller et al., 1985). The reason why the MBSS is not widely used may be due to the fact that it only measures a specific form of approach and avoidance, i.e. information-seeking versus information-avoidance, and that the situations or scenes included in it lack validity for various patient populations. The new, more sophisticated version of the Ways of Coping Checklist (WCC) also includes approach- and avoidance-like coping scales (Folkman et al., 1986). However, like the older version of the WCC, this measure assesses coping in general at a relatively micro-analytic level. In other words, the WCC aims at assessing specific forms of coping with 'general problems', which is exactly the opposite of what we are interested in, i.e. trying to assess basic forms of coping with specific stresses of illness. In conclusion, the existing measures for assessing approach and avoidance have not been specifically designed to assess coping with a specific disease.

An Approach-Avoidance Questionnaire for Coronary Patients

In order to achieve our objective of assessing how patients with coronary heart disease cope with the specific stresses of their illness, we developed a new questionnaire (Coping Questionnaire for Coronary Patients). In the development of this questionnaire we initially looked for situations which are relevant for coronary patients. Although many situations could be imagined, a too-detailed level of situation specificity would have affected the applicability of the questionnaire. Therefore, with the WHO's definition of health ("health is a state of complete physical, psychological and social well-being") in mind, we decided to operationalize situation specificity in terms of three different problem domains: (1) a medical problem situation, (2) a psychological problem situation, and (3) a social problem situation. More specifically, we asked patients: (1) how they behave when experiencing cardiac complaints, (2) how they behave when worrying about their heart, and (3) how they behave when their environment treats them as a patient. Each of these three problem situations was represented by 54 statements depicting possible ways of coping with the situation. The statements were selected on the basis of a comprehensive and critical review of the literature (Matheny et al., 1986) and practical experience with coronary patients. Each statement had to be rated on a 4 point scale, ranging from 'hardly ever' to 'almost always'. As we considered approach and avoidance basic modes of coping, we conducted a forced two-factor analysis for each of the three problem situations, the results of which are described below.

Subjects

The Coping Questionnaire for Coronary Patients was obtained from 174 coronary patients who participated in a research project supported by the Dutch Heart Foundation. In this study, patients completed several self-report questionnaires. They also participated in a semi-structured clinical interview. Patients were recruited after they had participated in a rehabilitation program. Most patients had suffered from one or more myocardial infarctions (71%), some patients had undergone coronary bypass surgery (9%), and some had suffered from myocardial infarction and undergone surgery (20%). The average time since the (last) cardiac incident was 5 years, ranging from 0 to 15 years. The average age of the patients was 57 years, with a range of 38 to 71 years. Ninety-three percent of the patients were males.

Scale Construction

For each of the three problem situations, a principal components analysis was carried out followed by an oblique rotation. In order to allow for analysis of the coping strategies according to a simple dichotomy, we used a two-factor solution.

Examination of the results of the two-factor solution indicated that, for each situation, one factor was predominantly approach-oriented and the other predominantly avoidance-oriented. Many of the items in the approach-oriented factor were directed toward the stressful situation. Representative items include: focussing on the problems, self-blame, and pessimism. Many of the items of the avoidance-oriented factor were directed away from the threat. Examples include items which represent withdrawal, distraction, active forgetting, and use of humour. We believe that these results show clear support for the dichotomous classification of coping strategies in terms of approach and avoidance.

On the basis of these results, we constructed two scales for each problem situation: an approach-oriented scale and an avoidance-oriented scale. The scale construction included two steps. First, the selection of items that loaded more than 0.35 on a factor, and second, the selection of the 8 highest loading items per factor.

Reliability Assessment

In order to assess the internal stability of the approach and avoidance scales we calculated Cronbach's alpha coefficient.

Table 1 *Cronbach's alpha coefficients for approach and avoidance scales*

problem situation	approach scale	avoidance scale
medical	0.78	0.84
psychological	0.87	0.79
social	0.79	0.83

As one can see in Table 1, all scales reveal rather strong internal consistency with coefficients ranging from 0.78 to 0.87.

Intercorrelations

The correlations between the situation specific approach and avoidance scales are shown in Table 2.

Table 2 *Intercorrelations between approach and avoidance scales(M=medical situation, P=psychological situation, S=social situation, Ap=approach, and Av=avoidance)*

	M-Ap	P-Ap	S-Ap	M-Av	P-Av	S-Av
M-Ap						
P- Ap	0.56***					
S- Ap	0.52***	0.76***				
M-Av	−0.16*	−0.33***	−0.27***			
P- Av	−0.02	−0.21**	−0.07	0.41***		
S- Av	−0.15*	−0.30***	−0.18**	0.38***	0.50***	

*$p<0.05$ **$p<0.01$ ***$p<0.001$ (one-tailed probabilities)

The intercorrelations between the three approach scales show a consistent pattern of moderate, positive values. This is also true for the three avoidance scales. On the other hand, the correlations between the approach and avoidance scales show a pattern of negative or non-significant correlations.

These data suggest that the scales of the Coping Questionnaire for Coronary Patients have a promising potential for measuring the two coping dimensions. As a consequence, we became interested in the possible relationship between approach and avoidance coping strategies and several other personality and behavioral variables in patients with coronary heart disease. In our study we administered the questionnaire along with a number of well-being measures, among which were: the trait version of the Dutch State-Trait Anxiety Inventory (Van der Ploeg et al., 1981) measuring anxiety, the trait version of the Dutch Depression Adjective Checklist (Van Rooijen, 1977) measuring depression, the trait version of the Dutch State-Trait Anger Scales (Van der Ploeg et al., 1982) measuring anger, and the Medical Psychological Questionnaire for Heart Patients (Erdman, 1982), which measures displeasure, feelings of invalidity, social inhibition, and well-being. By means of a semi-structured clinical interview in the presence of the spouse, we also collected data concerning stress-related health habits, e.g. the number of cigarettes and alcoholic drinks consumed daily. In addition, we collected data on the use of medical resources during this interview, e.g. the number of visits to a general practitioner or cardiologist during the last year and the amount of medicines used. Other interview questions pertained to employment status and angina pectoris symptoms.

Hypotheses

The following predictions were made:
1. Approach will be associated with a lower degree of well-being and avoidance with a higher degree of well-being. (Therefore, a positive correlation will be expected between approach and anxiety, depression, anger, displeasure, feelings of invalidity, and social inhibition and, conversely, a negative correlation between approach and well-being. On the other hand, a negative correlation will be expected between avoidance and anxiety, depression, anger, displeasure, feelings of invalidity, and social inhibition and, conversely, a positive correlation between avoidance and well-being).

2. Approach will be associated with more negative stress-related health habits and avoidance with fewer negative stress-related health habits. (Therefore, a positive correlation will be expected between approach and the number of cigarettes and alcoholic drinks consumed per day, and a negative correlation between avoidance and these consumption variables).
3. Approach will be associated with higher use of medical resources and avoidance with lower use of medical resources. (This will imply a positive correlation between approach and the number of visits to general practitioner or cardiologist during the last year and the amount of medicines used. In contrast, a negative correlation will be expected between avoidance and these medical consumption variables).
4. Patients who are employed will score lower on the approach scales and higher on the avoidance scales than patients who are unemployed.
5. Patients with angina pectoris symptoms will score higher on the approach scales and lower on the avoidance scales than patients without symptoms.

Results

The correlations between the situation-specific approach and avoidance scales and the well-being measures are shown in Table 3. All approach scales correlate positively with anxiety, depression, anger, displeasure, feelings of invalidity, and social inhibition, and negatively with well-being. Avoidance scales, however, show the reverse pattern.

As you can see in Table 4, approach is generally associated with more cigarettes, more visits to both general practitioner and cardiologist, and the use of more medicines, while avoidance is generally associated with fewer visits.

Table 5 indicates that patients who were unemployed scored generally higher on the approach scales than patients who were employed. For avoidance, although all values were in the expected direction, only one significant difference between the patient groups was found.

Table 3 *Correlations between approach and avoidance scales (M=medical situation, P=psychological situation, S=social situation, Ap=approach, and Av=avoidance) and well-being measures*

	anxiety	depres-sion	anger	displea-sure	invali-dity	social inhibi-tion	well-being
M-Ap	0.39***	0.32***	0.29***	0.44***	0.40***	0.06	−0.32***
P- Ap	0.53***	0.60***	0.25***	0.57***	0.41***	0.15*	−0.49***
S- Ap	0.50***	0.57***	0.28***	0.51***	0.46***	0.12	−0.44***
M-Av	−0.27***	−0.34***	−0.12	−0.31***	−0.18**	−0.12	0.27***
P- Av	−0.30***	−0.25***	−0.23**	−0.25***	−0.07	−0.22**	0.23**
S- Av	−0.40***	−0.35***	−0.17*	−0.34***	−0.22**	−0.23**	0.32***

*p<0.05 **p≤0.01 ***p≤0.001 (one-tailed probabilities)

Table 4 *Correlations between approach and avoidance scales (M=medical situation, P=psychological situation, S=social situation, Ap=approach, and Av=avoidance) and health behavior and use of medical resources*

	cigarettes per day	alcoholic drinks per day	visits general practioner	visits cardiologist	number of medicines used
M-Ap	0.23***	0.06	0.21**	0.16*	0.04
P- Ap	0.13	−0.11	0.24***	0.20**	0.25***
S- Ap	0.14*	−0.08	0.24***	0.19**	0.25***
M-Av	−0.06	0.09	−0.16*	−0.21**	−0.04
P- Av	−0.02	−0.02	−0.13	−0.12	0.02
S- Av	−0.04	0.04	−0.20**	−0.16*	−0.12

*p‹0.05 **p‹0.01 ***p≤0.001 (one-tailed probabilities)

Table 5 *t-tests on approach and avoidance scales (M=medical situation, P=psychological situation, S=social situation, Ap=approach, Av=avoidance) between patients with (n=49) and without (n=117) employment*

	mean		t
	patient group employed	unemployed	
M-Ap	11.71	13.23	2.41**
P- Ap	10.59	13.73	4.68***
S- Ap	12.02	14.15	3.21***
M-Av	24.61	23.80	−0.88
P- Av	19.52	21.32	2.02
S- Av	23.83	22.08	−1.93*

*p‹0.05 **p‹0.01 ***p≤0.001 (one-tailed probabilities)

Table 6 *t-tests on approach and avoidance scales (M=medical situation, P=psychological situation, S=social situation, Ap=approach, and Av=avoidance) between patients with (n=79) and without (n=87) angina pectoris symptoms*

	mean		t
	patient group with symptoms	without symptoms	
M-Ap	13.22	12.39	−1.33
P- Ap	13.73	11.95	−2.26*
S-Ap	14.41	12.71	−2.49**
M-Av	24.14	23.95	−0.22
P- Av	19.90	21.63	2.16*
S- Av	21.48	23.60	2.42**

*p‹0.05 **p‹0.01 (one-tailed probabilities)

Table 6 indicates that patients who did not have angina pectoris symptoms scored generally lower on the approach scales than patients with angina. For avoidance, significant differences between the patient groups were found in the reverse direction.

Discussion

This study suggests that the constructed approach and avoidance scales have many of the predicted relationships with well-being, stress-related health habits, use of medical resources, employment status, and the presence of angina pectoris symptoms in patients with coronary heart disease. As predicted, the approach scales correlated positively with anxiety, depression, anger, displeasure, feelings of invalidity and social inhibition, and negatively with well-being. The avoidance scales showed the reverse pattern. These findings are in agreement with existing empirical data, which consistently show that avoidance can be considered as a well-being strategy, while more vigilant forms of coping with illness can negatively affect well-being (Roth & Cohen, 1986; Suls & Fletcher, 1985).

As far as health behaviors are concerned, we only have data on cigarette and alcohol consumption. While significant positive correlations were found between the approach scales and cigarette consumption, no significant correlations exist between the avoidance scales and cigarette consumption. Alcohol consumption is neither significantly related to approach nor avoidance. Although the relationship between approach and cigarette consumption confirms our expectation, this finding needs at least a short comment. In fact two rival hypotheses can be formulated about the relationship between approach and avoidance on the one hand, and cigarette and alcohol consumption on the other. In our opinion, use of cigarettes and alcohol can be seen as forms of regulation of distress. As higher levels of distress are associated with approach-like forms of coping, we predicted a higher level of cigarette and alcohol consumption to be associated with the approach scales. However, one may also consider cigarette and alcohol consumption as behaviors which are opposed to medical recommendations. As other studies have shown that avoidance is related to non-compliance with medical recommendations (Croog et al., 1971; Levine et al., 1987), one could argue that avoidance should be associated with higher levels of cigarette and alcohol consumption.

Several significant positive correlations were found between the approach scales and the number of visits to both general practitioner and cardiologist during the last year, as well as the amount of medicines taken. As predicted, these findings illustrate that approach-like strategies result in a more intensive use of medical resources. The results for the avoidance scales confirm this pattern, since the significant correlations between the avoidance scales and the use of medical resources are in the opposite direction. Whether increased or decreased use of medical resources is good or bad is, however, a very different question. Apart from economical aspects, the answer depends on the reason for visiting a physician or taking medicines.

We reasoned that approach strategies would lead to an aggravation of the existing health problems and would , therefore, be found more frequently in the unemployed than the employed, and that avoidance strategies would show the reverse pattern. Although the hypothesis was confirmed for all the approach strategies, only one significant difference between the avoidance scales and employment was in the expected direction. These findings may reflect some controversial findings in the literature, since at least one study found detrimental (Croog et al., 1971) and another one beneficial effects (Stern et al., 1976) of denial on employment. Because many factors can influence employment (e.g. disease characteristics, occupation, age, sex), we plan to inspect our data further in order to formulate more specific hypotheses for a future study.

Last but not least, we compared patients with and without angina pectoris symptoms. As patients experiencing angina complaints are more frequently reminded of their illness, we hypothesized that these patients would be more likely to use approach-like (and less avoidance-like) coping strategies than patients not suffering from angina pectoris. This hypothesis was confirmed, which may reveal that specific medical characteristics of patients should be taken into account when studying the effects of coping with a specific illness. Many other disease characteristics may also influence possible relationships between modes of coping and outcome variables, e. g. having suffered from a myocardial infarction or not, the severity of the myocardial infarction, having undergone coronary bypass surgery or not, the frequency of myocardial infarctions or surgery, and the time elapsed since the cardiac accident.

This last aspect deserves careful consideration. On average the patients included in our study were investigated about 5 years after the last cardiac incident, the implication being that this study deals with relationships between approach and avoidance strategies and outcome variables in the long-term. It is quite imaginable that approach and avoidance strategies have other relationships with the variables under study at other stages of the illness, for example in the period when cardiac symptoms are initially experienced, but medical help has not yet been invoked, or in the period immediately after a heart attack (see also Suls & Fletcher, 1985). Future studies should, therefore, try to relate approach and avoidance strategies to the outcome variables during different stages of the illness.

Although these data suggest that approach and avoidance may be considered basic modes of coping in patients with coronary heart disease, there are also other basic modes of coping which can be taken into account when studying coping behavior in clinical populations. The most important among these is the difference between problem-oriented and emotion-oriented coping and the difference between cognitive and behavioral coping. Problem-oriented coping implies that the coping response is directed at the problem itself, while in the case of emotion-oriented coping, the coping response is oriented toward the emotional consequences of the stressor (Lazarus & Folkman, 1984). Cognitive coping aims at influencing the appraisal of a stressful event or its consequences, while behavioral coping implies undertaking action. Billings and Moos (1981) and Feuerstein and associates (1986) presented a framework which integrates these three modes of coping as illustrated in Table 7.

Table 7 makes clear that, if one looks at illness behavior from an approach and avoidance perspective only, other important aspects may be neglected. In other words, the relationship of approach strategies with relevant outcome variables may, for example, differ if an approach strategy is directed towards the problem itself or towards the emotional consequences. The same applies to the nature of the coping behavior (cognitive versus behavioral). In our current research we are trying to differentiate between various approach and avoidance strategies starting from these distinctions. We think that at least some of the contradictory results in the existing

Table 7 *Classification of coping responses (Billings & Moos, 1981; Feuerstein et al., 1986; Matheny et al., 1986)*

focus	method	
	approach	avoidance
problem-oriented	cognitive or behavioral	cognitive or behavioral
emotion-oriented	cognitive or behavioral	cognitive or behavioral

literature may be explained by the fact that these various components have not been taken into consideration.

Finally, it should be noted that in order to test the predictive power of our approach-avoidance questionnaire for coronary patients more studies should be carried out with different groups of coronary patients and at different stages of the illness.

References

Billings, A. G. and Moos, R. J. (1981). The role of coping responses and social resources in attenuating the impact of stressful events. *Journal of Behavioral Medicine, 4* 139–157.

Byrne, D. (1961). The repression-sensitization scale: rationale, reliability, and validity. *Journal of Personality, 29,* 334–349.

Chatrou, M. and Maes, S. (1984). *The effects of physiotherapy on anxiety and well-being in patients with coronary heart disease.* Internal Report. Tilburg: Tilburg University.

Cohen, F. and Lazarus, R. S. (1973). Active coping processes, coping dispositions and recovery from surgery. *Psychosomatic Medicine, 35,* 375–389.

Croog, S. H., Shapiro, D. S. and Levine, S. (1971). Denial among male heart patients. *Psychosomatic Medicine, 33,* 385–397.

Dimsdale, J. E. and Hackett, T. P. (1982) Effect of denial on cardiac health and psychological assessment. *American Journal of Psychiatry, 139,* 1477–1480.

Erdman, R. A. M. (1982). *Medisch Psychologische Vragenlijst voor Hartpatiënten.* [Medical Psychological Questionnaire for Heart Patients]. Lisse: Swets en Zeitlinger B. V..

Gentry, W. D., Foster, S. and Haney, T. (1972). Denial as a determinant of anxiety and perceived health status in the Coronary Care Unit. *Psychosomatic Medicine, 34,* 39–44.

Feuerstein, M., Labbé, E. E. and Kuczmierczyk, A. R. (1986). *Health Psychology: A psychobiological perspective.* New York: Plenum.

Folkman, S., Lazarus, R. S., Gruen, J. and Delongis, A. (1986). Appraisal, coping, health status and psychological symptoms. *Journal of Personality and Social Psychology, 50,* 571–579.

Hackett, T. P. and Cassem, N. H. (1974). Development of a quantitative rating scale to assess denial. *Journal of Psychosomatic Research, 18,* 93–100.

Heck, G. L. M. van (1981). *Anxiety: the profile of a trait.* Dissertation.Tilburg: Tilburg University.

Lazarus, R. S. (1983). The costs and benefits of denial. In S. Breznitz (Ed.), *The denial of stress* (pp. 1–30). New York: International Universities Press.

Lazarus, R. S. and Folkman, S. (1984). *Stress, appraisal, and coping.* New York: Springer.

Levenson, J. L., Kay, R., Monteferrante, J. and Herman, M. V. (1984). Denial predicts favorable outcome in unstable angina pectoris. *Psychosomatic Medicine, 46,* 25–32.

Leventhal, H., Nerenz, D. R. and Steele, D. J. (1984). Illness representations and coping with health threats In A. Baum, S. E. Taylor and J. E. Singer (Eds.), *Handbook of psychology and health. Vol. IV: Social psychological aspects of health* (pp. 219–525). New Jersey: Erlbaum.

Levine, J., Warrenburg, S., Kerns, R., Schwartz, G., Delaney, R., Fontana, A., Gradman, A., Smith, S. Allen, S. and Cascione, R. (1987). The role of denial in recovery from coronary heart disease. *Psychosomatic Medicine, 49,* 109–117.

Lipowsky, Z. J. (1970). Physical illness, the individual and the coping process. *International Journal of Psychiatry in Medicine, 1,* 91–102.

Matheny, K. B., Aycock, D. W., Pugh, J. L., Curlette, W. L. and Silva Cannella, K. A. (1986). Stress coping: a qualitative and quantitative synthesis with implications for treatment. *Counseling Psychologist, 14,* 499–549.

Miller, S. M. (1980). When is a little information a dangerous thing: coping with stressful events by monitoring versus blunting. In S. Levin and H. Ursin (Eds.), *Coping and health* (pp. 145–169). New York: Plenum.

Miller, S. M. (1987). Monitoring and blunting: validation of a questionnaire to assess styles of information seeking under threat. *Journal of Personality and Social Psychology, 52,* 345–353.

Miller, S. M. and Brody, D. S. (1985). *Coping with stress by monitoring versus blunting: implications for health.* Paper presented at the American Psychological Association. Los Angeles.

Miller, S. M., Brody, D. S., Leinbach, A., LaPorte, D. J. and Summerton, J. (1985). *Coping style in hypertensives: implications for treatment.* Paper presented at the Society for Behavioral Medicine. New Orleans.

Miller, S. M. and Mangan, C. E. (1983). Interacting effects of information and coping style in adapting to gynecologic stress: should the doctor tell all? *Journal of Personality and Social Psychology, 45*, 223–236.

Mullen, B. and Suls, J. (1982). The effectiveness of attention and rejection as coping styles: a meta-analysis of temporal differences. *Journal of Psychosomatic Research, 26*, 43–49.

Ploeg, H. M. van der, Defares, P. B. and Spielberger, C. D. (1981). *Zelf-Beoordelings Vragenlijst, Z.B.V.* [Dutch version of the State-Trait Anxiety Inventory by Spielberger et al. (1970)]. Lisse: Swets en Zeitlinger B. V..

Ploeg, H. M. van der, Defares, P. B. and Spielberger, C. D. (1982). *Zelf-Analyse Vragenlijst, Z. A. V.* [Dutch version of the State-Trait Anger Scales by Spielberger *et al.* (1980)]. Lisse: Swets en Zeitlinger B. V..

Rooijen, L. van (1977). *Enige gegevens over de VROPSOM-lijsten voor de bepaling van depressieve gevoelens.* [Some data with regard to the Dutch version of the Depression Adjective Checklist by Lubin and Levitt (1975)]. Amsterdam: Free University of Amsterdam.

Roth, S. and Cohen, L. J. (1986). Approach, avoidance and coping with stress. *American Psychologist, 41*, 813–819.

Shaw, R. E., Cohen, F., Doyle, B. and Palesky, J. (1985). The impact of denial and repressive style on information gain and rehabilitation outcomes in myocardial infarction patients. *Psychosomatic Medicine, 47*, 262–273.

Soloff, P. H. (1978). Denial and rehabilitation of the post-infarction patient. *International Journal of Psychiatry in Medicine, 8*, 125–132.

Stern, M. J., Pascale, L. and Ackerman, A. (1977). Life adjustment post myocardial infarction: determining predictive variables. *Archives of Internal Medicine, 137*, 1680–1685.

Stern, M. J., Pascale, L. and MacLoone, J. B. (1976). Psychosocial adaptation following an acute myocardial infarction. *Journal of Chronic Disease, 29*, 513–526.

Suls, J. and Fletcher, B. (1985). The relative efficacy of avoidant and nonavoidant coping strategies: a meta-analysis. *Health Psychology, 4*, 249–288.

Weinberger, D. A., Schwartz, G. E. and Davidson, R. J. (1979). Low-anxious, high-anxious and repressive coping styles: psychometric patterns and behavioral and physiological responses to stress. *Journal of Abnormal Psychology, 33*, 369–380.

The Value of Mental Stress Testing in the Investigation of Cardiovascular Disorders

Andrew Steptoe

Introduction

Mental stress testing in the laboratory involves the measurement of physiological reactions during the imposition of psychologically meaningful stimuli or the performance of information-processing tasks. The use of mental stress testing in the investigation of cardiovascular disorders is based on the assumption that reactions may elucidate the patterns of autonomic and neuroendocrine activation that are significant in the development of disease. In this respect, mental stress testing is somewhat analogous to physical exercise testing or neural regulation tests such as tilt or lower body negative pressure. The difference is that the reactions to mental stress testing are thought to reflect the involvement of cognitive and emotional processes in cardiovascular regulation, rather than the elicitation of basic reflex mechanisms.

Mental stress testing was first introduced systematically by Brod, Fencl, Hejl, and Jirka (1959) for the study of psychological factors in essential hypertension, but the last decade has witnessed a major expansion of the use of the method in cardiovascular research.

The research on hypertensives has developed to include studies of normotensives at high risk for future disease, and the investigation of neural and haemodynamic mechanisms. Work has also been conducted on patients with coronary heart disease, and on the interaction with physical risk factors for heart disease. In addition to these studies of etiology, mental stress testing has been utilised in order to shed light on the effects of behavioural interventions in cardiovascular disease (e.g. Irvine, Johnston, Jenner and Marie, 1986; Roskies, Seraganian, Oseasohn, Hanley, Collu, Martin and Smilga, 1986).

The basic technique of mental stress testing involves the imposition of arbitrary psychological stressors or tasks for brief periods (usually less than 30 minutes and sometimes as short as one or two minutes). Differences in the magnitude or duration of physiological reactions (generally expressed as changes from resting levels) are then analysed in relation to the factors under study. This methodology has been subject to many refinements concerning such aspects as the selection of tasks, the recording of suitable baselines, the motor component of responses to tasks, and the appropriate form of analysis (see Steptoe, Rüddel & Neus, 1985 and Matthews, Weiss, Detre, Dembroski, Falkner, Manuck & Williams, 1986 for detailed discussions of these issues).

Nevertheless, the technique has not been accepted unreservedly, and the value of conducting mental stress tests in the laboratory has been questioned. Weder and Julius (1985) provided a cogent critique, and their reservations are reflected in the writings of many other investigators (e.g, Mancia & Parati, 1987; Pickering & Gerin, 1988). The basic objections can be summarised as follows:

1. Mental stress tests produce physiological reactions that are unreliable and inconsistent, with poor repeat test reliability.

2. The reactions to mental stress tests are not consistently related to the variability or "reactivity" of cardiovascular parameters in real life.

3. Neurogenically-mediated phasic cardiovascular reactions do not lead to fixed hypertension, and are not predictive of future cardiovascular disease.

The purpose of the present chapter is to examine these criticisms in detail, so as to discover what value can be placed on mental stress testing in the investigation of cardiovascular disorders. It will be argued that some of these arguments have force and should rightly curb the investigation of trivial reactivity effects. However, a greater awareness of the methodological problems surrounding mental stress testing can lead to the elicitation of robust effects. In addition, many criticisms of mental stress tests underestimate the weight of evidence concerning the reliability and value of the procedure in cardiovascular research.

The Reproducibility of Reactions to Mental Stress Tests

The first issue concerns the reliability of mental stress testing. If reactions cannot be elicited in a robust and reproducible fashion, then it is difficult to understand how they could be relevant to an etiological process that may require repeated or sustained activation (possibly over many years) in order to promote cardiovascular disease.

There are two aspects to the problem of reproducibility. The first concerns consistency of reactions across tasks: do those people who show the greatest reactions to one task also react the most to other tests? The evidence on inter-task consistency is mixed, but this is not surprising (see Obrist, 1981; Manuck, Kasprowitz, Monroe, Larkin and Kaplan, 1989). The haemodynamic patterns underlying cardiovascular reactions vary with task demands. It has been argued, for example, that conditions eliciting active coping behaviour generate blood pressure reactions that are sustained predominantly by heightened cardiac sympathetic stimulation, while in conditions where there is little motor involvement, blood pressure increases are secondary to elevations in peripheral vascular resistance (Steptoe, 1981). Since only some of these reaction patterns may be relevant to the etiology of cardiovascular disorders, inter-task consistency would not be expected. It is true that even among so called 'active coping' tasks, consistency has been variable. It is probable however that this category is too general, and that the precise haemodynamic correlates of such tasks may vary. In addition, individual differences in inter-task consistency may themselves be etiologically relevant characteristics (Manuck et al., 1989).

The second and more serious aspect is test-retest reliability. Neus, v. Eiff, Friedrich, Heusch and Schulte (1981) found that hypertensives showed greater blood pressure reactions than normotensives during their first test, but these differences disappeared with retesting one week later. The problem that pervades much mental stress testing is that reactions tend to diminsh with repeated presentations, as subjects become more familiar with the task requirements and test procedure. However, the fact that the absolute size of reactions declines is unimportant, provided that individual rankings in response are maintained. The key issue is whether individual differences in reactivity are reproducible, not whether the magnitude of responses is stable.

Several studies have now been published related to this issue, and these are summarised in Table 1. In this Table, as in later parts of the chapter, "task level" will be taken to refer to the absolute values of cardiovascular parameters recorded during tasks, while "reactivity scores" are changes in activity, usually calculated by subtracting measures during base line from task values. Meta-analysis might be considered for evaluating these results, but is unlikely at present adequately to account for the large variation in experimental parameters, test-retest intervals and populations studied in these reports. It can be seen that test-retest intervals of between one day and two-and-a-half years have been studied in a variety of predominantly healthy groups. Many of these studies included measures other than blood pressure and heart rate, but for the sake of simplicity Table 1 is restricted to these basic cardiovascular parameters. A number of experiments have been excluded from Table 1, either because they only assessed responses to the cold pressor test (eg Lacey & Lacey, 1962), or because results have not been published in detail (eg Rombouts, 1982).

In general, it can be seem that correlations between cardiovascular measures taken on two test occasions tend to be significant, with greater consistency in systolic pressure and heart rate than for diastolic pressure. The difference is particularly striking in assessment of reactivity scores, where 26 out of 30 comparisons for systolic pressure (87%) and 30 out of 36 comparisons from heart rate (83%) were significant, but only 18 out of 30 comparisons for diastolic pressure (60%). By contrast, the majority of comparisons of diastolic pressure task levels (15 out of 18 or 83%) were significant. The implication is that for diastolic pressure, task levels are more stable than reactivity scores.

The "magnitude" columns in Table 1 indicate whether or not the absolute levels of activity (task level) or numerical reactivity scores are maintained across occasions, or diminish with repeat testing. Here the results are mixed, and may depend to some extent on the tasks employed. Nevertheless, contrary to the view frequently voiced in the literature, diminution of reactions is by no means the norm in mental stress testing paradigms. Twelve out of 23 studies of reactivity scores and 10 out of 17 studies of task levels showed unchanged responses on repeat testing. Of course, the significance of correlations depends on the sample size, and in large studies rather modest correlation will be reliable. However, considering the large number of confounding factors that are difficult completely to control in experiments repeated over extended periods (such as time of day, changes in exercise habits and physical fitness, use of nicotine, caffeine and other substances, mood, recent life experiences, maturational changes in children and hormonal status in women), the degree of consistency is impressive.

The experiments outlined in Table 1 are all assessments of repeat administration of the same or very similar tasks. Other investigators have analysed the reproducibility and stability of reactions to mental stress tests by employing different tasks on various occasions. The intervals between sessions have ranged from one week to four years, and the majority of these studies have also shown substantial stability of individual differences in reactivity (Glass, Lake, Contrada, Kehoe & Erlanger, 1983; Seraganian, Hanley, Hollander, Roskies, Smilga, Martin, Collu & Oseasohn, 1985; Lovallo, Pincomb & Wilson, 1986; Matthews, Rakaczky, Stoney &

Table 1. Test retest reliability of cardiovascular reactions to mental stress tests

Study	Interval	Subjects	Task	Level				Reactivity Score			
				SBP	DBP	HR	Magnitude	SBP	DBP	HR	Magnitude
Arena et al., 1983	1 day	Male & female students n = 15	Mental arithmetic			+					Note 1
			Stressful imagery			+					/
			Cold pressor			−					/
Ray et al., 1984	1 & 2 days	Male & female students n = 10	Multiple test performance battery			+	+				0
Drummond, 1985	1 & 2 days	Borderline hypertensives and normotensives n = 26	Mental arithmetic	+	+			+	+	−	0
			Reaction time	+	+			+	+	−	0
Manuck and Schaefer, 1978	1 wk	Male students n = 42	Concept formation	+	+			+	−	+	0
Giordani et al., 1981	1 wk	Male children n = 34	Concept formation	+	+			+	−	+	/
Carroll et al., 1984	1 wk	Male students n = 42	Mental arithmetic	+	+			+	+		/
			Video game	+	+			+	+		/

Table 1. *continued*

Study	Interval	Subjects	Task	Task Level				Reactivity Score				
				SBP	*DBP*	*HR*	*Magnitude*	*SBP*	*DBP*	*HR*	*Magnitude*	
Myrtek, 1985	1 wk	Male students n = 48	Reaction time	+	+	+	0	+	−	+	/	
			Cold pressor	+	+	+	0	+	+	+	/	
			Cognitive task	+	+	+	0	+	−	+	/	
Faulstich et al., 1986	2 wks	Male & Female students n = 48	Mental arithmetic	+	+	+	/	−	−	+	/	
			Quiz	+	+	+	/	−	−	−	/	
			Cold pressor					+	−	+	/	
Murphy et al., 1988	2 wks	Male & Female children n = 310	Video game					+	+	+	/	
Fahrenberg et al., 1987	3 wks	Male Students n = 58	Mental arithmetic	−	+	+		+	+	+		Note 2
			Cold pressor	+	−	+		+	−	+		
Giaconi et al., 1987	4 wks	Borderline hypertensives n = 20	Mental arithmetic					+	+	+	0	
			Cold pressor					+	+	−	0	
Van Egeren and Sparrow 1989	4 wks	Male & female adults n = 36	Mental arithmetic					+	+	+		
			Memory task					+	+	+		
			Cold pressor					+	+	+		
Langewitz et al., 1989	4 wks	Patients with 'fatigue' n = 134	Reaction time	+	+	+	0	+	+	+	0	Note 3
			Mental arithmetic	+	+	+	0	+	+	+	0	

Table 1. continued

Study	Interval	Subjects	Task	Level				Reactivity Score			
				SBP	DBP	HR	Magnitude	SBP	DBP	HR	Magnitude
McKinney et al., 1985	3 mths	Middle-aged males n = 60	Video game	+	+	+		+	+	+	+
			Reaction time	+	+	+		+	−	+	+
			Cold pressor	+	+	+		+	+	−	−
Matthews et al., 1987	10 mths	Female adolescents n = 18	Mental arithmetic	+	−	+	/	−	−	−	/
			Mirror drawing	−	+	+	/	−	+	+	/
Horvath et al., 1986	12 mths	Research workers n = 106	Stroop test					+	+	+	+
			Cold pressor					+	+	−	−
Neus and von Eiff, 1985	12 mths	Male children n = 60	Mental arithmetic				0	+	+	+	0
Manuck and Garland, 1980	13 mths	Male students n = 19	Concept formation					+	−	+	0
Allen et al 1987	2½ yrs	Male students n = 25	Reaction time	+	−	+	0	+	−	+	0
			Cold pressor	+	+	+	/	+	+	+	/

Table 1. *continued*

Legend: SBP = Systolic Pressure; DBP = Diastolic Blood Pressure; HR = Heart Rate; Task Level = Absolute level measured during task; Reactivity Score = Change score, usually between task and pre-task level

+ = Between – subject correlation across occasions is significant

– = Between – subject correlation across occasions is not significant

/ = Magnitude of responses is unchanged across occasions

0 = Magnitude of responses is reduced between the first and later occasions

Note 1 Longer test-retest intervals were assessed, but are not strictly comparable with other studies, owing to additional exposure to task conditions.

Note 2 Longer test-retest intervals were assessed, but behavioural interventions were carried out with a proportion of subjects Blood pressure was recorded after rather than during trials.

Note 3 Longer test-retest intervals were assessed, but the testing situation was changed.

'Manuck, 1987).

The literature reviewed in this section suggests that individual differences in reactions to mental stress tests are reproducible, and that the problems with this aspect of validity have been overstated. Reductions in the magnitude of reactions are frequently but not universally observed, and the factors that lead to maintenance of responses deserve further study. Clearly, there are many variables that may influence the course of cardiovascular responses, and temporal stability (or lack of it) may itself be important etiologically (Manuck et al, 1989). It is worth noting however that even "physical" test of autonomic regulation and reflex function in the cardiovascular system (such as phenylephrine injection, isometric handgrip and neck suction) show considerable variability across occasions (Parati, Pomidossi, Ramirez, Cessana & Mancia, 1985). This should not however discredit results from a single occasion, provided that the test is carefully carried out.

Mental Stress Tests and Cardiovascular Activity Outside the Laboratory

The second major criticism of mental stress testing is that it relates poorly with cardiovascular measures recorded outside the laboratory, while people go about their ordinary lives. If mental stress testing is designed to model processes that are significant for pathology in the long-term, there should clearly be some relationship between cardiovascular activity in the laboratory and field.

Two approaches have been taken to the issue of laboratory-field comparability, and these will be considered separately.

Ambulatory Monitoring versus Mental Stress Testing

The first strategy has been to compare stress reactions in the laboratory with the level and variability of blood pressure and heart rate recorded from the same individuals while they go about their everyday lives. The simplest type of study in this area involves comparisons between laboratory measures and self-monitored pressure. Steptoe, Melville & Ross (1984) found that mean systolic pressure recorded up to four times a day over a twelve day period was correlated with systolic and diastolic pressure reactions to active coping tasks (the Stroop test and a video game) in a group of mild hypertensives and age-matched normotensives. Variability in self-monitored diastolic pressure was significantly associated with reactions to these tasks. Similarly, Manuck, Corse & Winkleman (1979) showed that among middle-aged male attorneys, high pressure reactors in the laboratory had more variable casual systolic pressure readings over a six week period than did low reactors. But although these results demonstrate reliable associations, they are of limited value since the frequency of measurements in everyday life was low, and participants were able to select the time at which blood pressure was recorded.

The advent of electronic sphygmomanometers with automatic cuff inflation and data recording has greatly increased the information that can be obtained about ambulatory cardiovascular activity. The results of comparisons with mental stress testing in the laboratory have generally shown that while task levels are associated with ambulatory measures, reactively scores are not. For example, Morales-Ballejo et al. (1988) assessed hypertensive and normotensive subjects during a series of laboratory tasks, and then with automated cuff monitoring every thirty minutes for the waking day. Correlations of 0.78 were obtained between average mean blood pressure in working subjects over the working day and pressure levels recorded during mental arithmetic and video game tasks. Another study reported correlations ranging from 0.53 to 0.66 between systolic and diastolic pressure levels during mental arithmetic and video game tasks and measures recorded every fifteen minutes at work (Harshfield, James, Schlussel, Yee, Blank & Pickering, 1988). However, when reactivity scores for mental stress tests were computed, the correlations with ambulatory readings were no longer significant. A similar result has been described by Fredrikson, Blumenthal, Evans, Sherwood & Light (1989). To date, the only study to obtain reliable correlations between ambulatory readings and reactivity scores for laboratory tests is one involving adolescents (Southard, Coates, Kolodner, Parker, Padgett & Kennedy, 1986). Systolic pressure reactions to a series of tasks correlated with ambulatory averages over both awake and sleeping periods (r=0.44 and 0.39, n=28). The diastolic pressure effects were not significant. More recently, an assessment of factors associated with ambulatory pressure levels found that baseline pressure in the laboratory was the most consistent predictor, with reactions to the Type A Structured Interview or the cold pressor test accounting for only a modest additional portion of the variance (Ironson, Gellman, Spitzer, Llabre, Pasin, Weidler & Schneiderman, 1989).

These studies present a consistent picture. However, their limitations should be borne in mind. The most serious problem is the intermittent nature of the ambulatory readings obtained. There are typically between 3, 500 and 6, 500 cardiac cycles (and individual systolic and diastolic blood pressures) every hour, so the recording of two or four values provides a tiny amount of information. The pattern of variability is virtually impossible to estimate, yet variability may be much more important than average levels in comparisons with mental stress testing. Three reports have now been published in which ambulatory recordings were obtained using intra-arterial monitoring, so that beat-to-beat data could be analysed. Watson, Stallard, Flynn & Littler (1980) showed that systolic and diastolic pressure responses to the cold pressor test were correlated across individuals with blood pressure variability, while there was no association with blood pressure average levels. Floras et al. (1987) described significant correlation between the variability of mean blood pressure during waking hours and reactions to a mental arithmetic ($r = 0.26$) and a reaction time task ($r = 0.53$, $n = 56$). Finally, a study from Milan showed reliable associations between mean arterial pressure peak reactions to mental arithmetic and variability over waking hours ($r = 0.60$, $n = 22$), with a similar pattern for peak reactions to a mirror drawing task ($r = 0.74$, Parati, Pomidossi, Casadei, Ravogli, Groppelli, Cessana & Mancia, 1988). In contrast the correlations with reactions to the cold pressor test were not significant ($r = 0.14$).

A number of important points emerge from comparisons between ambulatory measures and responses to mental stress tests.

1. Major differences can be seen between the results obtained with continuous and intermittent ambulatory recordings. With continuous measures, significant correlations have been found between reactivity scores and measures of ambulatory blood pressure variability. These are particulary prominent with tasks involving active behavioural coping rather than passive stressors such as the cold pressor test. The data from intermittent recordings show associations between ambulatory means and task levels, but not reactivity scores. Intermittent blood pressure recorders may be adequate for assessing average levels, but are

poor at determining variability (Casadei, Parati, Pomidossi, Groppelli, Trazzi, Di Rienzo & Mancia, 1988). Attempts to relate variability in intermittent ambulatory recordings with laboratory measures have not been successful (Van Egeren & Sparrow, 1989). This pattern was clearly apparent in a study presented by Schmidt et al. (1989). Volunteers were divided into low and high reactors on the basis of responses to a reaction time task in the laboratory. Subsequently, subjects underwent ambulatory monitoring with blood pressure recorded every 15 minutes, while heart rate was measured continuously. No association was found between low and high reactor status in the laboratory and blood pressure in the field, or with heart rates recorded simultaneously with blood pressure. But when the continuous heart rates were examined, responses in the field were greater in high and low laboratory reactors. Schmidt et al point out that when ambulatory pressure is recorded, subjects are obliged to suspend ongoing activities and stay still, blunting individual differences in responsivity.

2. Careful attention needs to be paid to the selection of appropriate measures from mental stress testing sessions. It may be valuable to index reactions to mental stress tests not by average values during tasks but by assessing peak responses (Johnston, Anastasiades & Wood, in press). At the same time it is possible that the baselines obtained in the laboratory are unrepresentative measures, recorded only in the unusual situation of resting immobility in the laboratory during a working day (Krantz & Manuck, 1984).

3. Another major problem of interpretation lies in distinguishing cardiovascular variability that is a result of physical activity from fluctuations that are relevant to psycho-social factors. Clearly the major factor contributing to variations in blood pressure and heart rate over the day is the level of physical activity, with movement, posture, digestion and speaking all having cardiovascular correlates. Comparisons between summary measures of variability in ambulatory records and reactions to mental stress tests and therefore likely to underestimate the strength of the association with stress-related cardiovascular activity in the field. Indeed, Manuck et al., (1989) have argued that given the limited reliability of both laboratory reactivity estimates and ambulatory measures, correlations are almost inevitably low. An important step towards resolving this difficulty has recently been described by Johnston et al. (in press). They recorded an index of physical activity (low amplification muscle tension monitored from the thigh) together with 24 hour electrocardiograms, and then applied autoregressive time series analysis in order to remove the variability in heart rate that is accounted for by activity. In this way, it was possible to identify heart rate variability that was independent of concurrent motor activity, The use of such methods may improve the estimation of stress-related ambulatory cardiovascular variability. Other sophisticated developments in time series analysis of ambulatory recordings, which overcome the statistical limitations of using simple measures such as standard deviation with serially dependent data, have also been reported (Pagani, Lombardi, Guzzetti, Rimoldi, Furlan, Pizzinelli, Sandrone, Malfatto et al., 1986).

4. Finally, the nature of the relationship between reactivity to mental stress tests and ambulatory recordings must be considered. Krantz & Manuck (1984) have distinguished a "recurrent activation model", in which task reactions might be related to reactions or variability during everyday life, and the "prevailing state

model" in which people with larger task reactions may have higher cardiovascular activity throughout the day, without necessarily showing greater variability. Light (1987) and Pickering (1988) have argued that intermediate patterns may be more representative. These models have implications for the nature of the association between laboratory and field, and until the appropriate pattern is determined, predictions from reactions to mental stress tests are difficult to make.

Reactions to Real Life Stress

The second method of evaluating the representiveness of mental stress tests is to compare results with cardiovascular reactions to stressful experiences outside the laboratory. If no association betweeen the two situations were to be found, this would undermine the value of recording reactions to laboratory tasks. The real life stress that has been studied most frequently is public speaking, but the results have been inconsistent. Three high and three low heart rate reactors to laboratory tasks out of a sample of 24 were identified by Turner, Carroll, Dean & Harris (1987), and they were subsequently monitored during public speaking. The high reactors in the laboratory produced large heart rate increases during the field test, but then so did one of the low heart rate reactors. A more elaborate comparison involving adolescent volunteers was performed by Matthews, Manuck & Saab (1986). Blood pressure but not heart rate reactivity to laboratory tasks such as mental arithmetic and mirror drawing was associated with pressure levels measured during speech tests. By contrast, Van Doornen (1988) found that cardiovascular responses to laboratory tasks were relatively inconsistent predictors of physiological activity recorded during an important public speaking occasion, while Dimsdale (1984) found no association between catecholamine or electrodermal responses to mental arithmetic in the laboratory and reactions to public speaking in a small sample of physicians.

An alternative approach to comparisons between reactions to mental stress tests and real life stress is to study people who differ in their life stress experience. It may hypothesised that people who are testing during stressful episodes of their lives will be more labile psychophysiologically than those who are not stressed. Two experiments contrasting students who reported high and low levels of recent life event stress produced different patterns of results, so remain inconclusive (Pardine & Napoli, 1983; Cohen, Simons, Rose, McGowan & Zelson, 1986). More interesting was a comparison of cardiovascular reactions to a problem solving task in adults living in crowded or uncrowded conditions, as indexed by population density (Fleming, Baum, Davidson, Rectanus & McArdle, 1987). Chronic stress evidently had an impact on reactions to the laboratory test, with greater blood pressure and heart rate responses and slower recovery following termination of the task among those living in crowded as opposed to uncrowded streets.

These strategies for comparing mental stress tests and cardiovascular activity outside the laboratory have not yet been evaluated extenisvely. They may however provide valuable supplementry data, overcoming an important limitation of ambulatory studies, which is that the person being monitored may not encounter any serious psychological stressors during the observation period.

The Prediction of Future Disease

The third important aspect of mental stress testing is whether or not it predicts future hypertension or coronary heart disease. Critics of the technique rightly point out that mental stress testing is largely justified on the basis of hypothetical models and cross-sectional comparisons, rather than upon empirical demonstrations of increased disease risk among people with exaggerated cardiovascular reactions to laboratory tasks. Some proponents of mental stress testing have allied themselves closely with specific theories of cardiovascular disease etiology that do not have widespread currency (e.g. Obrist, Langer, Light & Koepke, 1983). This has led to objections based more on the models than upon the results of mental stress testing (Conway 1984; Weder & Julius, 1985). The study of mental stress tests in relation to hypertension has progressed from comparisons between hypertensives and normotensives to investigations of normotensive people at increased risk of future disorder. This strategy overcomes the problem of deciding whether heightened reactivity is secondary to hypertensive status, since exaggerated reactions have also been observed in normotensives with a positive family history (Fredrikson & Matthews, in press). However, it is a major step from these comparisons to the prediction of future hypertension, since only a small proportion of those at increased risk through family history or raised normal blood pressure actually progress to fixed hypertension themselves (Watt, 1986).

Inevitably, any test of the prognostic significance of cardiovascular reactions during mental stress testing is a long-term undertaking, since hypertension and coronary heart disease are disorders with extended aetiologies. Clinical manifestations are frequently not apparent until middle age, even though the disease process may have begun in childhood. Ideally, the predictive power of mental stress tests should be evaluated by testing large samples on several occasions early in life, then following them up for decades, evaluating cardiovascular health status along with associated risk factors. If mental stress tests have validity in this context, it would be argued that individuals producing consistently high cardiovascular and neuroendocrine reactions to stress tests are more likely than the less reactive to develop cardiovascular disease. Unfortunately, hypotheses concerning mental stress tests have reached a sophisticated stage of development only in the last 15 years. Consequently, studies in which testing was carried out sufficiently long ago and in large enough samples to be able to evaluate edaquate numbers of diagnosed patients, tended to involve testing procedures that are imprecise by modern standards. Results from three extended longitudinal studies have shown positive results in the prediction of coronary heart disease and hypertension using reactions to the cold pressor test (Keys, Taylor, Blackburn, Brozek, Anderson & Simonson, 1971; Wood, Sheps, Elveback & Schirger, 1984; Menkes, Matthews, Krantz, Lundberg, Mead, Qaqish, Liang, Thomas, Pearson, 1989). However, negative findings have also been described (Armstrong & Raftery, 1950; Harlan, Osborne & Graybiel, 1964), and many investigators would not consider the cold pressor to be a test likely to demonstrate great predictive power (see Steptoe, 1981, pp. 116–117).

Several other longitudinal studies are in progress, relying at present on weaker end points such as hypertension progression and blood pressure tracking as criteria of predictive power. These studies are summarised in Table 2. It can be seen that they tend to show favourable effects, with greater incidence of hypertension or tracking of blood pressure in those manifesting exaggerated pressor responsivity or delayed recovery to such tasks as mental arithmetic. Two additional features should be noted. Firstly, the prediction with mental stress testing in these studies was independent of blood pressure level, and was not simply a product of tonic effects. Secondly, reactions to mental stress tests appear to be particularly significant in the presence of other risk factors such as high body weight, family history of hypertension or disturbances of sodium metabolism. There may therefore be important interactions between propensity to exaggerated cardiovascular reactivity and biological risk in predisposing people to disease.

These data provide modest encouragement for believing mental stress testing may be of prognostic significance, and it is to be hoped that longitudinal studies currently under way will provide more definitive information. Even if the effects prove to be robust, it cannot of course be inferred that stress reactivity as indexed by tests in the laboratory is involved in the aetiology of essential hypertension. An alternative explanation is that stress reactivity is a marker, associated with future hypertension while not being causally significant. In support of this notion is the argument that heightened blood pressure variability in normotension is not prognostic, and that most patients do not pass through a labile phase as they progress towards fixed high blood pressure (Horan, Kennedy & Padgett, 1981; Julius & Schork, 1978). However, the only convincing way of discovering whether stress reactivity is important aetiologically or is only a marker would be to carry out an intervention trial, to determine whether reducing reactivity also lowers the likelihood of future hypertension. No such trial has yet been performed.

In this section, the issue of whether reactions to mental stress tests predict future disease has been addressed in relation to hypertension. One of the most important developments of recent years is the recognition that stress reactions may also be significant in cardiovascular disease independently of hypertensive status. Several lines of evidence are relevant.

1. A relationship has been found between the variability of blood pressure and target organ damage, or the pathological sequelae of hypertension, independent of blood pressure level. Parati et al. (1987) divided a large sample of hypertensives into quintiles of mean arterial pressure as determined by 24 hour intra-arterial monitoring. Within each category, a division was made into those with high and low blood pressure variability (average standard deviation of mean arterial pressure within each 30 minute epoch of the day). The extent of target organ damage increased with blood pressure level, as might be expected. In addition however, targer organ damage was higher in the subgroups with greater blood pressure variability. It is likely that much of this variability is related to psychosocial stimulation.

2. Evidence is accumulating for the importance of sympathetic nervous system activity in the development of atherosclerosis, again independently of hypertension (Ablad, Björkman, Gustafsson, Hansson, Ostlund-Lindqvist & Pettersson, 1988). For example, atherogenesis in rabbits fed cholesterol-rich diets was reduced by beta-adrenergic blockade, without altering cholestrol levels in the blood (Östlund-Lindqvist, Lindqvist, Bräutigan, Olsson, Bondjers & Nordborg, 1988). A recent trial of the beta-blocker metoprolol in the primary prevention of coronary heart disease showed that the drug produced similar anti-hypertensive effects to thiazide diuretics (Wikstrand, Warnold, Olsson, Tuomeliehto, Elmfeldt, & Berglund, 1988). However, mortality was reduced to a greater extent in the metoprolol group. In primates, Manuck, Kaplan and

Table 2. *Longitudinal prediction studies*

Study	Sample	Duration	Outcome	Predictor test
Von Eiff et al., 1985	Adolescents	1 year	Blood pressure tracking	Heart rate reactions to mental arithmetic
Aivazyan et al., 1988	Adult hypertensives	1 year	Hypertension progression	Diastolic pressure reactions to mental arithmetic and computer games, and delayed recovery in blood pressure following tasks
Falkner et al., 1981	Adolescents with high normal blood pressure	1.5 years on average	Hypertension progression	Blood pressure and heart rate reactions to mental arithmetic
Parker et al., 1987	Children with high normal blood pressure	4 years	Blood pressure tracking	Diastolic pressure reactions to the cold pressor test and handgrip
Borghi et al., 1986	Young borderline hypertensives	5 years	Hypertension progression in subgroup with high intralymphocyte sodium	Delayed recovery in diastolic pressure following mental arithmetic

Clarkson (1983) demonstrated that heart rate reactivity to a standardised psychological challenge predicted coronary atherosclerosis in animals fed moderately atherogenic diets. The beta blocker propranolol lowered the degree of coronary atherosclerosis induced by a combination of psychological stress and moderately atherogenic diet, but again the effect was not directly related to the blood pressure lowering response to the drug (Kaplan, Manuck, Adams, Weingand & Clarkson, 1987).

3. Sympathetically-mediated cardiovascular reactivity may also be significant in promoting acute dangerous clinical episodes of myocardial ischaemia and ventricular fibrillation in people with established coronary heart disease. Rozanski et al. (1988) studied 39 coronary patients with sophisticated cardiac imaging techniques during a series of mental stress tests. Myocardial wall motion abnormalities and transient coronary stenosis were observed in 21 patients during mental stress. Experiments with animals have demonstrated that the threshold for ventricular fibrillation is reduced by stress induced aversive classical conditioning or aggressive challenge (Lown, Verrier & Corbalan, 1973; Verrier, Hagestod & Lown 1987). These patterns may be relevant to the neurogenic processes involved in sudden cardiac death (Lown, DeSilva, Reich & Murawski, 1980).

It can be seen that strong evidence is becoming available attesting to the importance of cardiovascular and neuroendocrine reactions to mental stress at several stages of atherogenesis and heart disease. Whether or not mental stress testing is predictive of hypertension, the technique has considerable potential for the evaluation of mechanisms relating psychological and social factors with serious diseases of the heart.

Conclusions

Several factors related to mental testing in the investigation of cardiovascular disorders have been discussed. To some extent, the value of mental stress testing may have been overstated in the past. Future work would benefit from closer attention to the nature of the tasks employed, the standardisation of precedures for determining baselines, and the relationships between reactions in the laboratory and field. The need for longitudinal studies is paramount, while associations between mental stress tests and atherosclerosis deserve fuller investigation. However the evidence in favour of the technique is growing, and it is apparent that robust effects can be elicited. Mental stress testing in the laboratory has the inestimable advantage of permitting investigations in which the psychological demands upon the individual are established in a quantifiable fashion, while sophisticated physiological and endocrine monitoring is carried out. It therefore holds a vital place in the array of strategies used to investigate psychosocial factors in cardiovascular disease, bringing the gap between physiological studies on the the one side and psychosocial epidemiology on the other.

Acknowledgements
    This chapter has benefitted from discussions that have taken place within the CEC Medical and Health Research Programme Concerted Action on Quatification of Parameters for the Study of Breakdown in Human Adaptation.

References

Ablad, B., Björkman, J.-A., Gustafsson, D., Hansson, G., Östlund-Lindqvist, A.-M., and Pettersson, K. (1988). The role of sympathetic activity in atherogenesis: effects of β-blockade. *American Heart Journal, 116*, 322–327.

Aivazyan, T. A., Zaitsev, V. P., Khramelashvili, V. V., Golanov, E. V. and Kichkin, V. I. (1988). Psychophysiological interrelations and reactivity characteristics in hypertensives. *Health Psychology, 7* (Suppl.), 139–144.

Allen, M. T., Sherwood, A., Obrist, P. A., Crowell, M. D., and Grange, L. A. (1987). Stability of cardiovascular reactivity to laboratory stressors: a two and a half year follow-up. *Journal of Psychosomatic Research, 31*, 639–645.

Arena, J. G., Blanchard, E. B., Andrasik, F., Cotch, P. A. and Myers, P. E. (1983). Reliability of psychophysiological assessment. *Behaviour Research and Therapy, 21*, 447–460.

Armstrong, H. G. and Raftery, J. A. (1950). Cold pressor test follow-up study for seven years on 166 officers. *American Heart Journal, 39*, 484–490.

Borghi, C., Costa, F. V., Boschi, S., Mussi, A. and Ambrosini, E. (1986). Prediction of stable hypertension in young borderline subjects: a five-year follow-up study. *Journal of Cardiovascular Pharmacology, 8* (Suppl. 5) S138–S141.

Brod, J., Fencl, V., Hejl, Z., and Jirka, J. (1959). Circulatory changes underlying blood pressure elevation during acute emotional stress in normotensive and hypertensive subjects. *Clinical Science, 18*, 269–279.

Carroll, D., Turner, J. R., Lee, H. J., and Stephenson, J. (1984). Temporal consistency of individual differences in cardiac response to a video game. *Biological Psychology, 19*, 81–94.

Casadei, R., Parati, G., Pomidossi, G., Grolpelli, A., Trazzi, S., Di Rienzo, M., and Mancia, G. (1988). 24 hour blood pressure monitoring: evaluation of Spacelabs 5300 monitor by comparison with intra-arterial blood pressure recording in ambulant subjects. *Journal of Hypertension, 6*, 797–803.

Cohen, L. H., Simons, R. F., Rose, S. C., McGowan, J., and Zelson, M. F. (1986). Relationship among negative life events, physiological reactivity, and health symptomatology. *Journal of Human Stress, 12*, 142–148.

Conway, J. (1984). Hemodynamic aspects of essential hypertension in humans. *Physiological Reviews, 64*, 617–660.

Dimsdale, J. E. (1984). Generalizing from laboratory studies to field studies of human stress physiology. *Psychosomatic Medicine, 46*, 463–469.

Drummond, P. D. (1985). Cardiovascular reactivity in borderline hypertension during behavioral and orthostatic stress. *Psychophysiology, 22*, 621–628.

Fahrenberg, J., Schneider, H.-J., and Safian, P. (1987). Psychophysiological assessments in a repeated measurement design extending over a one year interval: trends and stability. *Biological Psychology, 24*, 49–66.

Falkner, B., Kushner, H., Onesti, G., and Angelakos, E. T. (1981). Cardiovascular characteristics in adolescents who develop essential hypertension. *Hypertension, 3*, 521–527.

Faulstich, M. E., Williamson, D. A., McKenzie, S. J., Duchmann, E. G., Hutchinson, K. M. and Blouin, D. C. (1986). Temporal stability of psychophysiological responding: a comparative analysis of mental and physical stressors. *International Journal of Neuroscience, 30*, 65–72.

Fleming, I., Baum, A., Davidson, L. M., Rectanus, E., and McArdle, S. (1987). Chronic stress as a factor in psychological reactivity to challenge. *Health Psychology, 6*, 221–237.

Floras, J. S., Hassan, M. O., Jones, J. V. and Sleight, P. (1987). Pressor responses to laboratory stresses and day-time blood pressure variability. *Journal of Hypertension, 5*, 715–719.

Fredrikson, M., and Matthews, K. A. (in press). Cardiovascular responses to behavioral stress and hypertension: a meta-analytic review. *Annals of Behavioral Medicine*.

Fredrikson, M., Blumenthal, J. A., Evans, D. D., Sherwood, A., and Light, K. C. (1989). Cardiovascular responses in the laboratory and in the natural environment. *Journal of Psychosomatic Research, 33*, 753–762.

Giaconi, S., Palombo, C., Genovesi-Ebert, A., Marabotti, A., Mezzasalma, L., and Ghione, S. (1987). Medium-term reproducibility of stress tests in borderline arterial hypertension. *Journal of Clinical Hypertension, 3*, 654–660.

Giordani, B., Manuck, S. B. and Farmer, J. F. (1981). Stability of behaviorally induced heart rate change in children after one week. *Child Development, 52*, 533–537.

Glass, D. C., Lake, C. R., Contrada, R. J., Kehoe, K., and Erlanger, L. R. (1983). Stability of individual differences in physiological responses to stress. *Health Psychology, 2*, 317–341.

Harlan, W. R., Osborne, R. K., Graybiel, A. (1964). Prognostic value of the cold pressor test. *American Journal of Cardiology, 13*, 832–837.

Harshfield, G. A., James, G. D., Schlussel, Y., Yee, L. S., Blank, S. G., and Pickering, T. G. (1988). Do laboratory tests of blood pressure reactivity predict blood pressure changes during every day life? *American Journal of Hypertension, 1*, 168–174.

Horan, M. J., Kennedy, H. C., and Padgett, N. E. (1981). Do borderline hypertensive patients have labile blood pressure? *Annals of Internal Medicine, 94*, 466–468.

Horvath, M., Frantik, E., and Slaby, A. (1986). Psychophysiologic testing of cardiovascular response to physiologic and psychological challenge: analysis of intraindividual stability. In T. H. Schmidt, T. M. Dembroski, and G. Blümchen (Eds.), *Biological and Psychological Factors in Cardiovascular Disease* (pp. 315–322). Berlin: Springer.

Ironson, G. H., Gellman, M. D., Spitzer, S. B., Llabre, M. A., Pasin, R., Weidler, D. J. and Schneiderman, N. (1989). Predicting home and work blood pressure measurements from resting baselines and laboratory reactivity in black and white Americans. *Psychophysiology, 26*, 174–184.

Irvine, J., Johnston, D. W., Jenner, D., and Marie, G. V. (1986). Relaxation and stress management in the treatment of essential hypertension. *Journal of Psychosomatic Research, 30*, 437–450.

Johnston, D. W., Anastasiades, P., and Wood, C. (in press). The relationship between cardiovascular response in the laboratory and in the field. *Psychophysiology*.

Julius, S. and Schork, M. A. (1978). Predictors of hypertension. *Annals of the New York Academy of Sciences, 304*, 38–52.

Kaplan, J. R., Manuck, S. B., Adams, M. R., Weingand, K. W., and Clarkson, T. B. (1987). Propranolol inhibits coronary atherosclerosis in behaviorally predisposed monkeys fed an atherogenic diet. *Circulation, 76*, 1364–1372.

Keys, A., Taylor, H. L., Blackburn, H., Brozek, J., Anderson, J. T., and Simonson, E. (1971). Mortality and coronary heart disease among men studied for 23 years. *Archives of Internal Medicine, 128*, 201–214.

Krantz, D. S. and Manuck, S. B. (1984). Acute psychophysiologic reactivity and risk of cardiovascular disease: a review and methodologic critique. *Psychological Bulletin, 96*, 435–464.

Lacey, J. I. and Lacey, B. C. (1962). The law of initial values in the longitudinal study of autonomic constitution: reproducibility of autonomic responses and response patterns over a four year interval. *Annals of the New York Academy of Science, 98*, 1257–1290.

Langewitz, W., Rüddel, H., Noack, H., and Wachtarz, K. (1989). The reliability of psychophysiological examinations under field conditions: Results of repetitive mental stress testing in middle-aged men. *European Heart Journal, 10*, 657–665.

Light, K. C. (1987). Psychosocial precursors of hypertension: experimental evidence. *Circulation, 76*, (Suppl. I), 167–176.

Lovallo, W. R., Pincomb, G. A. and Wilson, M. A. (1986). Heart rate reactivity and Type A behavior as modifiers of physiological response to active and passive coping. *Psychophysiology, 23*, 105–112.

Lown, B., Verrier, R., and Corbalan, R. (1973). Psychologic stress and the threshold for repetitive ventricular response. *Science, 183*, 834–836.

Lown, B., DeSilva, R. A., Reich, P., and Murawski, B. J. (1980). Psychophysiologic factors in sudden cardiac death. *American Journal of Psychiatry, 137*, 1325–1335.

McKinney, M. E., Miner, M. H., Rüddel, H. McIlvain, H. E., Witte, H., Buell, J. C., Eliot, R. S., and Grant, L. B. (1985). The standardised mental stress test protocol: test-retest reliability and comparison with ambulatory blood pressure monitoring. *Psychophysiology, 22*, 453–463.

Mancia, G., and Parati, G. (1987). Reactivity to physical and behavioral stress and blood pressure variability in hypertension. In S. Julius and D. S. Bassett (Eds), *Handbook of Hypertension*, vol. 9: *Behavioral Factors in Hypertension* (pp. 104–122). Amsterdam: Elsevier.

Manuck, S. B., and Schaefer, D. C. (1978). Stability of individual differences in cardiovascular reactivity. *Physiology and Behavior, 21*, 675–678.

Manuck, S. B., Corse, C. D. and Winkelman, P. A. (1979). Behavioral correlates of individual differences in blood pressure reactivity. *Journal of Psychosomatic Research, 23*, 281–288.

Manuck, S. B., and Garland, F. N. (1980). Stability of individual differences in cardiovascular reactivity: a 13-month follow-up. *Physiology and Behavior, 24*, 621–624.

Manuck, S. B., Kaplan, J. R., and Clarkson, T. B. (1983). Behaviorally induced heart rate reactivity and atherosclerosis in cynomolgus monkeys. *Psychosomatic Medicine, 45*, 95–108.

Manuck, S. B., Kasprowicz, A. L., Monroe, S. M., Larkin, K. T. and Kaplan, J. R. (1989). Psychophysiologic reactivity as a dimension of individual differences. In N. Schneiderman, S. M. Weiss and P. G. Kaufmann (Eds.), *Handbook of Research Methods in Cardiovascular Behavioral Medicine*. New York: Plenum.

Matthews, K. A., Weiss, S. M., Detre, T., Dembroski, T. M., Falkner, B., Manuck, S. B., and Williams, R. B., (1986). *Handbook of Stress, Reactivity and Cardiovascular Disease*. New York: Wiley-Interscience.

Matthews, K. A., Manuck, S. B., and Saab, P. G., (1986). Cardiovascular responses of adolescents during a naturally occuring stressor and their behavioral and psychophysiological predictors. *Psychophysiology, 23*, 198–209.

Matthews, K. A., Rakaczky, C. J., Stoney, C. M., and Manuck, S. B. (1987). Are cardiovascular responses to behavioral stressors a stable individual difference variable in childhood? *Psychophysiology, 24*, 464–473.

Menkes, M. S., Matthews, K. A., Krantz, D. S., Lundberg, U., Mead, L. A., Qaqish, B., Liang, K-Y., Thomas, C. B., and Pearson, T. A. (1989). Cardiovascular reactivity to the cold pressor test as a predictor of hypertension. *Hypertension, 14*, 524–530.

Morales-Ballejo, H. N., Eliot, R. S., Boone, J. L., and Hughes, J. S. (1988). Psychophysiologic stress testing as a predictor of mean daily blood pressure. *American Heart Journal, 116*, 673–681.

Murphy, J. J., Alpert, B. S., Willey, E. S., and Somes, G. W. (1988). Cardiovascular reactivity to psychological stress in healthy children. *Psychophysiology, 25*, 144–152.

Myrtek, M. (1985). Adaptation effects and the stability of physiological responses to repeat testing. In A. Steptoe, H. Rüddel, and H. Neus (Eds.), *Clinical and Methodological Issues in Cardiovascular Psychophysiology* (pp. 93–106). Berlin: Springer

Neus, H., and Von Eiff, A. W. (1985). Selected topics in the methodology of stress testing: time course, gender and adaptation. In A. Steptoe, H. Rüddel, and H. Neus (Eds.), *Clinical and Methodological Issues in Cardiovascular Psychophysiology* (pp. 78–92). Berlin: Springer-Verlag.

Neus, H., von Eiff, A. W., Friedrich, G., Heusch, G., and Schulte, W. (1981). Das Problem der Adaptation in der klinisch-therapeutischen Hypertonieforschung [The problem of adaptation in clinical-therapeutical research on hypertension]. *Deutsche Medizinische Wochenschrift, 196*, 622–624.

Obrist, P. A. (1981). *Cardiovascular Psychophysiology, New York: Plenum*

Obrist, P. A., Langer, A. W., Light, K. C., and Koepke, J. P. (1983). *A cardiac-behavioral approach in the study of hypertension.* In T. M. Dembroski, T. H. Schmidt, and G. Blümchen (Eds.), *Biobehavioral Bases of Coronary Heart Disease* (pp. 290–303). Basel: Karger.

Östlund-Lindqvist, A. M., Lindqvist, P., Bräutigan, J., Olsson, G., Bondjers, G., and Nordborg, C. (1988). The effect of metoprolol on diet-induced artherosclerosis in rabbits. *Atherosclerosis, 8*, 40–45.

Pagani, M., Lombardi, F., Guzzetti, S., Rimoldi, O., Furlan, R., Pizzinelli, P., Sandrone, G., Malfatto, G., et al. (1986). Power spectral analysis of heart rate and arterial pressure variabilities as a marker of sympathovagal interaction in man and conscious dog. *Circulation Research, 59*, 178–193.

Parati, G., Pomidossi, G., Ramirez, A. J., Cessana, B., and Mancia, G. (1985). Variability of the haemodynamic responses to laboratory tests employed in assessment of neural cardiovascular regulation. *Clinical Science, 69*, 533–540.

Parati, G., Pomidossi, G., Albani, F., Malaspina, D., and Mancia, G. (1987). Relationship of 24-hour blood pressure mean and variability to severity of target-organ damage in hypertension. *Journal of Hypertension, 5*, 93–98.

Parati, G., Pomidossi, G., Casadei, R., Ravogli, A., Groppelli, A., Cessana, B., and Mancia, G. (1988). Comparison of the cardiovascular effects of different laboratory stressors and their relationship with blood pressure variability. *Journal of Hypertension, 6*, 481–488.

Pardine, P., and Napoli, A. (1983). Physiological reactivity and recent life-stress experience. *Journal of Consulting and Clinical Psychology, 51*, 467–469.

Parker, F. C., Croft, J. M., Cresanta, J., Freedman, D. S., Burke, G. L., Webber, L. S., and Berenson, G. S. (1987). The association between cardiovascular response tasks and future blood pressure levels in children: Bogalusa Heart Study. *American Heart Journal, 113*, 1174–1179.

Pickering, T. G. (1988). The study of blood pressure in everyday life. In T. Elbert, W. Langosch, A. Steptoe, and D. Vaitl (Eds), *Behavioural Medicine in Cardiovascular Disorders* (pp. 71–85). Chichester: John Wiley.

Pickering, T. G., and Gerin, W. (1988). Ambulatory blood pressure monitoring and cardiovascular reactivity testing for the evaluation of the role of physical factors and prognosis in hypertensive patients. *American Heart Journal, 116*, 655–672.

Ray, R. L., Brady, J. B., and Emurian, H, H, (1984). Cardiovascular effects of noise during complex task performance. *International Journal of Psychophysiology, 1*, 335–340.

Rombouts, R. (1982). The reproducibility of cardiovascular reactions during cognitive tasks. *Activitas Nervosa Superior*, (Suppl. 3), pt 2, 283–294.

Roskies, E., Seraganian, P., Oseasohn, R., Hanley, J. A., Collu, R., Martin, M., and Smilga, C., (1986). The Montreal Type A intervention project: major findings. *Health Psychology, 5*, 45–69.

Rozanski, A., Bairey, M., Krantz, D. S., Friedman, J., Resser, K. J., Morell, M., Hilton-Chalfen, S., Hestrin, L., Bietendorf, J., and Berman, D. S. (1988). Mental stress and the induction of silent myocardial ischaemia in patients with coronary artery disease. *New England Journal of Medicine, 318*, 1005–1012.

Schmidt, T. H., Klingmann, I., and Albus, C. (1989). *Cardiovascular reactivity during laboratory tasks and during daily life.* 10th Annual Proceedings of the Society of Behavioral Medicine.

Seraganian, P., Hanley, J. A., Hollander, P. J., Roskies, E., Smilga, C., Martin, N. D., Collu, R., and Oseasohn, R. (1985). Exaggerated psychophysiological reactivity: Issues in quantification and reliability. *Journal of Psychosomatic Reasearch, 29*, 393–406.

Southard, D. R., Coates, T. J., Kolodner, K., Parker, F. C., Padgett, N. E., and Kennedy, H. L. (1986). Relationship between mood and blood pressure in the natural environment: an adolescent population. *Health Psychology, 5*, 469–480.

Steptoe, A. (1981). *Psychological factors in cardiovascular disorders*. London: Academic Press.
Steptoe, A., Melville, D., and Ross, A. (1984). Behavioral response demands, cardiovascular reactivity and essential hypertension. *Psychosomatic Medicine, 45*, 33–48.
Steptoe, A., Rüddel, H., and Neus, H. (1985). *Clinical and methodological issues in cardiovascular psychophysiology*. Berlin: Springer.
Turner, J. R., Carroll, D., Dean, S., and Harris, M. G. (1987). Heart rate reactions to standard laboratory challenges and a naturalistic stressor. *International Journal of Psychophysiology, 5*, 151–152.
Van Doornen, L. J. P. (1988). *Physiological Stress Reactivity*. Proefschrift Vrije Universiteit Amsterdam.
Van Egeren, L. F. and Sparrow, A. W. (1989). Laboratory stress testing to assess real-life cardiovascular reactivity. *Psychosomatic Medicine, 51*, 1–9.
Von Eiff, A. W., Gogolin, E., Jacobs, V., and Neus, H. (1985). Heart rate reactivity under mental stress as a predictor of blood pressure development in children. *Journal of Hypertension, 3*, (Suppl. 4), S89–S91.
Verrier, R. L., Hagestod, E. L., and Lown, B. (1987). Delayed myocardial ischaemia induced by anger. *Circulation, 75*, 249–254.
Watson, R. D. S., Stallard, T. J., Flynn, R. M., and Littler, W. A. (1980). Factors determining direct arterial pressure and its variability in hypertensive men. *Hypertension, 2*, 333–341.
Watt, G. (1986). Design and interpretation of studies comparing individuals with and without a family history of high blood pressure. *Journal of Hypertension, 4*, 1–7.
Weder, A. B., and Julius, S. (1985). Behavior, blood pressure variability and hypertension. *Psychosomatic Medicine, 47*, 406–414.
Wikstrand, J., Warnold, I., Olsson, G., Tuomeliehto, J., Elmfeldt, D., and Berglund, G. (1988). Primary prevention with Metoprolol in patients with hypertension. Mortality results from the MAPHY. *Journal of the American Medical Association, 259*, 1976–1982.
Wood, D. L., Sheps, S. G., Elveback, L. R., and Schirger, A. (1984). Cold pressor test as a predictor of hypertension. *Hypertension, 6*, 301–306.

Type A Behaviour, Anxiety, and the First-Year Prognosis of a Myocardial Infarction

Juhani Julkunen, Ulla Idänpään–Heikkilä and Timo Saarinen

Introduction

While most of the work done with the Type A construct deals with its role as a primary risk factor , there are some studies reporting interesting differences in the reactions to the acute myocardial infarction (MI) between Type A and Type B patients. For example, Keefe, Castell and Blumenthal (1986) report that Type A cardiac patients were more likely to be classified as having more severe pain and functional limitation on the NYHA scale (New York Heart Association, 1964), although there was no difference in the severity of cardiac disease or in anxiety. In another report, Type A patients have been described as more active, more alert, friendlier but more emotionally withdrawn and, in addition, as remaining more anxious/depressed during post-MI recovery (Genrey et al, 1983).

Recently, the prognostic value of Type A behavior after a heart attack has been critically debated because of a series of negative findings (e.g. Case et al., 1985; Shekelle, Gale, & Norusis, 1985). These studies were based on large samples and follow-up times ranging from 1 to 3 years. However, they were unable to show any correlation between the Type A score as measured by the Jenkins Activity Survey (JAS) (Jenkins et al., 1971) and the risk of recurrent coronary events. These results are in contrast to the earlier findings of Jenkins, Zyzanski and Rosenman (1976). Furthermore, in a recent report (Ragland & Brand, 1988) it has demonstrated that in a long-term follow-up of the Western Collaborative Group Study the Type B persons had higher cardiac mortality as compared to Type A's. On the other hand, evidence of the San Francisco Recurrent Coronary Prevention Project shows that a decrease in Type A behavior was associated with a decrease in recurrent cardiac events (Friedman et al., 1984).

The clinical significance of anxiety for the treatment of the MI is widely recognized (see e.g. Shine, 1984), but still today there are only a few systematic surveys on the prevalence of anxiety in coronary patients during the acute phase or studies on the possible prognostic significance of reactive anxiety (Cassem & Hackett, 1973; Hanses, 1988).

As Haynes and Matthews (1988) in their review conclude, the question of the role of Type A behavior as a secondary risk factor according to our present knowledge seems rather debatable; the need for further studies is evident. It seems also necessary to direct research into more specific problems concerned with the psychological process of recovery after MI and into the possible differences between Type A's and Type B's in that process.

This study is a part of a larger project aimed at clarifying the role of some psychological factors (e.g. Type A behavior, aggression/hostility, anxiety, depression, and coping with illness) in the process of recovery and the prognosis of

331

Table 1 *Mean values of Type A and anxiety measures for men and women, baseline results and 3-month follow-up.*

Measure	men (n = 76) M	men (n = 76) SD	women (n = 16) M	women (n = 16) SD	t	df
baseline:						
Type A	39.76	6.97	43.69	6.93	2.05*	90
Anxiety-total[a]	33.97	13.13	35.50	14.98	0.41	87
Cognit. worry[a]	17.43	6.94	20.31	10.04	1.38	87
Auton.–emot.[a]	16.55	6.87	15.19	5.92	0.47	87
3-month follow-up:						
Anxiety-total[b]	36.57	14.84	36.19	13.59	0.09	84
Cognit. worry[b]	18.63	8.01	19.13	9.37	0.22	84
Auton.–emot.[b]	17.94	7.56	17.06	5.20	0.56	84

Note. [a] Missing data (questionnaire not completed): 3 men.
 [b] missing data (questionnaire not completed): 3 men and 3 cases of death in men.
 *p = 0.04 (two-tailed t-test)

of the MI. This first report is limited to an analysis of the interaction between Type A behavior and anxiety and of their impact on the prognosis during the first year after the MI.

Method

Design

The design of the main study is presented in Figure 1. The baseline questionnaires were administrated during the last days of hospital care, usually 8 to 10 days after the occurence of the MI. The follow-up data reported here were collected at clinic visits three and twelve months after the MI. At the 12-month follow-up missing data in cases of death were collected from hospital records. Essential information on survival and causes of death were able to be collected from the entire sample.

Subjects

The sample comprises a consecutive series of patients who were hospitalized because of their first MI and survived the acute phase (N = 123). A total of 16 patients were excluded from the sample because of problems in filling in the questionnaires due to other complicating illnesses or language difficulties, or social problems. Furthermore, 15 patients refused to participate in the program. In the age or sex distribution these 31 patients did not differ significantly from those (N = 92) who were able to participate.

The mean age was 53, 16 years (range 38–64 years); there were 76 men (82,6%) and 16 women (17,4%) in the sample.

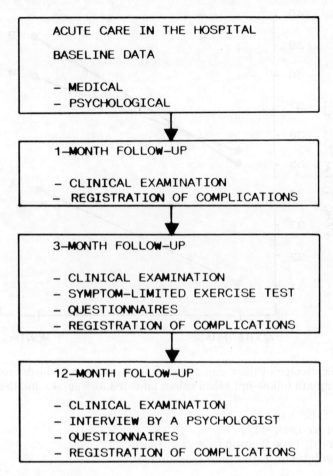

ACUTE CARE IN THE HOSPITAL

BASELINE DATA

- MEDICAL
- PSYCHOLOGICAL

1-MONTH FOLLOW-UP

- CLINICAL EXAMINATION
- REGISTRATION OF COMPLICATIONS

3-MONTH FOLLOW-UP

- CLINICAL EXAMINATION
- SYMPTOM-LIMITED EXERCISE TEST
- QUESTIONNAIRES
- REGISTRATION OF COMPLICATIONS

12-MONTH FOLLOW-UP

- CLINICAL EXAMINATION
- INTERVIEW BY A PSYCHOLOGIST
- QUESTIONNAIRES
- REGISTRATION OF COMPLICATIONS

Figure 1 Design of the study.

Measures

Type A behavior was measured with a self-report scale developed by Järvikoski and Härkäpää (1987). The sum of 14 items covers components of time urgency, impatience, competitiveness, efficiency, and inability to relax. The reliability of the scale is satisfactory (Cronbach's alpha =0.69), and the 14-item sum significantly differentiates persons with symptoms indicating coronary heart disease (Järvikoski & Härkäpää, 1987). It has further been shown to correlate significantly (r = 0.65, p = 0.001) with the Type A score of the JAS and to differentiate coronary patients from controls (Julkunen, unpublished data). The patients were asked to answer the questions according to how they used to live and behave before the present illness. Anxiety was measured by the Present Affect Reactions Questionnaire (PARQ IV) developed by Endler et al. (1985) to measure state anxiety. The scale is composed of two subscales, "cognitive-worry" (C–W) and "autonomic-emotional" (A–E), 10 items in each. The scale has been shown to be a highly reliable and valid measure of

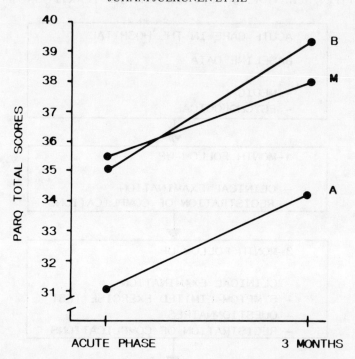

Figure 2. The change of the mean anxiety scores in Type A thirds from an acute phase to a 3-month follow-up. Mean values adjusted for age, sex and the severity of MI.
A = highest Type A (n = 27)
M = medium group (n = 27)
B = lowest third, Type B group (n = 26)
PARQ = Present Affect Reactions Questionnaire.

state anxiety (Endler et al., 1985). The extension of the MI (transmural vs. nontransmural) and the occurence of left ventricular failure in the acute phase were used to indicate the severity of the infarction.

Results

Table 1 summarizes the mean values of Type A and anxiety scores at the baseline and the anxiety scores at the 3-month follow-up for men and women. There is only one significant sex difference, i.e. women score higher on the Type A scale.

The interaction of Type A scores with changes in anxiety up to the 3-month follow-up was studied by using an analysis of covariance for repeated measures controlling for age, sex and severity of the MI. Figure 2 illustrates the changes of the total anxiety scores in Type A thirds. As to the whole sample, there is a significant increase in anxiety, $F(1,77) = 4.00$, $p = 0.05$. There is a tendency in the top Type A's to be less anxious at both time points, but none of the differences between the groups is significant.

The distribution of the observed complications during one year is presented in Table 2. Women tend to be more often hospitalized because of angina, but otherwise there are no significant sex differences. For further analysis the end-point categories 2 and 3 (hospitalization due to angina, angioplasty, or bypass operation) were combined and also the categories 4 and 5 (reinfarction or cardiac death) because of their relatively small frequencies.

Table 2 *Complications registered during the 1-year follow-up for men and women.*

complication	men		women		all	
	n	%	n	%	n	%
1. no complications	51	67.1	7	43.8	58	63.0
2. hospitalization due to angina pectoris	5	6.6	5	31.3	10	10.9
3. hospitalization due to angioplasty or bypass surgery	13	17.1	3	18.8	16	17.4
4. re-infarction	4	5.3	1	6.3	5	5.4
5. cardiac death	3	3.9	0	0.0	3	3.3
total	76	100.0	16	100.0	92	100.0

Note. The classification into different complications (end-point groups) is mutually exclusive. In cases with several complications only the most severe one according to the order indicated in the Table is registered here.

There were no other causes of death in this sample.

The association of the Type A scores and baseline anxiety with the prognosis were analyzed by COANOVAs by comparing the three end-point groups. Figure 3 illustrates these results indicating a significantly higher, $F(2,82) = 3.61$, $p = 0.03$, level of anxiety for the patients who will suffer a fatal or non-fatal cardiac event during the year after their first infarction.

The non-significant, $F(2,87) = 0.31$, association of the Type A scores with the prognosis was further controlled by using the social class and level of education as covariates. No essential change could be observed in the results.

Discussion

In this study we were not able to show that Type A behavior as measured with a self-report scale has any significant correlation with the one year prognosis of the first MI. This result is in line with most of the recent results obtained with the JAS or Structured Interview in larger samples (Case et al., 1985; Shekelle et al., 1985; Ragland & Brand, 1988).

What the results do suggest is that reactive anxiety during the phase of acute care, i. e. during the first week after the infarction, is an important indicator of a poor prognosis. The result was not affected by a statistical control for age, sex, or the severity of the MI as indicated by the left ventricular failure and/or transmural

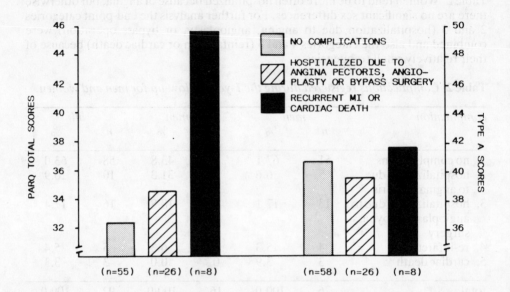

Figure 3. Baseline anxiety and Type A mean values in the three end-point groups (one-year follow-up). Mean values of Type A adjusted for age and sex. Mean values of anxiety adjusted for age, sex and severity of MI. (PARQ =Present Affect Reactions Questionnaire).

infarction diagnosed by a cardiologist. These prospective results indicate that after a MI, at least during the first year, reactive disorders like anxiety are more closely associated with the prognosis than is the Type A behavior.

The results also indicate that anxiety in post-MI patients increases after discharge from hospital up to the 3-month follow-up. This result confirms clinical experience and results in earlier resports (Kaufhold, 1987).

The data presented in this report do not justify a conclusion that anxiety has an independent causal role in the prognosis, although it is known that anxiety can produce undesirable physiological effects (e.g. arrhythmias) and thus affect survival from a heart attack (Shine, 1984).

It is also possible that the level of anxiety is an indicator of a poor coping style thus reflecting a more general inability to cope successfully with the crises caused by a serious, life-threatening illness. Data regarding coping was collected at the three-month follow-up and will be reported together with the continued follow-up of the whole sample.

Acknowledgements
This study was supported by a grant from the Signe and Ane Gyllenberg Foundation to the first author. Grateful acknowledgement is due to Inkeri Revitzer for assistance in collecting the psychological data.

References

Case, R. B., Heller, S. S., Case, N. B., Moss, A. J., and The Multicenter Research Group. (1985). Type A behavior and survival after acute myocardial infarction. *The New England Journal of Medicine, 312*, 737–741.

Cassem, N. H., and Hackett, T. P. (1973). Psychological rehabilitation of myocardial infarction patients in the acute phase. *Heart & Lung, 2*, 382–388.

Endler, N. S., Edwards, J. M., and Vitelli, R. (1985). *Situation-Response General Trait Anxiety Inventroy (S–R GTA) and Present Affect Reactions Questionnaire (PARQ IV): A manual for state and trait anxiety measures.* Research Report 152, Department of Psychology, York University, Toronto.

Friedman, M., Thoresen, C. E., Gill, J. J., Powell, L. H., Ulmer, D., Thompson, L., Price, V. A., Rabin, D. D., Breall, W. S., Dixon, T., Levy, R., and Bourg, E. (1984). Alteration of Type A behavior and reduction in cardiac recurrences in postmyocardial infarction patients. *American Heart Journal. 108*, 237–248.

Gentry, D. W., Baider, L., Oude-Weme, J. D., Musch, F., and Gary, H. E. (1983). Type A/B differences in coping with acute myocardial infarction: Further considerations. *Heart & Lung, 12*, 212–214.

Hanses, O. (1988). *Anxiety and psychological intervention in the rehabilitation of patients with myocardial infarction*, Kansaneläkelaitoksen julkaisuja ML:79, Turku.

Haynes, S. G., and Matthews, K. A. (1988). Area review: Coronary-prone behavior: Continuing evolution of the concept. *Annals of Behavioral Medicine, 10*, 47–59.

Jenkins, C. D., Zyzanski, S. J., and Rosenman, R. H. (1971). Progress toward validation of a computer-scored test for the Type A coronary-prone behavior pattern. *Psychosomatic Medicine, 33*, 193–202.

Jenkins, C. D., Zyzanski, S. J., and Rosenman, R. H. (1976). Risk of new myocardial infarction in middle-aged men with manifest coronary heart disease. *Circulation, 53*, 342–347.

Järvikoski, A., and Härkäpää, K. (1987). A brief Type-A scale and the occurance of cardiovascular symptoms. *Scandinavian Journal of Rehabilitation Medicine, 19*, 115–120.

Kaufhold, G. (1987). Zur Bedeutung des Typ-A Verhaltensmusters für die Herzinfarktrehabilitation [Type A behavior and the rehabilitation of coronary heart disease]. In B.Badura, G. Kaufhold, H. Lehman, H. Pfaff, T. Schott, and M. Waltz (Eds.), *Leben mit dem Herzinfarkt* (pp. 286–320) Berlin: Springer.

Keefe, F. J., Castell, P. J., and Blumenthal, J. A. (1986). Angina pectoris in type A and type B cardiac patients. *Pain, 27*, 211–218.

New York Heart Association, the Criteria Committee (1964). *Diseases of the heart and blood vessels. Nomenclature and criteria for diagnosis.* Boston: Little, Brown and Co.

Ragland, D. R., and Brand R. J. (1988). Type A behavior and mortality from coronary heart disease. *The England Journal of Medicine, 318*, 65–69.

Shekelle, R. B., Gale, M., and Norusis, M. (1985). Type A score (Jenkins Activity Survey) and risk of recurrent coronary heart disease in the Aspirin Myocardial Infarction Study. *American Journal of Cardiology, 56*, 221–225.

Shine, K. I. (1984). Anxiety in patients with heart disease. *Psychosomatics, 25*, 27–31.

Borderline Hypertension and Relaxation Training

Jan Vinck

Essential hypertension is a multifactorially determined health risk. One of the factors that are involved is behavior. WHO therefore recommends using behavioral methods as an adjunct or even as an alternative to pharmacological treatment in mild hypertension (WHO, 1986). Apart from the possible role of smoking and diet, it is commonly assumed that the experience of stress plays some role in the etiology of essential hypertension (e.g. McCaffrey & Blanchard, 1985). If the experience of stress is implicated in the etiology of hypertension, relaxation training should be a valid treatment approach for this condition, and we see that it is indeed among the frequently used behavioral treatment modalities for essential hypertension. The results of relaxation training are, however, generally moderate and for a considerable number of subjects insufficient (Vaitl, 1982; Cottier, Shapiro & Julius, 1984). One of the possible reasons for this relative weakness of relaxation training as a means of treating hypertension is that its effect is different in different subjects. We see that the effect is indeed, highly variable. Group means may mask strong effects in different directions in individual subjects. This implies that relaxation training may be an effective treatment, but only for some patients.

In this paper, a number of studies is reviewed exploring two ways in which the effect of relaxation training on blood pressure (BP) could be enhanced:
– by finding out how the effect of relaxation training on blood pressure can be predicted, so that it is possible to select "good" candidates for relaxation training, given this variability of the effect;
– by trying to understand the mechanism of the effect of relaxation training on BP; when this is known, it will be possible to focus on the active elements of the training.

Prediction of the Effect of Relaxation Training on BP

Our first efforts to predict the effect of relaxation training on BP were done with students. We developed regression equations for the prediction of two measures of the effect of the training: the therapeutic effect (THERAP: the difference between the BP readings before the first and before the last training session) and the training effect (TRAIN: BP decrease during relaxation in the first as compared to the last training session)(Vinck, Arickx & Hongenaert, 1987a). These regression equations are as follows:
for systolic BP

> THERAP : 101.185 – 0.828 initial BP + 5.811 male
> TRAIN : 5.242 – 0.747 initial BP change

for diastolic BP

> THERAP : 59.22 – 0.757 initial BP + 0.33 initial BP change
> TRAIN : –2.109 – 0.941 initial BP change – 0.399 NS + 0.109 E

"male" = 1 for male, 0 for female subjects; NS and E being both scales from the ABV: NS: neuroticism expressed in somatic complaints and E: extraversion, both comparable to EPI variables (Wilde, 1970).

Given observed values for the predictors in these regression equations, one can predict a specific outcome .

When we predicted BP response to relaxation training in a second group of students (N=104) with these regression equations, we found highly significant differences in mean BP changes between groups with predicted decrease and groups with predicted increase of their BP. This was also the case in a third group of students (N=96), where subjects were randomly assigned to progressive relaxation or to autogenic training (Table 1).

Table 1. *Mann-Whitney U tests on observed BP changes (mm Hg) after Autogenic Training (AT) and Progressive Relaxation (PR) between groups with predicted increase (Inc) and groups with predicted decrease (Dec) in BP*

			AT			PR	
Outcome	Predicted direction	N	Observed median	$p<$	N	Observed median	$p<$
THERAP							
SBP	Inc	26	+ 1	0.0005	12	+ 4.5	NS
	Dec	13	−13		25	− 8	
DBP	Inc	23	+ 4	0.0001	15	+12	0.0006
	Dec	16	−20		22	− 8	
TRAIN							
SBP	Inc	17	+ 9	0.0003	16	+ 9	0.0001
	Dec	22	− 7.5		21	− 6	
DBP	Inc	18	+14.5	0.0001	21	+ 8	0.0006
	Dec	21	− 8		16	−13	

From Vinck et al. (1987a). Copyright by A. P. A. Reprinted by permission.

Using the same method, we then predicted BP responses of the subjects from the English and Baker (1983) study (N=24). The correlations between predicted and observed BP responses range from 0.52 to 0.81 and are all significant.

It appears that this method can reliably predict immediate BP response to relaxation training in normotensives. The finding that higher initial BP is related to a larger (THERAP) effect is repeatedly reported for hypertensives (Jacob, Kraemer & Agras, 1977; Peters, Benson & Peters, 1977; Godaert, 1986). While initial BP is the most important element in the THERAP regression equation, we find the same relation in normotensives. The fact that initial success is inversely related to the TRAIN effect is rather unexpected. Also, the relative absence of psychological predictors in these regression equations is striking.

We also examined the relation between expectation of the effect of relaxation training on BP in another student sample. Agras, Horne and Taylor (1982) reported a relation between the belief in an immediate or in a delayed effect of relaxation training and the effect of training. In our study, however, we found strong correlations between expectation and initial BP (female group: $r = 0.46$, $p<0.01$; male group: $r = 0.26$, $p<0.05$), so that any correlation between expectation and the effect of relaxation training might be an artifact of this correlation between expectation and initial BP (Vinck, Arickx & Hongenaert, 1987b). Recently, Wittrock, Blanchard, McCoy, Musso, Berger, McCaffrey, Aivasyan, Khramelashvili, and Salenko (1988) found no relation between expectancy and outcome.

The possibility of predicting the effect of relaxation training on BP in *borderline hypertensives* is more important from a clinical point of view than the possibility to do so in students.

34 borderline hypertensives (5 female, 29 male; mean age 49.5 years; BP over 140/90 on at least two occasions; mean pre-training BP 146.32/98.2 mm Hg) were recruited from a large company and were given progressive relaxation during 9 one-hour sessions (Vinck, Van de Broeck, Vertommen & Props, 1987).

Blood pressure response to relaxation training was assessed in two different settings: in the training situation ("*laboratory effect*") and in the medical department of the company ("*clinical effect*").

Blood pressure response was predicted using the same regression equations as we used with our student samples. Furthermore two indices for BP reactivity were taken: *task reactivity* was measured using the Stroop Color Word Interference test; *Situational reactivity* was measured as the difference between initial BP readings in the clinical and in the training situation.

Prediction of the Short-Term Effect (Pre-Post)

Regression Equations and Cardiovascular Reactivity

The laboratory effect appeared to be strongly related to the predictions by means of the regression equations ($r=0.68$ for SBP and 0.69 for DBP) (Figure. 1:Post).

The clincal effect was only slightly related to the predictions on the basis of the regression equations ($r=-0.32$ for SBP and 0.21 for DBP); this clinical effect is, however, strongly related to BP reactivity: we find correlation of 0.40 (SBP, $p<0.10$) and 0.53 (DBP, $p<0.02$) with the magnitude of situational reactivity and of $-.73$ (SBP, $p<0.001$) and -0.36 (DBP, $p<0.10$) with the magnitude of task reactivity.

The direction of the effect of situational reactivity is as expected (Manuck & Krantz, 1984): greater reactivity goes with larger BP response to treatment. The direction of the effect of task reactivity is, however, opposite to expectation: larger reactivity to the task goes with *smaller* effects of the training. This relation is difficult to interpret. The same unexpected relation has been reported by Godaert (1986).

Representation of Illness

– hypertension as a somatic problem: we asked our subjects to indicate what, in their opinion, was the cause of their hypertension. About 2/3 of the sample was convinced that stress was the primary cause of their illness. 24% told us their hypertension was caused by a physical problem (although they had been medically screened so that no secondary hypertensions were included in the sample). It appeared that the clinical effect for the systolic BP correlated 0.51 ($p<0.05$) with this conviction that their hypertension was a physical problem; for diastolic BP the correlation was nonsignificant ($r = 0.25$). So those who are convinced that their hypertension is essentially a physical problem benefits less from relaxation training.

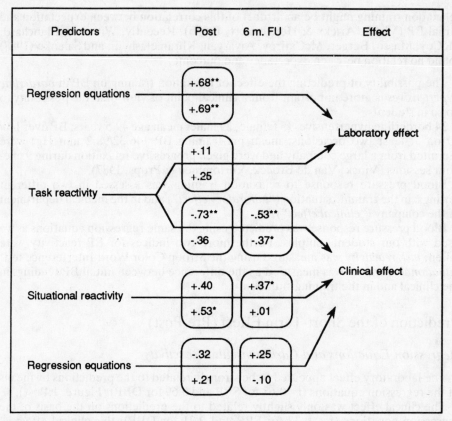

Figure 1. Pearson correlations between cardiovascular reactivity and effects of relaxation training on BP; correlations above the line refer to systolic, under the line to diastolic BP; correlations between regression equations and effects are correlations between predicted and observed BP changes $p < 0.10$; ** $p < 0.05$.

– the experiencing of symptoms: our subjects indicated, before the training, whether or not they could feel when their BP was high. Mean systolic BP reductions are larger in subjects perceiving symptoms, as can be seen from Table 2. Differences for diastolic BP are in the same direction but not significant. The fact that BP actually goes up in subjects without symptom perception is impressive.

Table 2. *Mean BP reductions for subjects with perception of symptoms*

| Effect | | Perception of symptoms | | |
		Yes	No	p
Laboratory	SBP	−5.00	+ 7.33	‹0.10
	DBP	−2.50	+ 3.00	NS
Clinical	SBP	−8.23	+ 12.66	‹0.05
	DBP	−4.47	− 0.66	NS

Prediction of the Effect after 6 months

After 6 months, we assessed BP only in the clinical situation. The predictions made with the regression equations correlated only slightly with the observed effect: $r = -0.25$ and 0.10 for systolic and diastolic BP respectively (Figure.1: 6m. FU). The correlations with cardiovascular reactivity were again higher and were in the same direction as with the immediate effect: for task reactivity: $r = -0.53$ ($p<0.01$) and -0.37 ($p<0.05$); for situational reactivity: $r = 0.37$ ($p<0.05$) and 0.01 (NS).

These results confirm the relation between the clinical effect of relaxation training on BP in borderline hypertensives and cardiovascular reactivity. Especially task reactivity is quite consistently related to the effect of the training: subjects with smaller BP reactions to the task show larger effects. Subjects with larger situational reactivity show larger effects.

In conclusion, we can say that, when they are measured in a non-clinical situation, BP changes after relaxation training can be predicted with the regression equations we presented, in normotensives as well as in borderline hypertensives. The fact that initial BP is an important factor in the prediction of the THERAP effect is not surprising: relations between initial BP and effect of relaxation training have been repeatedly reported (Jacob, Kraemer & Agras, 1977; Peters, Benson & Peters, 1977; Godaert, 1986). For the TRAIN effect we find that larger initial effects go with less changes after training.

Effects in the clinical situation are related to cardiovascular reactivity and to the representation of the illness in borderline hypertensives. Similar to the results reported by Godaert (1986), we find a relation in the expected sense for situational reactivity and in the opposite sense for task reactivity. The latter finding is difficult to interpret. As far as the role of representation of illness is concerned, it seems reasonable that when such representation fits with the rationale of relaxation training, compliance with instructions to keep practicing will be higher (Leventhal, Nerenz & Steele, 1984). Later on we will see that continued practice is usually related to the effect of relaxation training.

Further investigation will have to look at the possibility of using physiological correlates of emotion (Utz, Bernal, Higgins, Woerner & McGrady, 1984; Cottier, Shapiro & Julius, 1984) and of measures of coping style (Godaert, 1986) to predict BP changes.

The Mechanism of the Effect of Relaxation Training on BP

In another series of studies, we tried to find out *how* relaxation training affects BP. Is the effect of relaxation training on BP related to specific changes during the training? If this mechanism, which is not well known (Johnston, 1986), could be detected, we would be in a position to strengthen the effect by focusing on the active ingredients of the technique.

We have considered the possible role in this respect of psychophysiological and of psychological variables.

Psychophysiological Mechanisms

Again, we first looked at this possibility in students. In the first instance we explored the possibility that BP is affected by relaxation training via some physiological component of the relaxation response (Vinck, Arickx, Hongenaert, Grossman, Vertommen & Beckers, 1988). Three of these physiological changes, muscle relaxation, peripheral temperature and respiration, held our attention, because they are well-known elements of the relaxation response, because they had been related to the effect of relaxation training on BP (McCaffrey & Blanchard, 1985; Blanchard, McCoy, McCaffrey, Musso, Wittrock, Berger, Gerardi, Pangburn, Khramelashvili, Aivasyan & Berger, 1988a; Grossman & Defares, 1984) and because they can be specifically trained.

When we trained students to specifically alter these physiological parameters, we did not find stronger decreases of their BP than in control groups. For the muscle relaxation and the temperature groups this may be caused by the fact that our training was not very effective; in the respiration group, however, we see marked changes in respiratory pattern and no extra BP reduction. Given this failure to produce condition-specific effects, we decided to look at the correlations of the variations in these parameters and the variations in BP. If one of these variables is mediating BP change after relaxation training, it is to be expected, indeed, that large variations in BP will go with larger variations in this specific variable. There was, however, no such correlation between BP and any of the parameters concerned.

Finally, we looked at the possible role of changes in vagal activity, operationalized in terms of changes in respiratory sinus arrhythmia (RSA) in the production of BP changes: RSA appeared to be correlated to systolic BP at the beginning of the test session but not to BP changes (Hongenaert, Arickx & Vinck, 1985).

So, without being conclusive in any way, we clearly have not found the physiological mediator of the BP lowering effect of relaxation training.

In our group of borderline hypertensives, we examined the role of changes in cardiovascular reactivity. Cardiovascular reactivity is, as has been said, considered to be an important variable in the etiology and maintenance of essential hypertension. We therefore examined the hypothesis that changes in cardiovascular reactivity during the training would be related to the amount of change in BP. In accordance with the original hypothesis of an association between stronger cardiovascular reactivity, higher BP and stronger effects of relaxation training, we expected that in successful subjects, we would find a decrease in cardiovascular reactivity over the training period.

Table 3. *Mean BP changes (clinical effect) of subjects with task reactivty*

	increased		decreased	
	post	FU	post	FU
SBP				
N	8	8	15	14
Mean	−15.7	−14.4	+ 2.2	− 4.9
S.D	13.2	4.4	12.7	17.5
DBP				
N	7	6	15	14
Mean	−11.3	−15	− 1	− 4.8
S.D	8.1	4.4	6.7	7.1

As one can see from Table 3, the effects of relaxation training are much larger in subjects whose task reativity *increased* than in subjects whose cardiovascular reactivity decreased during the training. All differences of BP changes between groups with increased and groups with decreased reactivity are significant ($p<0.05$), except for the difference at follow-up for systolic BP. This is contrary to (at least our) expectation, but is consistent with the reported relation between smaller initial task reactivity and larger effects. It is also consistent with the increase in BP reactivity that Blanchard, McCoy, McCaffrey, Wittrock, Musso, Berger, Aivasyan, Khramelashvili and Salenko (1988b) found in their treated patients, much to their surprise and disappointment. As in the Blanchard et al. study, one must, of course, be cautious with these results because they are based on small numbers of observations. The consistency of the finding is, however, intriguing.

Psychologocial Mechanisms

Not only physiological changes occur when subjects learn to relax. All kinds of psychological changes are produced as well, and, as Johnston (1986) has argued, these could equally well play a role in the BP lowering effect of relaxation training. If the experience of stress is related to BP elevation, and if relaxation training can make subjects feel calm, or adopt a different outlook on life so that they experience less stress, this feeling of subjective relaxation might explain that after relaxation training BP goes down generally, and maybe explain that in some subjects it does not. Other changes could be added here but were not examined in our study.

Subjective Relaxation

In one study (Vinck, Arickx & Hongenaert, 1987b) we asked our students to rate on a visual analogue scale how relaxed they felt during the post-treatment relaxation test. We also had them fill out a number of personality questionnaires before and after the training. As far as subjective relaxation is concerned, we find a significantly negative correlation between subjective relaxation and change in systolic BP over the test session ($r = -0.225$, $p<0.05$). The direction of this relation is opposite to expectation: subjects who feel more relaxed show less systolic BP reduction. Again, however, this result may be an artifact of the even stronger correlation between subjective relaxation and initial systolic BP: subjects with lower systolic BP at the start of the test feel subjectively calmer during the session ($r = -0.235$, $p<0.01$). And this lower initial pressure is, as we have seen, related to lower BP reduction in this population.

Personality Changes

Correlations between changes in personality scale scores and changes in BP over the training period were, in our student sample, generally low. There is one notable exception: in the active training condition, we find a strong positive correlation between change in neuroticism and change in systolic BP ($r= 0.418$, $p<0.01$). The positive correlation means that – in this active group and not in the control group – a change in the direction of greater emotional stability is associated with greater BP reduction and vice versa. This finding cannot be interpreted as meaning that relaxation training leads to a reduction of neurotiscism: the mean N-score in this group does not change over the training period. But clearly the training is responsible for the association between both variables. Cottier, Shapiro and Julius (1984) report a similar finding of decreased anxiety over the training period in successfully-treated patients only.

Continued Practice

Most studies report larger effects for subjects that continue to practice relaxation after the training phase or trends in this direction (Charlesworth, Williams & Baer, 1984; Wadden, 1983). Godaert (1986) found no difference between subjects that were asked to continue and subjects that were asked to stop active training. In our sample of borderline hypertentives we had self-reported information on the amount of active use of the relaxation technique after the end of the training for 18 subjects. This variable correlated negatively with the clinical effect after 6 months: SBP $r = -0.43$ ($p < 0.10$); DBP $r = -0.46$ ($p < 0.05$). So subjects continuing to practice the relaxation tend to have more BP reduction after the 6 month follow-up.

It is possible that subjects continue practicing when they consider their problem as a stress-problem (and not as a somatic problem) and/or when they perceive symptoms that can be alleviated by relaxation training.

Summarizing the results of this section, we have found no evidence for a mediating role of psychophysiological variables in the effect of relaxation training on BP, except for the role of cardiovascular reactivity: a rise in cardiovascular reactivity may be related to stronger BP reductions after training. As far as psychological variables are concerned, the possible role of subjective relaxation could not be confirmed, but a change in emotional stability as measured by the N-scale may accompany better results of training. In the borderline group, continued practice appears to favour better outcome.

It must be stressed that in this section on mechanisms, we did not find any relation with diastolic pressure and that the results reviewed in this section await replication, which is not the case for the most important results of the "prediction" section.

Conclusion

If one of the starting points of this research program was the hypothesis that the effects of relaxation training on BP are highly variable, this has been amply confirmed. There is much situational and individual variability.

This variability of effect appears to be predictable to some extent. When the effect is assessed in a non-clinical situation, the effect can be predicted fairly well with the regression equations we presented. The clinical effect is related to cardiovascular reactivity and to the representation of the BP problem by the patient. While less is known about the mechanism behind this effect, changes in emotional stability, changes in cardiovascular reactivity and continued practice of the training might be implicated.

Many of the results we presented remain to be confirmed in replications. At the time of writing we are assessing the one-year follow-up results in a second group of borderline hypertensives. Important questions that remain have to do with the role of cardiovascular reactivity, as well with the role of task reactivity (that was inversely related to success and was enlarged in successful patients) as with that of situational reactivity. In connenction with this role of cardiovascular reactivity, the importance of physiological correlates of stress, anger and Type A behavior and the role of coping remain to be explored. One of the specific questions in this respect is whether continued practice is an effective form of coping and whether this is related to the representation of the problem, as our data suggest. Finally, the role of a family history of hypertension in this picture may not be overlooked.

From a clinical point of view, it will be important to set up controlled clinical trials where the results from this and other studies are incorporated to find out if clinical outcome is favorably affected by selection of patients using the predictors we described. Also the results from our studies suggest a number of potentially important treatment variables, like the representation of the problem and continued practice. It seems worthwhile to examine whether a treatment approach that is focused on these variables adds to the effet of relaxation training on BP.

Footnotes

(1) Parts of this research program have been supported by the Ministry of Health, and by the National Fund for Scientific Research. The collaboration of Dr. Pollefeyt, Med. Dept Belgische Boerenbond is also gratefully acknowledged.
(2) At different stages M. Arickx, J. Beckers, P. Grossman, M. Hongenaert, K. Lagrou, A. Props, M. Van de Broeck and H. Vertommen have collaborated in these studies.

References

Agras, W. S., Horne, M. and Taylor, C. B. (1982). Expectation and the blood-pressure-lowering effects of relaxation. *Psychosomatic Medicine, 44*, 389–395.

Blanchard, E. B., McCoy, G. C., McCaffrey, R. J., Musso, A., Wittrock, D., Berger, M., Gerardi, M., Pangburn, L., Khramelashvili, V., Aivasyan, T., and Salenko, B. (1988a). The USSR-USA collaborative cross-cultural comparison of autogenic training and thermal biofeedback in the treatment of mild hypertension. Presented 19th Annual Meeting of the Biofeedback Society of America, Colorado Springs.

Blanchard, E. B., McCoy, G. C., McCaffrey, R. J., Wittrock, D., Musso, A., Berger, M., Aivasyan, T., Kramelashvili, V., and Salenko, B. (1988b). The effects of thermal biofeedback and autogenic training on cardiac reactivity: the Joint USSR-USA Behavioral Hypertension Treatment Project. *Biofeedback and Self-Regulation, 13*, 25–38.

Charlesworth, E. A., Williams, B. J., and Baer, P. E. (1984). Stress management at the worksite for hypertension: compliance, cost-benefit, health care and hypertension related variables. *Psychosomatic Medicine, 46*, 387–397.

Cottier, C., Shapiro, K. and Julius, S. (1984). Treatment of mild hypertension with progressive muscle relaxation. Predictive value of indexes of sympathetic tone. *Archives of Internal Medicine, 144*, 1954–1958.

English, E. H., and Baker, T. B. (1983). Relaxation training and cardiovascular response to experimental stressors. *Health Psychology, 2*, 239–259.

Godaert, G. (1986). *Hoge bloeddruk en relaxatie. Klinisch psychologische en psychofysiologische aspekten.* (Hypertension and relaxation.) Doctoral dissertation, Free Univ. Amsterdam.

Grossman, P., and Defares, P. (1984). Breathing to the heart of the matter. Effects of respiratory influences upon cardiovascular phenomena. In C. D. Spielberger and I. Sarason (Eds.), *Stress and anxiety. Vol 10*. Washington, DC: Hemisphere.

Hongenaert, M., Arickx, M., and Vinck, J. (1985). Vagal activity during relaxation and its relation to blood pressure. Presented 15th Annual Meeting of the European Association for Behavior Therapy, Munich.

Jacob, R. G., Kraemer, H. C., and Agras, W. S. (1977). Relaxation therapy in the treatment of hypertension: a review. *Archives of General Psychiatry, 34*, 1417–1427.

Johnston, D. (1986). How does relaxation training reduce blood pressure in primary hypertension? In T. H. Schmidt, T. M. Dembroski, and G. Blumchen (Eds.), *Biological and psychological factors in cardiovascular disease*. Berlin: Springer.

Leventhal, H., Nerenz, D. R., and Steele, D. J. (1984). Illness representations and coping with health threats. In A. Baum, S. E. Taylor, and J. S. Singer (Eds.), *Handbook of Psychology and Health. Vol. IV. Social psychological aspects of health*. Hillsdale, N. J.: Erlbaum.

Manuck, S. R., and Krantz, D. S. (1984). Psychophysiologic reactivity in coronary heart disease. *Behavioral Medicine Update, 6*, 11–15.

McCaffrey, R. J., and Blanchard, E. B. (1985). Stress management approaches of the treatment of essential hypertension. *Annals of Behavioral Medicine, 1*, 5–12.

Peters, R. K., Benson, H., and Peters, J. M. (1977). Daily relaxation response breaks in a working population: II. Effects on blood pressure. *American Journal of Public Health, 6*, 954–959.

Utz, S. H., Bernal, G. A. A., Higgins, J., Woerner, M., and McGrady, A. (1984). Predictors of success in hypertensives treated with biofeedback-assisted relaxation. *Biofeedback and Selfregulation, 9* (1), 187–188.

Vaitl, D. (1982). *Essentielle Hypertonie. Psychologisch-medizinische Aspekte* [Essential hypertension. Psychological and medical aspects]. Berlin: Springer.

Vinck, J., Arickx, M., and Hongenaert, M. (1987a). Predicting interindividual differences in blood pressure response to relaxation training in normotensives. *Journal of Behavioral Medicine, 10*, 395–410.

Vinck, J.,. Arickx, M., and Hongenaert, M. (1987b). On the mechanisms explaining blood pressure decrease after relaxation training. In W. Huber (Ed.), *Progress in Psychotherapy Research*. Louvain-La-Neuve: Presses Universitaires de Louvain.

Vinck, J., Van de Broeck, M., Vertommen, H., and Props, A. (1987). Cardiovascular reactivity and the effect of relaxation training on blood pressure. Presented First International Conference on Biobehavioral Self-Regulation and Health. Honolulu, Hawaii.

Vinck, J., Arickx, M., Hongenaert, M., Grossman, P., Vertommen, H., and Beckers, J. (1988). Can psychophysiological changes explain the blood pressure lowering effect of relaxation training? In T. Elbert., W. Langosch., A. Steptoe and D. Vaitl (Eds.)., *Behavioral Medicine in Cardiovascular Disorders*. London: Wiley.

Wadden, T. A. (1983). Predicting treatment response to relaxation therapy for essential hypertension. *Journal of Nervous and Mental Disease, 171*, 683–689.

Wilde, G. J. S. (1970). *Neurotische labiliteit, gemeten met de vragenlijstmethode*. [Neurotic lability measured by questionnaire]. Amsterdam: Van Rossen.

Wittrock, D. A., Blanchard, E. B., McCoy, G. C., McCaffrey, R. J., and Khramelashvili, V. K. (1988). Stress management procedures in the treatment of essential hypertension: relationship of patient expectancies to treatment outcome. Presented 19th Annual Meeting of the Biofeedback Society of America, Colorado Springs.

World Health Organisation (1986). 1986 Guidelines for the treatment of mild hypertension: Memorandum from a WHO/ISH meeting. *Bulletin of the World Health Organisation, 64*, 31–35.

Section 7

Beliefs and Perceptions of Chronic Illness

Psychological Determinants of Diabetic Self-Care: The Role of Knowledge, Beliefs and Intentions

Liesbeth J. M. Pennings-Van der Eerden

The central theme of this study is the prediction of self-care behaviour in patients with Insulin-Dependent Diabetes Mellitus (IDDM). Diabetes mellitus is a chronic metabolic disease characterized by an absolute or relative insufficiency of insulin, a pancreatic hormone. Without administration of insulin, normalization of blood glucose levels in IDDM patients cannot take place. The view that normalization of blood glucose levels leads to fewer medical complications (e.g. blindness, renal failure, amputation, heart attack) has received increasing empirical support. Normalization of metabolic function therefore constitutes the goal of treatment with emphasis upon maintenance of relatively normal blood glucose levels. Because blood glucose levels fluctuate throughout the day, self-care behaviour by diabetic patients is vital in the treatment of the illness.

Self-care behaviours include taking medication, following dietary prescriptions, physical exercise, foot care, testing urine and blood glucose, making notes and preventing hypoglycaemia and hyperglycaemia. According to the theory of reasoned action (Ajzen, 1985), a person's intention to perform (or not to perform) self-care behaviour is the immediate antecedent of that behaviour. The intention, in turn, can be a function of other functions, such as internal locus (Schlenk & Hart, 1984), knowledge (Wysocki, Czyzyk, Slonska, Krolewski & Janeczko, 1978), self-efficacy expectations (McCaul, Glasgow & Schafer, 1987), health beliefs (Wilson, Ary, Biglan, Glasgow, Toobert & Campbell, 1986) and social support (Glasgow & Toobert, 1988). A satisfactory knowledge score does not always imply good self-care behaviour (e.g. Beggan, Cregan & Drury, 1982), which is why the relationship between knowledge and diabetic self-care behaviour is probably not a direct one.

Until now hierarchial regression techniques have been used to determine several powerful predictors of self-care behaviour. McCaul et al. (1987) found that motivational (e.g. self-efficacy expectations and environmental support) rather than knowledge factors were better predictors of self-care behavior (e.g. insulin administration and glucose testing), accounting for 20% of the variance. The results of Wilson et al. (1986) also revealed that psychosocial variables accounted for 25% of the variance in diabetic self-care behaviour. The variables most predictive of self-care behaviour are health beliefs, social support, knowledge, anxiety and depression. In a study by Glasgow et al. (1988), social environment was the strongest predictor of self-care behaviour among predictors such as stress and medical care satisfaction. Bloom-Cerkoney and Hart (1980) found that health belief motivators (e.g. perceived severity, perceived susceptibility, treatment benefits, barriers to carry out self-care behaviour and cues to action), accounted for 25% of the variation in self-care behaviour. It should be noted, however, that predictions from studies using regression procedures are confounded by the uncontrolled effect of correlated error terms. No attempt has been made to validate a diabeters-related behaviour model by the use of a more powerful technique that avoids this problem, such as structural equation modeling. In an attempt to determine a model of self-care behaviour, the present study applies LISREL-analysis (Jöreskog & Sörbom, 1983). It is intended to trace predictors and to model self-care behaviour.

Method

Sample

Seven-hundred and twenty diabetic patients were recruited from the population of members of the Dutch patient association, 'Diabetes Vereniging Nederland', 546 of whom responded (response rate 76%). All persons received and returned a questionnaire by post. Only IDDM patients (n = 475) were selected for the investigation under report in order to obtain a homogeneous group. Subjects' ages ranged from 18 to 65; 246 were male and 229 female. The average duration of diabetes was 14.0 years (range 0–51 years). The education level varied from low (16%), low-middle (39%) and middle (20%) to middle-high (17%) and high (8%).

Measures

The level of self-care behaviour was measured by a self-report inventory, the Self-care Behaviour Checklist (SCBC), designed to measure 14 components of diabetes self-care. Three functional groups of components were distinguished: (a) following basic medical prescription (supply of insulin; dietary intake; physical exercise), (b) self-observation (self-monitoring of urine and blood glucose; inspection of the feet; body weight; making notes) and (c) self-regulation (correction of hypoglycaemia or hyperglycaemia; variation of dietary intake; preparing a holiday; self-regulating activities in case of physical exercise; viral infection and environmental stress). A 5-point scale with endpoints "never" and "always" was used for each item. Cronbach's alpha reliability for the inventory is 0.76.

Intention to Self-Care Behaviour (ISCB) was a 14-item inventory designed to measure the degree to which patients attempt to exhibit the 14 self-care behaviours mentioned above. A 5-point scale with endpoints "extremely unlikely" and "extremely likely" was used for each item. Cronbach's alpha reliability for this inventory is 0.85.

The Self (vs. Physician) Motivation Scale (SPMC) was developed to assess the extent to which a patient views himself/herself as responsible for controlling the illness, as opposed to the physician. The scale comprised 9 diabetes specific statements with 5 point subscales ("strongly agree" and "strongly disagree"), such as "Only the physician can regulate my blood sugar" (negative) and "I can monitor my blood sugar" (positive). Cronbach's alpha reliability for this scale is 0.71.

The Locus (internal vs external) Scale (LS) consisted of six situations such as "Imagine, you are at home with friends and you follow dietary prescriptions", with two response alternatives: "(a) Is this because you can easily skip snacks" (internal) "or (b) is it just by chance" (external). Cronbach's alpha for the scale is 0.61.

The Controllability (effort vs. ability) Scale (CS) consisted of seven situations, such as 'Imagine, that you don't inspect your feet well at home", with two response alternatives: "(a) Is this because you cannot inspect your feet" (lack of ability, i. e. uncontrollable), "or (b) is this because you don't make the effort (lack of effort; i. e. controllable). Cronbach's alpha for this scale is 0.76.

Knowledge of the Disease (KD), a 10-item multiple-choice test, was hypothesized to measure general knowledge of diabetes. Cronbach's alpha for this test is 0.69.

The sum score of the Health Condition Questionnaire (HCQ) resulted from nine perceived manifestations of diabetic health condition such as the level of trembling, tiredness and nausea (negative) and the level of vivacity, activity and fitness (positive). This 9-item questionnaire contained 5-point scales with endpoints "always" and "never". Cronbach's alpha for this questionnaire is 0.79.

Barriers in Daily Life due to Illness (BDLI) measured the perceived level of interference due to the illness in five daily life situations: carrying out daily activities, leasure activities, sport activities, having parties or going out and spending holidays. A 5-point scale with endpoints "always" and "never" was used for each item. Cronbach's alpha for this scale is 0.81.

Design and Data Analysis

The study was designed to examine whether self-care behaviour is related to trait-like variables which seemed promising in other studies and a pilot study (Pennings-van der Eerden, 1984). For the reason of space limitation, only one self-care behaviour model will be presented (Figure. 1). The social environment was not included in this study. Other excluded variables were age, sex and illness duration, of which age correlated only slightly with the behaviour measures (r = −0.19). The dependent variables in the model were intention and self-care behaviour. The predictor variables in this study were six independent variables, grouped in three sets of latent variables: motivation, knowledge and the perception of physical health. Indicators of the latent variable 'motivation' are 'internal locus' (LS), 'self motivation' (SPMC) and 'controllability' (CS), and indicators of latent variable 'the perception of physical health' and 'health condition' (HCQ) and 'barriers in daily life' (negative) (BDLI). Intention, self-care behaviour and knowledge were directly measured by the means of the measures ISCB, SCBC and KD.

To obtain a thorough understanding of the data, the statistical procedure of LISREL was used. LISREL models can be recursive and nonrecursive. Recursive means that the latent variable have unidirectional relations, while non-recursive means that reciprocal causal effects could be identified. LISREL also allows the researcher to estimate effects of latent (unobservable) constructs (for an introduction to the LISREL-approach, see: Saris & Stronkhorst, 1984). Analyses were based on the General Model of Jöreskog (1979) and performed with the LISREL VI programme (Jöreskog & Sörbom, 1983). Errors of measurement are present because of imperfections in the various measuring instruments. The errors of measurement of the variables are discounted in the model by including alpha-reliability coefficients of the different measures.

Results

The resulting model is shown in Figure. 1. The overall goodness-of-fit test of the final LISREL model is 0.996, indicating a high degree of fit between the observed covariance matrix and the covariance matrix derived from the estimated effects (X^2 = 8.27, df = 9, p = 0.507). This means that the model fits the data. The amount of variance accounted for in self-care behaviour by the variables in the model is 81%. In Figure 1, the various measures are enclosed in squares while the latent variables or factors are enclosed in ovals. Straight arrows indicate the direction of influence, and the estimates of parameters for the arrows may be interpreted as standardized regression coefficients (i.e. beta weights). A bidirectional arrow indicates correlation, without any assumption of causality.

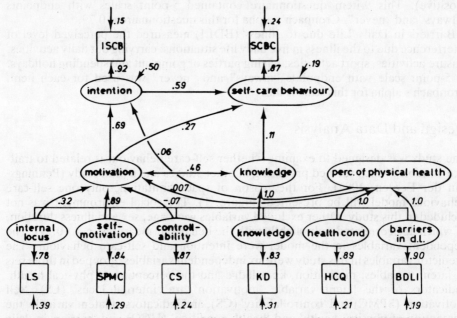

Figure 1. Psychological determinants of diabetic self-care, performed by LISREL VI.

Giving primary attention to the regression coefficients of the paths linking the ovals in the upper-half of the model, one can see that self-care behaviour is strongly determined by the latent variables 'intention to perform self-care behaviour' (0.59), less by 'motivation' (0.27), and slightly by 'knowledge' (0.11). In turn, intention, as a moderator, is strongly determined by motivation (0.69) and very slightly by the perception of physical health (0.06). Knowledge of diabetes mellitus is chiefly an indirect predictor of self-care behaviour through motivation (r = 0.46). The latent variable, the perception of physical health, is indirectly, but extremely slightly related to motivation (0.007) and to intention (0.06).

Discussion

Intention appears to be a good moderator between behaviour and the other latent variables. What was surprising in this study is that knowledge of the illness chiefly predicts self-care behaviour indirectly: only if a person is motivated does knowlege result in enhanced self-care behaviour. Possessing knowledge with a certain degree of motivation led to only slightly better scores on self-care behaviour. In the model, the latent variable 'the perception of physical health', showed scarcely any relationship to the other latent variables in the model. This means that perceived health condition does not predict self-care behaviour.

Motivation acquires a central role in this self-care model. One important feature of motivation is the perception of subjects that they are relatively independent of medical practioners in controlling the illness (0.89). This result seems not consistent with the results of several studies, which used Wallston and Wallstons' MHLC (cf. Wallston & Wallston, 1982; Schlenk et al., 1984), wherein the powerful other scales (PHLC) predicts diabetic self-care behaviour. These contradictory findings may be accounted for more extreme formulation of the SPMC items in the study under report, where patients are differentiated by (blindly) following their physicians in the treatment as opposed to acting (fully) independently.

In addition, patients with high self-care scores in this study consider themselves to be rather responsible for their treatment. In actual practice however, it is evident that medical practitioners must create the opportunity for patients to be active and self-responsible participants. For instance, Stewart (1984) found a positive effect on patient self-care behaviour and patient satisfaction when physicians explicitey requested patients' opinions and helped patients to express their own opinions.

Another feature of motivation is internal locus (0.32). Internal patients tend to exhibit higher levels of self-care behaviour as compared with patients who attribute self-care actions to chance or interference of the social environment. These data are consistent with several other studies (Wierenga, 1980; Schlenk et al., 1984; Holstein, Jörgenson & Sestoft, 1986).

Finally, controllability,as an important third feature of motivation does not contribute to the latent variable (–0.07). Perhaps, Weiner's (1980) suggestion of a dichotomeously measurement of 'lack of ability' and 'lack of effort', i.e. uncontrollable vs. controllable, which was applied in this study, is conceptually wrong, because both 'lack of ability' and 'lack of effort' can be controllable if – as in this case – learning is possible (cf. Weiner, 1985).

The fact that there is hardly any relationship between the latent variable 'perceived health condition' and the other factors in the model probably can be attributed to the fact that physical symptoms of diabetes may operate earlier as barriers (e.g. attempts to lower blood glucose could increase the frequency of hypoglycaemic episodes).

This study indicates that diabetic self-care behaviour can be particularly enhanced by an increase of knowledge, if patients view themselves as responsible for their health and as actors in controlling the illness. However, they should be encouraged in these perceptions by their health care provider. Diabetes education programmes should do more than merely provide factual information about diabetes. Knowledge of what a patient is supposed to do is neccesary, but not sufficient condition for enhancing self-care behaviour.

Acknowledgements

The author wishes to acknowledge her thanks to W. E. Saris, Ph. D., Professor in the Methodology of Social Science Research, University of Amsterdam, for valuable guidance of LISREL data analysis.

This research was supported by the Dutch patient association, 'Diabetes Vereniging Nederland'.

References

Ajzen, I. (1985). From Intentions to actions, a theory of planned behavior. In J. Kuhl and J. Beckmann (Eds.), *Action control: from cognition to behavior* (pp. 11–40). Heidelberg: Springer.

Beggan, M. P., Cregan, D., and Drury, M. I. (1982). Assessment of the outcome of an educational programme of diabetes self-care. *Diabetologia, 23*, 246–251.

Bloom-Cerkoney, K. A. B., and Hart, L. K. (1980). The relationship between health belief model and compliance of persons with diabetes mellitus. *Diabetes Care, 3*, 594–598.

Glasgow, R. E., and Toobert, D. J. (1988). Social environment and regimen adherence among type II diabetic patients. *Diabetes Care, 11*, 377–386.

Holstein, B. E., Jörgensen, H. V., and Sestoft, L. (1986). Illness-behaviour, attitude and knowledge in newly diagnosed diabetics. *Danish Medical Bulletin, 33*, 165–171.

Jöreskog, K. G. (1979). Structural equation models in the social sciences: specification, estimation and testing. In K. G. Jöreskog and D. Sörbom (Eds.), *Advances in factor analysis and structural equation models* (pp. 105–128). Cambridge: Adt Books.

Jöreskog, K. G., and Sörbom, D. (1983). *LISREL VI Users guide*. Upsala: Department of Statistics, University.

McCaul, K. D., Glasgow, R. E., and Schafer, L. C. (1987). Diabetes regimen behaviors. *Medical Care, 25*, 868–881.

Pennings-Van der Eerden, L. J. M. (1984). *Zelfzorg en motivatie bij patiënten met diabetes mellitus* [Self-care and motivation with diabetic patients]. Unpublished manuscript. Utrecht: RUU/AGE, 84. 16.

Saris, W., and Stronkhorst, H. (1984). *Causal modeling in nonexperimental research*. Amsterdam: Sociometric Research Foundation.

Schlenk, E. A., and Hart, L. K. (1984). The relationship between health locus of control, health value and social support and compliance of persons with diabetes mellitus. *Diabetes Care, 7*, 566–74.

Stewart, M. H. (1984). What is a successful doctor-patient interview? A study of interactions and outcomes. *Social Science Medicine, 10*, 167–175.

Wallston, K. A., and Wallston, B. S. (1982). Who is responsible for your health? The construct of health locus of control. In G. S. Sanders, and J. Suls (Eds.), *Social Psychology of health and illness* (pp. 65–95). Hillsdale: Erlbaum.

Weiner, B. (1980). An attributional theory of behavior. In B. Weiner (Ed.), *Human Motivation* (pp. 327–406). London: Holt, Rinehart and Winston.

Weiner, B. (1985). An attributinal theory of achievement motivation and emotion. *Psychological Review, 92*, 548–573.

Wierenga, M. E. (1980). The interrelationship between multidimensional health locus of control, knowledge of diabetes, perceived social support, self-reported compliance and therapeutic outcomes six weeks after the adult patient has been diagnosed with diabetes mellitus. *Dissertation Abstracts International, 40*; 5610B.

Wilson, W., Ary, D. V., Biglan, A., Glasgow, R. E., Toobert, D. J., and Campbell D. R. (1986). Psychosocial predictors of self-care behaviors (compliance) and glycemic control in non-insulin-dependent diabetes mellitus. *Diabetes Care, 9*, 614–622.

Wysocki, M., Czyzyk, A., Slonska, Z., Kronlewski, A., and Janeczko, D. (1978). Health behavior and its determinants among insulin-dependent diabetics: results of the Diabetes Warsaw Study. *Diabetes & Metabolism, 4*, 117–122.

Changes in Patient Perceptions of Chronic Disease and Disability with Time and Experience

Marie Johnston, Theresa Marteau, Cecily J. Partridge and
Penny Gilbert

Introduction

In studies of chronic disease, coping strategies and disease/disability representations have been predictive of the outcomes of the disease in terms of emotional, disease and disability outcomes (e. g. Smith, Peck, Milano & Ward, 1988; Felton, Revenson & Hinrichsen, 1984; Meyer, Leventhal & Gutman, 1985; Partridge & Johnston, 1989). In each case, predictions were independent of the state of disease or disability. Smith et al. (1988) found that for patients with rheumatoid arthritis, depression was related to the degree of cognitive distortion, especially arthritis related distortion, even when disability level had been allowed for; cognitive distortion also predicted concurrent disability scores. In Felton et al.'s (1984) study measures of positive and negative affect in patients with different diseases (hypertension, diabetes mellitus, cancer and rheumatoid arthritis) were unrelated to the patient's disease, but were predictable from the coping strategies used; positive affect was associated with cognitive strategies while negative affect was associated with emotional strategies.

While the above two studies deal with simultaneous measures, other studies demonstrate that future disease/disability can be predicted from current views of the condition. Meyer et al. (1985) and Partridge & Johnston (1989) found that current perceptions of the condition were predictive of subsequent hypertension and disability respectively. In Partridge & Johnston's (1989) study of stroke and wrist fracture patients, perceived personal control over recovery predicted recovery from disability, even when the association between current perceptions and current disability was allowed for. In both studies the authors suggest that patients' representations determine their coping behaviours which in turn lead to the outcomes observed. Meyer et al. (1985) confirmed this hypothesis, finding that patients' adherence to anti-hypertensive drug regimens was consistent witht their expectations of the duration of the condition. Patients who perceived hypertension to be a chronic condition complied with medication recommendations and achieved blood pressure reductions whereas those who thought it was an acute state failed to persist with medication and their blood pressure remained uncontrolled.

Models of stress and coping place considerable emphasis on the representation or appraisal of the threat (Leventhal, Nerenz & Steele, 1984; Lazarus & Folkman, 1984). Leventhal et al.'s (1984) self-regulatory model (Figure 1) proposes two parrellel processes, one dealing with objective danger and the other with fear. Within each, a process of representation of threat, coping responses and the evaluation of that coping result in different outcomes. This model includes multiple feedback loops and implies that each element of the model is modified by the experience of every other.

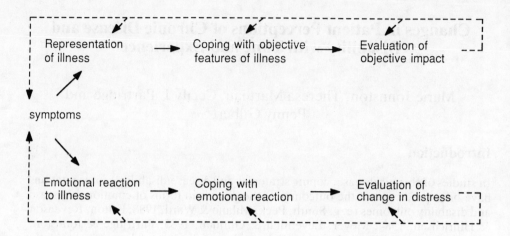

Figure 1. Self-regulatory model (adapted from Leventhal, Nerenz & Steele, 1984)

Implicit in this model, and explicit in these feedback loops, is the implication that all of the main components will alter with time. A different presentation of the model makes this longitudinal time dimension more explicit. Figure 2 describes the coping process as it changes over time. It now becomes clear that a cumulative process is occuring.

While cross-sectional studies such as Smith et al.'s (1988) and Felton et al.'s (1984) throw light on the relationships between the elements and examine whether relationships are consistent with the model at one time point, they do not explore the longitudinal or causal aspects. For example, Felton et al.'s finding that patients who adopt cognitive strategies have better adjustment than those who adopt emotion focussed strategies may be due to:

1. Cognitive coping resulting in better adjustment
2. Better adjustment resulting in less emotional and more cognitive strategies or
3. Some other factor e.g. progress of their illness or social support available, resulting in both better adjustment and more cognitive strategies.

All three are entirely consistent with current knowledge of the relationship between cognition and emotion.

Prospective studies such as Meyer et al.'s (1985) or Partridge and Johnston's (1989) elucidate one aspect of the time line, namely the power of one element to predict or influence the next element. This is important in determining possible causal directions between representations, coping responses and outcomes. In Partridge and Johnston's (1989) study, the finding that perceived control at the beginning of physiotherapy predicted gains made over the course of treatment gives more support to a causal hypothesis than a cross-sectional study could have achieved.

However, none of these studies takes account of longitudinal changes in each component of the model, nor do they examine how the critical components become established at the time of the onset of the condition. Changes in attributions about

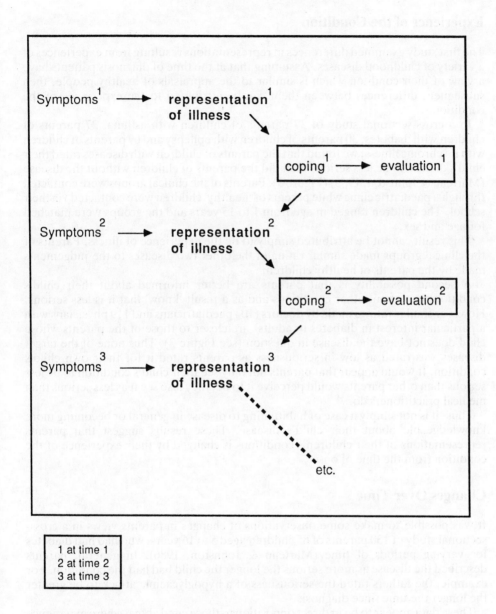

Figure 2. Self-regulatory model: changes in representations

illness over time have been noted (Turnquist, Harvey & Anderson, 1988). The current paper describes a series of studies which focus on the patient's or relatives' representations and how they change over time from the point of onset or diagnosis. Two aspects of the representations are considered: perceived seriousness and perceives controllability.

Experience of the Condition

The first study examined differences in representations resulting from experiences of a variety of childhood diseases. Assuming that at the time of diagnosis patients have a view of their conditon which is similar to the appraisals of healthy people, then subsequent differences between them can be attributed to the experience of the condition.

In a cross-sectional study of 37 parents of children with asthma, 37 parents of children with diabetes, 30 parents of children with epilepsy and 69 parents of children with no chronic illness, we found that the parents of children with diseases rated their child's disease to be less serious than did the parents of children without the disease (Marteau & Johnston, 1986) (Figure 3). Parents of the clinical groups were contacted through a paediatric clinic while parents of 'healthy' children were contacted via their school. The children ranged in age from 1 to 15 years and the groups were matched for age and sex.

This result cannot be attributed simply to be the experience of illness. Parents of the clinical groups made similar rating of the other two diseases to the judgements made by the parents of healthy children.

A second possibility is that parents are better informed about their child's condition than about other conditions and as a result 'know' that it is less serious. However similar ratings made by doctors (104 paediatricians and 119 physicians with a particular interest in diabetes in adults) are closer to those of the parents whose child does not have the disease in question (see Figure 3). Thus none of the target diseases was rated as low in seriousness as parents rated it for their own child's condition. It would appear that parents not only see their child's condition to be less serious than other parents would perceive it to be, they also see it as less serious than medical practitioners do.

Thus, it is not simply a case of habituating to disease in general or becoming more knowledgeable about their child's disease. These results suggest that parents representations of their children's conditions is changed by their experience of the condition from the time of onset.

Changes Over Time

It was possible to make some observations of changes in parents views in a cross-sectional study of 130 parents of 65 children aged 5 to 16 years, who had had diabetes for varying periods of time (Marteau & Johnston, 1986). In general, parents described the disease as more serious the longer the child had had the condition. For example, the fathers rated the seriousness of a hypoglycaemic attack to be greater the longer the time since diagnosis.

These data appear to be in direct opposition to those cited above where experience of the condition *lessened* rather than increased its perceived seriousness. However, they give no indication of what happens immediately after diagnosis or at the time of onset of the condition.

Rank order of seriousness of 3 childhood illnesses by 4 groups
of parents (based on mean ratings of 11 childhood illnesses).

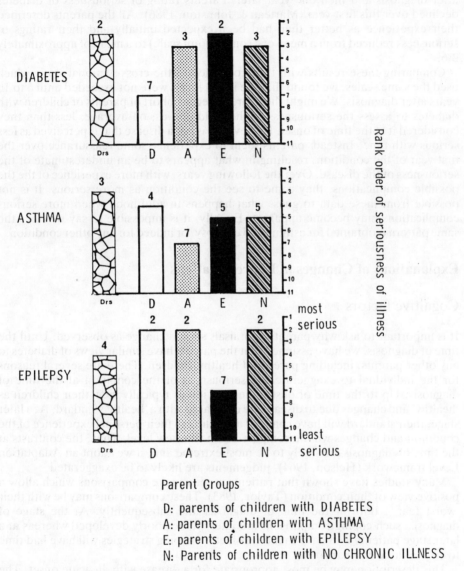

Parent Groups

D: parents of children with DIABETES
A: parents of children with ASTHMA
E: parents of children with EPILEPSY
N: Parents of children with NO CHRONIC ILLNESS

Figure 3. Seriousness of childhood illnesses: ratings by parents and doctors

Onset of the Condition

It seems unlikely that the onset or diagnosis of a disease results in instantaneous
changes in the perceptions of the seriousness of the disease. Thus, it is necessary to
observe changes over time in these appraisals, from the time when the disease is first

recognised, in order to establish the full pattern.

In a small scale study, we have observed a group of 13 diabetic children two weeks after diagnosis and then one year later. Parents rating of seriousness of diabetes declined over this first year (Marteau & Johnston, 1986). All the parents described their experience as better than had been expected initially and their ratings of seriousness reduced from a mean of 4 (on a 6 point scale) to a mean of approximately 2.6.

Comparing these results with those obtained in the cross-sectional study which used the same scales, we found that the initial levels were not exceeded until 6 to 10 years after diagnosis. We might therefore expect a cohort of parents of children with diabetes to assess the seriousness of the condition as, on average, less than they considered it at the time of onset. However, it is not a disease that is perceived as less serious with time. Instead, parents seem to experience some reassurance over the first year of the condition, resulting in what appears to be an underestimate of the seriousness of the disease. Over the following years, with more experience of the the possible complications, they come to see the condition as more serious. It is not possible from these data to guess what happens in adulthood when more serious complications may become apparent. Equally, it is impossible to say whether the same pattern is obtained for asthma and epilepsy, or indeed for any other condition.

Explanations of Changes in Representations

Cognitive factors

It is important to ask why parents appraisals should change as observed. Until the time of diagnosis, we have assumed that the parents have similar views of diabetes to any other parents, including parents of healthy children. There are several reasons for the individual to exaggerate the seriousness of the condition at the time of diagnosis. Up to the time of onset, the individuals typically view their children as 'healthy' and changes due to disease are compared with a 'health' standard. At a later stage, their standard will have changed according to their personal experience of the condition and changes will be compared with this new level. Thus, the contrasts at the time of diagnosis are likely to be most extreme and, if we adopt an Adaptation Level framework (Helson, 1964), judgements are likely to be exaggerated.

Many studies have shown that patients readily make comparisons which allow a positive view of their condition (Taylor, 1983). These comparisons may be with their 'worst fears', both at the time of diagnosis and subsequently. At the stage of diagnosis, such coping comparisons are likely to be poorly developed whereas at a later stage patients who have found satisfactory coping strategies will have had time to evolve these comparisons.

This description may be most appropriate for a disease with an acute onset. The process may be quite different where the condition has a gradual or uncertain onset. In these conditions, patients might already have fears or fantasies based on their symptoms and on the response of their medical practitioners before the condition is diagnosed. In this case, these notions will be the standard against which the eventual diagnosis is judged. The patient who fears that the symptoms are predictive of death within weeks or months may be reassured to get a diagnosis of multiple sclerosis, whereas someone believing the symptoms were temporary and due to overwork will have quite a different experience of the diagnosis. In a disease like multiple sclerosis where the onset is uncertain, the diagnosis problematic and the progress variable, cognitive coping resources are likely to prove valuable. Foley. Bedell, LaRocca, Scheinberg and Reznikoff (1987) have found that stress inoculation training facilitates coping in patients with multiple sclerosis.

Another factor which may contribute to an exaggerated perception of change with the onset of the condition is Unrealistic Optimism. Weinstein (1982) has observed that on average, people see themselves as less vulnerable to a wide range of conditions than they are in reality. This optimism has been found to be associated with negative views of the condition (Mahatane & Johnston, 1989). Finding oneself to be ill when one has both a belief in invulnerability to the disease and a negative view of the disease may add to the sense of catastrophe.

One's beliefs or knowledge about the disease may also be misleading, especially for conditions which are invisible. For conditions like diabetes, asthma and epilepsy, the sufferer is indistiguishable except when having an attack or when having treatment for the condition. We frequently learn that someone has diabetes if the person goes into a coma, or has epilepsy if they have a seizure, especially if they are not personally known to us and cannot therefore disclose the information. Thus, our information is inevitably biassed when we try to bring to mind examples of occasions when we encountered someone with epilepsy, asthma or diabetes. We would recall a disproportionate number of problem incidents, being unaware of the many occasions when we meet the sufferers behaving 'normally'. Recent attempts to use the phase 'people with' diabetes, a disability or a mental illness rather than referring to 'diabetics', 'the disabled' or the 'mentally ill' attempt to redress this balance by placing some emphasis on the normality of the individual rather than their deviant status. However, the way we process information is likely to exaggerate the number of problem incidents, and using Kahneman and Tversky's (1973) availability analysis, influence the judgement of seriousness of the disease or condition.

The effects of availability may be quite different for a familiar condition. Here the critical factors would appear to be the nature of the experience we have of the condition. In the first year after the diagnosis of juvenile onset diabetes, the child is likely to be relatively well compared with the initial onset experience and this might therefore result in the reductions in perceived seriousness observed. As noted above, at the end of the first year, all the parents in our prospective study described it as much better than they had expected.

Social Influences

In a condition with a familial element the experience of relatives with the condition may colour initial views. In a study of 130 parents of 65 diabetic children, we found no difference between those parents who had a relative with diabetes and those who had not in their views of the seriousness of the condition. However, the state of the relatives health was important. If the relative's health was good, parents viewed diabetes as less serious in terms of vulnerability to complication and expected seriousness in 20 years time than if the relative was in average or poor health (Marteau & Johnston, 1986).

A further source of patients' perceptions of their conditions is their communication with the health care system. Nerenz and Leventhal (1984) found that, in patients having chemotherapy for cancer, the symptom which was associated with worry was tiredness. Hair loss and nausea were not associated with such distress. It would appear that these latter symptoms had been clearly explained to patients and could therefore be attributed to the chemotherapy. Tiredness on the other hand, was perceived as a sign of possible progression of the disease and not a side effect of treatment, and was therefore seen to be of more concern.

Undoubtedly, health care staff and the health care system play an important role in determining what patients believe about their condition. In a recent study of women having screening tests in pregnancy, we found that younger women were more likely than older women to have a sustained pattern of raised anxiety on receiving a positive result (Marteau et al., 1988). We suggest that these findings are due to the manner in which tests are introduced to pregnant women, with older women being alerted right from the start about the possibility that the test might be positive and that they might be carrying an abnormal foetus.

Many studies have demonstrated that communications with patients can alter their knowledge and understanding of their condition and can facilitate their adherence to complex treatment regimens (Ley, 1988). We have explored the possibility that altering communications can influence critical perceptions patients have about their condition and its treatment.

Our observation (Partridge & Johnston, 1989) that patients perceived control over recovery from disability predicted the progress made led us to hypothesise that the rehabilitation environment could serve to increase or diminish the patient's belief in personal control. Clinical observations of the style of delivery of care in rehabilitation settings frequently reveals a situation in which dependency is encouraged. This is well illustrated in a study by MacDonald and Butler (1974) in which use of a wheelchair in a resident capable of walking was contingently reinforced by care staff. Reversal of the contingencies increased walking and reduced the use of the wheelchair.

We hypothesised that the normal mode of introducing the patients to the physiotherapy rehabilitation department served to reduce perceived personal control as physiotherapists frequently encouraged their patients to 'depend on me'. We therefore investigated the effects of an introductory paragraph added to the regular appointment letter (Johnston, Gilbert, Partridge & Collins, in preparation). The paragraph emphasized the patient's role in participating in treatment and carrying out any homework assignments. Seventy-one patients (27 men and 44 women; mean age 47.6 years) coming for their first visit to the physiotherapy department were randomly allocated to receive either the routine appointment letter or the experimental letter with the additional paragraph. One week after commencing treatment their perceived personal control was assessed using the measure we had developed to assess control over recovery from disability (Partridge & Johnston, 1989). The resulting effects are shown in Figure 4.

The experimental group showed a significant increase in perceived control. These results, combined with the finding that perceived control predicts recovery, suggests that it may be possible to contribute to better outcomes of physiotherapy by altering these beliefs, using different methods of introducing the patients to rehabilitation such as the experimental letter.

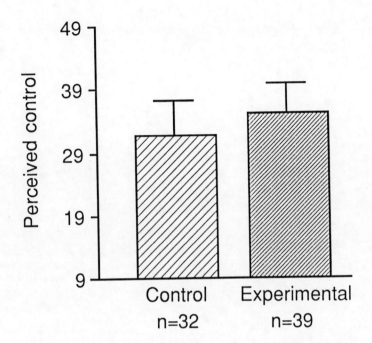

Figure 4. Perceived control over disability: effects of altering appointment letter to patients

Conclusions

Models of coping with chronic disease have drawn attention to the primary appraisal or representation of the disease as an important determinant of coping and coping outcomes. However, these appraisals will change over time. Thus, the threat against which patients and their families pit their coping resources is not constant. The threat may be changed if the nature of the disease or its symptoms changes. Additionally, there are psychological processes which result in changing perceptions.

. Parents of children with chronic disease perceived their own child's disease to be less serious than did doctors or other parents. The most likely explanation lies in their experience of the disease and in turn the way this experience is processed cognitively. Social processes, including communications between patients and health care staff, may also influence representations. In a study of rehabilitation patients, it was possible to alter patients' perceptions by altering the initial communication to patients coming for physiotherapy.

Any attempt to understand changes in coping in chronic disorders must take account not only of changes in the condition but also of changes in the patients' representations of the condition. Studies predicting later coping or adjustment from initial appraisals might achieve more predictive power by taking account of changes in appraisals also.

References

Felton, B., Revenson, T. A., and Hinrichsen, R. L. (1984). Stress and coping in the explanation of psychological adjustment among chronically ill adults. *Social Science and Medicine, 18*, 889–898.

Foley, F. W., Bedell. J. R., LaRocca, N. G., Scheinberg, L. C., and Reznikoff, M. (1987). Efficacy of stress-inoculation training in coping with multiple sclerosis. *Journal of Consulting and Clinical Psychology, 55*, 919–922.

Helson, H. (1964). *Adaptation-Level Theory*. New York: Harper and Row.

Kahneman, D., and Tversky, A. (1973). On the psychology of prediction. *Psychological Review, 80*, 237–251.

Johnston, M., Gilbert, P., Partridge, C., and Collings, J. (in preparation). *Altering perceived control in rehabilitation patients*.

Lazarus, R. S., and Folkman, S. (1984). *Stress, appraisal, and coping*. New York: Springer.

Leventhal, H., Nerenz, D. R., and Steele, D. J. (1984). Illness representations and coping with health threats. In A. Baum, S. E. Taylor and J. E. Singer (Eds.), *Handbook of Psychology and Health* (Vol. IV, pp. 219–252). Hillsdale, N. J.: Erlbaum.

Ley, P. (1988). *Communication with patients*. London: Chapman and Hall.

MacDonald, M. L., and Butler, A. K. (1974). Reversal of helplessness: producing walking behaviour in nursing home wheelchair residents using behavior modification procedures. *Journal of Gerontology, 29*, 97–101.

Mahatane, J., and and Johnston, M. (1989). Unrealistic optimism and attitudes towards mental health. *British Journal of Clinical Psychology, 28*, 181–182.

Marteau, T. M., and Johnston, M. (1986). Determinants of beliefs about illness: A study of parents of children with diabetes, asthma, epilepsy and no chronic illness. *Journal of Psychosomatic Research, 30*, 673–683.

Marteau, T. M., Kidd, J., Cook, R., Johnston, M., Michie, S., Shaw, R. W., and Slack, J. (1988). Screening for Down's syndrome. *British Medical Journal, 297*, 1469.

Mayer, D., Leventhal, H., and Gutman, M. (1985). Common-sense models of illness: the example of hypertension. *Health Psychology, 4*, 115–136.

Nerenz, D. R., and Leventhal, H. (1984). Psychological aspects of cancer chemotherapy. International Review of Applied Psychology, *33*, 521–529.

Partridge, C., and Johnston, M. (1989). Perceived control of recovery from physical disability: Measurement and prediction. *British Journal of Clinical Psychology, 28*, 53–59.

Smith, T. W., Peck, J. R., Milano, R. A., and Ward, J. R. (1988). Cognitive distortion in rheumatoid arthritis: relation to depression and disability. *Journal of Consulting and Clinical Psychology, 56*, 412–416.

Taylor, S. E. (1983). Adjustment to threatening events. *American Psychologist, 38*, 1161–1173.

Turnquist, D. C., Harvey, J. H., and Anderson, B. (1988). Attributions and adjustment to life threatening illness. *British Journal of Clinical Psychology, 27*, 55–65.

Weinstein, N. (1982). Unrealistic optimism about susceptibility to health problems. *Journal of Behavioral Medicine, 5*, 441–460.

Self-Attribution of Coping and its Social Adaptability in Patients Operated for Lumber Disc Herniation

Ladislav Valach, Klaus-Friedrich Augustiny, Jiri Dvorak,
Peter Fuhrimann, Andreas Blaser, Waltraud Tschaggelar, and
Edgar Heim

Introduction

Low back pain is a serious economic and social problem. Its psychosocial aspects have been recognized for many years (Luck, 1946) and .."are now believed to equal, if not exceed, in importance physiopathologic abnormalities." (Pheasant, 1977). Although the simple idea that a person with particular psychological features or specific conflicts is predisposed to develop a particular illness has been abandoned in psychosomatic medicine. The majority of research work on psychosocial aspects of low back pain investigate personality measures, mainly using the MMPI, in order to improve the prediction of a successful operation (Herron & Pheasant, 1982; Garron & Leavit, 1983; Bradley & Van der Heide, 1984). Research on social aspects of low back pain is far less common, although low back pain is primarily seen as a social problem (Schuler, 1981). Social consequences of various illnesses and injuries have been described but in low back pain patients the question of psychosocial cause seems to be more fascinating (Holmes & Rahe, 1967; Leavitt, Garron & Bielauskas, 1978; Feuerstein, Sult & Houle, 1985; Krüskemper, Degner, Krämer & Wilke, 1986).

Unfortunately, relating low back pain, psychological (e.g., personality) and social aspects does not permit any dynamic conceptualization of these processes. The approaches using the concept of 'skills', 'strategies', and 'coping' seem to be more appropriate representing these processes. The coping concept has advanced far beyond nonempirical theorizing. A number of studies on coping have been conducted with various health and other problems such as laryngectomy (Natvig, 1983), hypertension (Linden & Feuerstein, 1981), breast cancer (Heim et al., 1988), chronic pain (Rybstein-Blinchik, 1979; Philips, 1987) and also with low back pain (Schmermelleh-Engel & Kies, 1986; Turner, Clancy & Vitaliano, 1987). In the majority of these studies the outcomes which were related to coping, were closely connected with the actual health problems (Rosenbaum 1980; Schmermelleh-Engel & Kies, 1986). However, introducing the criteria of the quality of life into the evaluation of medical treatment, the possibility of improving any accessible parts of the psychosocial processes in a patient's history will also become important.

In this article we have attempted to deal with this issue. We believe that certain forms of coping are associated with better social adaptation in low back pain patients. We would like to present the results of a study on self-attributions of coping occurring in interviews between physicians and patients, who had been operated on for low back, pain, about the patients' history and complaints. This self-attributed coping by the patients is compared with the extent of the patient's social adjustment in an attempt to discover which types of coping self-attributions are adaptive and which are maladaptive.

Methods

Our study was conducted as a part of a large follow up investigation by the Department of Neurology of the University of Berne. The hospital records of all patients who were operated there in 1965, 1970, 1974 and 1975 for disc herniation were analyzed (n = 672) (Dvorak et al., 1988a). 8–19 years after their operation 423 (63%) patients answered a questionnaire on their present occupational situation, their ability to work and their pain. These patients do not differ in their sociodemographic characteristics nor in the duration of their complaints and length of hospitalization or in their preoperative or postoperative findings (see Valach et al., 1988 for more details on the comparison of these two populations).

Sixty-eight pensioned patients after surgery for low back pain responded to the questionnaire and were asked to participate. Forty-four of them did take part in the study (group III). Fifty one patients without pain (group I) were chosen and matched in age, gender and year of operation with 40 patients with pain but without pension (group II) from the remaining 355 patients. These three groups of patients were examined further. There were no differences between these three groups with regard to gender, age at the time of the operation, age at the time of the examination, duration of the preoperative complaints, length of the stay in hospital, neurological findings at the time of the operation, level of the operation and the neurological findings immediately after surgery. However, the three groups did differ in some relevant somatic aspects (e.g. paravertebral muscle spasm, laseque) and therefore the patient's pain experience could be supported by somatic findings even if not in the expected extent (see Valach et al., 1988).

The psychosocial assessment was performed at the time of the follow-up examination at the Dept. of Neurology 8 to 19 years after the operation. A semistructured interview was conducted in which the patients were asked about self-attributions for coping and their social adjustment was evaluated. The modes of coping were identified and labeled according to the formulation of Heim (Heim et al., 1986). Social adaptation was assessed using a modification of Barabee's concept (Barabee et al., 1955; Heim et al., 1982). Fourteen aspects in five life areas were evaluated in detail: (I. Occupation: a.) number of working hours, b.) constancy of work, c.) changes of job, d.) relation to others at work, e.) affective atitude to work. II. Finances: a.) financial situation, b.) affective attitude to financial situation. III. Family life: i.) marriage-family: A1.partnership, A2.parent/child relationship, A3. fulfilling of family responsibilities, ii.) Family of origin: B1. relation to parents, B2. relation to siblings. IV.a.) social contacts, b.) social activity.

Results

Social Adaptation

The patients without complaints described their occupational and financial situation as being better than that of the patients with complaints. They also reported better partnership and marriage than the pensioned. Also their social life – going out, seeing others – seemed to be more satisfying (see Dvorak et al., 1988b).

Some patients (10 patients with complaints without pension (25%), could not work the same amount as before the onset of low back pain because of their complaints: 'I worked in a supermarket with vegetables..had to lift boxes and realized that I stumbled with my right leg..I had pain also after surgery. I had to reduce my working hours and worked only half a day as a helper. I stopped working six years ago, I could not do it any more. The work was too difficult, I had pain. Now I look after the household of my daughter. She works. But ironing and vacuuming is the most difficult. I cannot stand or lift my arms. I live with my daughter so that I don't have to do my own housework.' (Mrs. N. 52 years, widow, operated nine years ago.)

The back complaints after an operation not only made the patients give up their jobs or reduce their working hours but were also reasons for long and frequent absences: 'for fifteen weeks I haven't been able to work. I have such pain now that I can't do anything. I can't get up in the morning. I have been certified unable to work for an unlimited length of time. Before that I never stayed at home from work.' (Mr. J., 59 years, operated 19 years ago, civil servant.)

Another patient described a whole series of job changes resulting in a job he considers humiliating: 'Fourteen years ago the pain worsened. I had to give up my job. I am a qualified blacksmith, worked later as a foreman and was even later independently in charge of an enterprise and became chief of a warehouse. I had to stop because I couldn't stand or lift or even sit down. Therefore, I qualified as an insurance consultant. For five years everything went fine and then it was all over. I couldn't walk and didn't have any feeling in my left leg. After surgery everything went well but later it became a bit harder. I was constantly in pain..A year ago I was manoeuvered out of the insurance job because I couldn't go on any more. There was nothing else left for me but to give notice. For two years I have been working freelance for the insurance company but this is not possible any more. At my age, where do you want to look for a job, who is going to employ you as a more or less invalid person? I got a part time job last week..as a helper. I clean the machinery for the apprentices. Previously I was a chief and now I am even lower than an apprentice..On the side I am still working for the insurance company.' (Mr. C., 58 years, operated 10 years ago.)

Some other patients stayed in their jobs, although they were in pain, but complained that their boss does not show any understanding for their situation: '..but my boss does not understand my problems (low back pain) at all..I went to him and said: 'Listen, I shouldn't be doing this and that any more'' and asked whether there would be another possibility for me to work on a less physically strenuous task. I could see some possibilities in longer terms. The only answer I've got was: "Listen, if you can't do it then you are not acceptable for us." This after I worked for the same firm for 21 years.' (Mr. C., electrician, 48 years, operated 15 years ago, married.)

Consequently, in some patients the back complaints led to a negative attitude to work: 'Lately, I was more or less..how should I say it.. depressive. I had enough of everything. I woke up early in the morning, walked up and down in the corridor, could not sleep and was tired in the morning. The housework wasn't progressing and I was fed up with it.' (Mrs. L., 52 years, operated 1975, housewife, widow, two children.)

Many patients (28%) suffered a financial cut either due to their job change, reduction of working time or to their loss of job: 'My family doctor told me that he applied for a disability pension for me. I received a letter recently that I will not get anything because it isn't a satisfactory reason for a disability pension..That it isn't enough..Now I've got to make sure that I'll get by. But if I have to have somebody to help me with my housework I don't know how to pay for it. Thank God, I have a widows pension..but I can't spend very much. It is sufficient, but I have to cut down and plan well.' (Mrs. S. 52 years, widow, housewife, operated 1975.) Some patients also report problems in their marriage. Several of them have been living in a difficult relationship for a while which suffered additionally through their back complaints: 'My husband didn't have any patience. The healing should have been quicker. His reaction made me sad..At the beginning he was sexually always impatient..He was also unfaithful at that time. It was not the first time but now, I found, I could not do anything like this.. particularly at this time..I've tried hard but something like this was really mean.' (Mrs. T. 42 years, housewife, 3 children, operated 5 and 11 years ago.)

These statements illustrate that some patients with complaints described social problems and that they are not very well socially adapted. We found similar and even worse situations with pensioned patients which shows that receiving a pension does not outweigh all social difficulties and that apart from financial problems there are a number of other burdens which have to be dealt with by other means. We postulate that an important way of overcoming these social problems is coping by the patients. We would like to present here some correlational data which illustrate the hypothesis of improved social adaptation through appropriate coping. However, as the data stem from self-attribution of coping their relevance for coping processes has to be based on theoretical conceptions.

Self-Attribution of Coping and its Social Adaptivity

Correlating the coping modalities of all patients with their described degree of social adaptation (split in half by median of all patients) the following coping modalities were attributed by patients who described better social adaptation: TACKLING, OPTIMISM, PRESERVING COMPOSURE, ACCEPTANCE, THOUGHT AS DIVERSION, ACTIVITY AS DIVERSION. This means that patients describing these coping modalities also describe better social adaptation and that they therefore understand these coping modalities as socially adaptive. COMPENSATION, PASSIVE COOPERATION, RESIGNATION, SOCIAL WITHDRAWAL, RUMINATION, SELF-ACCUSATION and VALORIZATION were attributed by patients who described worse social adaptation and understand these coping modalities as being socially maladaptive.

Sixty-two patients (46%) self-attributed one to five adaptive but no maladaprive coping modalities. Adaptive coping modalities were used more often. Sixty-six patients (49%) attributed three to five adaptive and no more than one maladaptive coping modalits. This group is described as patients with adaptive coping strategies. As there are less patients who attributed themselves maladaptive coping modalities, the group of patients with maladaptive coping strategies consists of patients with more maladaptive than adaptive coping modalities (N=38). Patients who gave self-attributions of adaptive coping strategies differ from those with maladaptive coping strategies neither in gender, occupation, age at time of the assessment nor in their marital status.

Fifteen of the 40 patients with complaints but without pension gave socially adaptive and 13 maladaptive coping strategies. They do not differ in gender, occupation, age and marital status. In this group the following self-attributed coping modalities correlate with a socially adaptive strategy: ACTIVITY AS DIVERSION, THOUGHT AS DIVERSION, ACCEPTANCE, PRESERVING COMPOSURE, OPTIMISM, ATTENTION AND CARE. On the other hand REVOLT, PASSIVE

COOPERATION, PROBLEM ANALYSIS, SOCIAL WITHDRAWAL and RUMINATION correlate with the self-attribution of maladaptive coping strategy.

The group of operated patients with a pension contains 14 patients with a socially adaptive and 24 with a socially maladaptive coping strategy. They also do not differ in gender, occupation, age and marital status. THOUGHTS AS DIVERSION, ACCEPTANCE, PRESERVING COMPOSURE, ATTENTION AND CARE are the self-attributed modalities of coping which correlate with a socially adaptive coping strategy in this group. A maladaptive coping strategy correlates with COMPENSATION, RUMINATION and SELF-ACCUSATION.

Patients with pension included ACTIVITY AS DIVERSION AND OPTIMISM less often in their social adaptive coping strategy. They also attributed themselves a specific social maladaptive coping strategy containing COMPENSATION and SELF-ACCUSATION. The following step presents the configuration of individual aspects of social adaptation for the socially adaptive and socially maladaptive coping strategies which the patients attributed to themselves. Kendall's Tau b coefficients of the aspects of social adaption for the 38 patients who attributed a maladaptive coping strategy were ordered spatially by a Multidemensional Scaling Method: Smallest Space Analysis (MINISSA). It was also performed with the 66 patients who attributed an adaptive coping strategy.

Table 1. *Correlation matrix of social adaptation (SAS) 1–14: adaptive coping strategy, (Kendall's Tau b)*

SAS	SAS 1	SAS 2	SAS 3	SAS 4	SAS 5	SAS 6	SAS 7	SAS 8	SAS 9	SAS 10	SAS 11	SAS 12	SAS 13
2	0.32												
3	0.22	0.17											
4	0.40	0.67	0.30										
5	0.45	0.39	0.27	0.40									
6	0.55	0.36	0.26	0.43	0.32								
7	0.34	0.49	0.18	0.37	0.42	0.61							
8	0.20	−0.03	0.11	−0.19	0.22	0.10	0.04						
9	0.21	0.08	−0.10	0.04	−0.04	0.28	0.07	0.38					
10	0.44	0.27	0.21	0.42	0.12	0.30	0.21	−0.07	0.30				
11	0.12	0.08	−0.05	0.40	−0.12	−0.12	0.09	−0.23	0.06	−0.04			
12	0.02	−0.10	0.22	0.31	−0.11	−0.02	0.11	0.04	−0.01	0.14	0.38		
13	0.10	0.06	0.23	0.37	0.06	0.17	0.30	0.03	0.21	0.25	0.18	0.47	
14	0.20	0.20	0.11	0.31	0.23	0.16	0.23	0.03	−0.08	0.15	0.07	0.24	0.44

The organization of relations of individual aspects of social adaptation calls for a three dimensional-presentation (Stress Dhat 0.10 and 0.11). However, as we performed the analysis without dimensional assumptions we will use the two-dimensional solution (Stress Dhat 0.19 in both cases). The patients with the adaptive coping strategy show a configuration with the working area in a center, their external social relations on one side and their family life on the other. The configuration of the individual dimensions of social adaptation of patients with a maladaptive coping strategy builds a center with a family life and the affective area. The financial situation and the social life form the periphery. We could conclude that the two configurations differ in part. In each case there is a new center and also new areas are separated.

Table 2. *Correlation Matrix of social adaptation (SAS) 1–14: maladaptive coping strategy, (Kendall's Tau b)*

SAS													
2	0.77												
3	0.30	0.45											
4	−0.05	0.38	0.04										
5	−0.05	0.14	0.35	0.07									
6	0.45	0.53	0.48	0.02	−0.13								
7	0.01	0.20	0.64	0.07	0.17	0.47							
8	0.07	0.19	0.09	0.63	0.19	−0.07	0.20						
9	0.02	0.08	−0.07	0.40	−0.14	0.37	0.52	0.53					
10	0.35	0.58	0.13	0.61	0.09	0.12	0.01	0.16	0.25				
11	−0.50	−0.17	−0.51	0.77	0.00	−0.55	0.07	0.26	0.42	0.29			
12	−0.18	−0.16	−0.11	0.07	0.09	0.05	0.25	0.26	0.18	0.08	0.52		
13	−0.36	−0.18	0.28	0.26	0.13	0.02	0.27	−0.02	−0.05	−0.09	0.20	0.26	
14	−0.17	0.14	0.15	0.29	0.09	−0.14	0.07	−0.02	−0.05	0.28	0.25	0.30	0.51

SAS 1 SAS 2 SAS 3 SAS 4 SAS 5 SAS 6 SAS 7 SAS 8 SAS 9 SAS 10 SAS 11 SAS 12 SAS 13

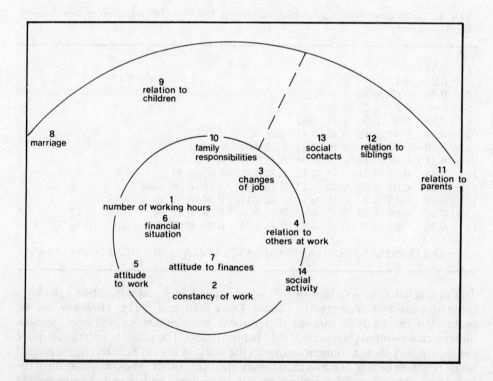

Figure 1. MINISSA of social adaptation (areas 1–14) for patients with socially adaptive coping strategy.

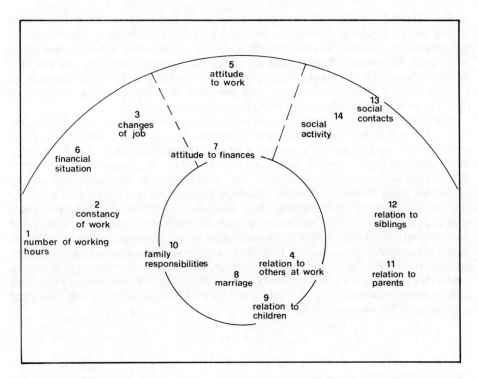

Figure 2. MINISSA of social adaptation (areas 1–14) for patients with a socially maladaptive coping strategy.

There were no differences in questionnaire data on pain between the patients with adaptive and maladaptive coping strategies in both groups. The only exception was 'headache' which was mentioned more often by patients with pension who attributed themselves a maladaptive coping strategy. There are only a few differences in the somatic findings which are related to the social adaptability of the attributed coping strategy. As they are also different in each group we could conclude that there is no systematic relation between the social adaptability of coping and somatic findings.

Discussion

This inquiry is a part of a cross-sectional study which was conducted as part of an extensive neurological and neurosurgical follow-up study. We cannot therefore make any statements on psychosocial processess, influences or effects. The aim of our data analysis was to illustrate and to differentiate the hypothesis that a number of patients attribute to themselves a coping strategy which is either socially adaptive or maladaptive and also to prepare some material for a prospective study. We were able to work out these hypotheses in detail. Although the patients of each group do not differ in their sociodemographic and physical characteristics and their complaints, some of their self-attributed coping modalities show a connection with social adaptation. The relevance of these findings could be questioned in regard to the

functionality of coping for social adaptation as we are relating self-attribution of
coping and a subjective description of social adaptation. Obviously this cannot be
interpreted as a causal relation between coping or its self-attribution and social
adaptation. But as our interest in coping and its functionality is mainly accompanied
by interventionistic intentions, these doubts are not decisive. Often, reformulating
social problems in terms of coping and therefore offering an active modality of
problem awareness makes a supporting intervention easier.

Heim (1988) addressed the subject of adaptability of coping in cancer patients. He
stressed that it is necessary to interpret processes of coping in a finalistic way. As
more people participate in a patient's illness career there will also be several
interpretations and several goals which have to be considered. Another
differentiation he suggested regards the situational specificity. Some coping
modalities were discussed in several studies as adaptive and seemed to be more
general, others were more specific. In a comparison of various coping processes
several perspectives, goals, situations, phases in illness trajectory and, finally, also
the specificity of an illness have to be accounted for. A cross-sectional study cannot
fulfil a number of these demands. In order to answer the questions on the systematic
relation between coping and social behavior, on the specific use of the coping
modalities in a particular situation as well as the question how future plans and
expectations influence action and how they develop, other methodological
approaches must be used.

References

Barrabee, P., Barrabee E. L. and Finnesinger, J. E. (1955). A normative social adjustment scale. *American Journal of Psychiatry, 112*, 252–259.

Bradley, L. A., and Van der Heide, L. H. (1984). Pain-related correlates of MMPI profile subgroups among back pain patients. *Health Psychology, 3*, 157–174.

Dvorak, J., Gauchat, M., Valach, L., and Heim, E. (1988a). The outcome of operation for lumber disc herniation: A 4–17 years follow-up with emphasis on somatic aspects. *Spine, 13*. 1418–1422.

Dvorak, J., Valach, L., Fuhrimann, P., and Heim, E. (1988b). The outcome of operation for lumber disc herniation: A 4–17 years follow-up with emphasis on psychosocial aspects. *Spine, 13*, 1423–1427.

Feuerstein, M., Sult, S., and Houle, M. (1985). Environmental stressors and chronic low back pain: life events, family and work environment. *Pain, 22*, 295–307.

Garron, D. C., and Leavitt, F. (1983). Chronic low back pain and depression, *Journal of Clinical Psychology, 39*, 486–493.

Heim, E. (1988). Coping und Adaptivität: gibt es geeignetes oder ungeeignetes Coping? [Coping and adaptation: Is there good and bad coping?]. *Psychotherapie, Psychosomatik, Medizinische Psychologie, 38*, 8–18.

Heim, E., Adler, R., and Moser, A. (1982). Beeinträchtigung der psychosozialen Anpassung durch terminal Krankheit. [Psychosocial adaptation in terminal disease]. *Zeitschrift für Psychosomatische Medizin, 28*, 347–362.

Heim, E., Augustiny, F. K., Blaser, A., Bürki, C., Schaffner, L., and Valach, L. (1986). *Manual zur Erfassung der Krankheitsbewältigung: Die Berner Bewältigungsformen (BEFO)*. [Manual of the Berner Coping Questionnaire]. Unpublished manuscript. Psychiatrische Universitätspoliklinik, Bern.

Heim, E., Augustiny, F. K., Blaser, A., Bürki, C., Kühne, D., Rothenbühler, M., Schaffner, L., and Valach, L. (1988). Bewältigung von Brustkrebs – eine longitudinale Studie. [A longitudinal study of coping with breast cancer]. In W. Steffens, and H. Kächele (Eds.), *Abwehr und Bewältigung – zur Psychologie und Psychotherapie schwerer körperlicher Krankheiten* (pp. 133–160). Heidelberg: Springer.

Herron, L. D., and Pheasant, H. C. (1982). Changes in MMPI profiles after low back surgery. *Spine, 7*, 591.

Holmes, T. H., and Rahe, R. H. (1967). The social readjustment rating scale. *Journal of Psychosomatic Research, 11*, 213–218.

Krüskemper, G. M., Degner, F. L., Krämer, J., and Wilcke, A. (1986). Chronischer Rückenschmerz, life events und Verhaltensmodifikation. [Chronic back pain, life events, and behaviour modification]. In A. Schorr (Ed.), *Bericht über den 13. Kongress für Angewandte Psychologie. Band II.* (pp. 213–215). Bonn: Deutscher Psychologen Verlag.

Leavitt, F., Garron, D. C., and Bieliauskas, L. A. (1978). Stressing life events and the experience of low back pain. *Journal of Psychosomatic Research, 23*, 49–55.

Linden, W., and Feuerstein, M. (1981). Essential hypertension and social coping behavior. *Journal of Human Stress, 7*, 28–34.

Luck, J. V. (1946). Psychosomatic problems in military orthopaedic surgery. *Journal of Bone Joint Surgery, 28*, 213–228.

Natvig, K. (1983). Study No. 1: Social, personal, and behavioral factors related to present mastery of the laryngectomy event. *The Journal of Otolaryngology, 12*, 155–162.

Pheasant, H. C. (1977). The problem back. In J. P. Ahstrom (Ed.), *Current practice in orthopaedic surgery*, Volume 7 (pp. 89–115). Saint Louis: The C.V. Mosby Company.

Philips, H. C. (1987). Avoidance behaviour and its role in sustaining chronic pain. *Behavior Research and Therapy, 25*, 273–279.

Rosenbaum, M. (1980). Individual differences in self-control behaviors and tolerance of painful stimulation. *Journal of Abnormal Psychology, 89*, 581–590.

Rybstein-Blinchik, E. (1979). Effects of different cognitive strategies on chronic pain experience. *Journal of Behavioral Medicine, 2*, 93–100.

Schmermelleh-Engel, K., and Kies, N. (1986). Copingstrategien von Patienten mit chronischen Rückenschmerzen. [Coping of patients with chronic back pain]. In A. Schorr (Ed.), *Bericht über den 13. Kongress für Angewandte Psychologie. Band II.* (pp. 216–222). Bonn: Deutscher Psychologen Verlag.

Schuler, C. (1981). Soziale Aspekte der Rückenerkrankungen. [Social aspects of back diseases]. *Therapeutische Umschau, 38*, 681–685.

Turner, J. A., Clancy, S., and Vitaliano, P. P. (1987). Relationship of stress, appraisal and coping to chronic low back pain. *Behavior Research and Therapy, 25*, 281–288.

Valach, L., Augustiny, K. F., Dvorak, J., Blaser, A., Fuhrimann, P., Tschaggelar, W., and Heim, E. (1988). Coping von Rücken-Operierten Patienten. [Coping of patients with back surgery]. *Psychotherapie, Psychosomatik, Medizinische Psychologie, 38*, 28–36.

Section 8

Coping with Chronic Disease and Stressful Medical Procedures

Coping With Life-Threatening Disease: Some Research Problems and Selected Findings

Sigrun-Heide Filipp, Thomas Klauer, Dieter Ferring, and
Elke Freudenberg

For many years there has been profound interest in critical life events and their role as "change agents" across the life span (for an overview, see e. g., Callahan & McCluskey, 1983). Many studies have used physical health status as a central criterion in estimating the impact of critical life events on the individual, and quite a few results have shown this to be worth-while (see Maddi, Bartone & Puccetti, 1987). However, this research approach has blurred our view of the fact that deterioration of physical health status in itself is one of the most critical experiences in human lives, and the onset of chronic disease can be even conceived of as a prototype of critical life events.

In addition, the diagnosis of chronic disease, such as cancer, seems to be highly illustrative of what has been called "ill-defined" or "weakly scripted" situations elsewhere (Abelson, 1981). This term nicely indicates that we are not normally prepared via "anticipatory socialization" to handle situations of that kind and that most of us do not have behavioral routines available in times of health-related stress.

Accordingly, one might even conceive of the onset of chronic disease as a situation, in which behavioral differences between individuals are maximized. Thus, the issue of how individuals cope with chronic disease and the question of how adaptive their coping behaviors prove to be with regard to various criteria, represent extremely important research agendae. They are, at the same time, still in need of further empirical clarification.

Because of its central importance, we will start out with a few comments on how to define the concept of "coping"; we will then outline related basic research agendae; finally, we will describe our own research work with cancer patients, and report findings on two selected topics, namely the issue of temporal stability in coping behaviors and the issue of variations in coping effectiveness across coping modes and times of observation.

The Nature of Coping with Chronic Disease

Coping is frequently described in terms of all (overt and covert) behaviors aimed at preventing an individual from being "over-whelmed" by the perceived demands of a particular "stressful" life situation (e.g., Pearlin & Schooler, 1978). Unfortunately, however, that kind of *nominal* definition aimed at describing "coping" more precisely, itself contains a variety of weaknesses which becomes clear when coping is to be defined *operationally*. The problems inherent in that rather global definition are, at least, twofold.

First, behaviors referred to as "coping" are conceptually linked to a particular demanding situation, such as the diagnosis of chronic disease. Thus coping is seen as a *relational* concept having a logical counterpart in terms of what has to be coped with. This, however, does imply that a given behavioral act, such as seeking affiliation, may be "coping" at one time (when dealing with a stressful situation), yet not be "coping" in different situational circumstances. Accordingly, coping behaviors do not, by definition, differ from "non-coping" behaviors in terms of their phenomenological quality. Which behaviors should one, then, select as "coping" responses? Are all behaviors in the face of chronic disease to be referred to as "coping"? Many researchers probably would not accept this.

Secondly, and as a consequence, coping behaviors often are equated with behaviors serving some "protective" function for the individual, and are thus connotatively related to "mastery" (or similar notions). While this, at first glance, seems to be a rather plausible restriction, it turns out to create problems when coping behaviors are to be studied empirically. For example, do we, on a priori grounds, know which behaviors do exert "beneficial" effects for the individual and which criteria should we take into consideration when evaluating their "protective" function? In the light of empirical evidence, indicating that a single coping mode may be considered "adaptive" when taking one criterion, yet, be completely maladaptive with regard to another, this approach can produce quite ambiguous results.

It seems obvious that we cannot rely on a "list" of coping behaviors to be included in our questionnaires when this definition is applied. Rather, we will always have to await a posteriori measurements of "coping" effectiveness with regard to various criteria. Thus, whether the various behaviors deserve to be included under the rubric of "coping", turns out to be a purely *empirical* rather than a *conceptual* issue, when adopting such a view.

There are quite a few ways out of this dilemma. Some researchers, for example, have focused upon single, narrowly defined coping responses like information seeking as one of the most often studied modes of coping with health-related problems (see Meyerowitz, Heinrich & Schag, 1983). Other researchers have conceived of coping with chronic disease in terms of broad and highly abstract behavioral categories, in particular "approach vs. avoidance", that can be related to fundamental processes of attentional distribution (see, e.g., Roth & Cohen, 1986). Still other researchers have simply listed a variety of coping responses without relating them to any theoretical concept or without explaining the rationale by which their selection of coping behaviors had been guided (e.g., Weisman, 1979).

We believe, however, that psychology can offer a rich repertory of conceptual tools that might be used to reconstruct "coping" in theoretical terms, and which, in turn, should allow for more sophisticated ways to measure coping behaviors (e.g., attribution theory, Taylor, Lichtman & Wood, 1984; social comparison theory, Festinger, 1954; models of problem-solving, Turk, Sobel, Follick & Youkilis, 1980).

Research Agenda in the Study of Coping with Chronic Disease

We will now turn to a brief overview of research agenda in the study of coping with chronic disease, for which our knowledge is still far from being sufficient. Three types of research agenda (which also serve as a guideline for our own research) will be addressed.

The first one is related to the problem of how to conceptualize and measure coping behaviors in the face of chronic disease. One can adopt various theoretical perspectives in the study of coping, as was just outlined; yet, whether coping *with chronic disease* is adequately represented by the various paradigms is a research question still awaiting answers. For example, attempts to reformulate coping in terms of causal reasoning ("Why me?") have become fairly prominent; nevertheless, one could doubt whether causal reasoning is indeed spontaneous and salient inside patients' heads rather than simply induced by researchers' questions (cf. Gotay, 1985).

More generally spoken, the problem is to what degree various modes of coping, either derived from a given theoretical framework or already studied in the context of other stressful life situations, are applicable to and appropriate for the description of how patients cope with chronic disease. For example, the "Ways of Coping Checklist" (Folkman & Lazarus, 1980) had been applied to the study of highly diverse stressful situations and proved to yield meaningful results also when related to chronic disease (Felton & Revenson, 1984). Nevertheless, whether particular conceptions of "coping" can be applied somewhat universally to possibly all types of stressors or should be specifically suited to the study of coping with chronic disease, is an open question.

The second research issue deals with the question of what determines individual differences in coping with chronic disease. First of all, one would presumably expect medical factors (e.g., type of chronic disease) to promote certain coping responses, while suppressing others. Felton, Revenson, and Hinrichsen (1984) found, however, that differences in coping strategies tended to be minimally explained by the type of disease (hypertension, diabetes mellitus, cancer, and rheumatoid arthritis). On the other hand, Kneier and Temoshok (1984) found cancer patients to score higher than patients suffering from coronary heart diseases in "repressive" coping; Feifel, Strack, and Nagy (1987) found that patients suffering from highly life-threatening diseases used "confrontative" strategies more frequently.

Only a few studies have investigated differences in medical status between patients having the same medical diagnosis and related them to coping behaviors. Histological grade and initial clinical stage, however, were found to be unrelated to coping behavior in cancer patients (Pettingale, Burgess & Greer, 1988).

One might speculate that subjective illness representations (i.e., the severity, cause, and outcome) are more important in determining coping responses than objective medical status (Moos & Schaefer, 1984); but evidence from studies is still scarce.

While the role of illness-related factors in shaping coping responses is still unproven, personality variables have long been thought of as powerful determinants based on two lines of reasoning. First, a focus on individual trait-like *styles* of coping with stress (e. g., contrasting "repressors vs. sensitizers" or "monitors vs. blunters") was introduced (e. g., Bell & Byrne, 1978; Miller & Mangan, 1983). Second, a variety of individual difference variables has been taken into consideration as predictors of coping behaviors. For example, locus of control has been shown to differentiate "confronters vs. non-confronters" in a sample of cancer patients (Burgess, Morris & Pettingale, 1988), internals using more confronting strategies than externals. Similarly, health locus of control was related to "self-blame" as a coping strategy in the study by Felton and Revenson (1987), while being completely unrelated to "information seeking" and "emotional expression".

Despite other individual factors there are also more general objections towards the assumption that coping responses are linked to personality variables. In contrast, it had been claimed that coping continuously changes and unfolds over time (Folkman & Lazarus, 1985) as well as varies across types of stressors to which individuals are exposed (Pearlin & Schooler, 1978).

The third type of research agenda is related to the issue of coping effectiveness and the question of which coping behaviors can be regarded "successful", and under which (personal and/or situational) circumstances they might prove to be effective. A closer look at these questions reveals that their importance, from an applied as well as from a basic research perspective, is matched by the difficulty of finding answers for them. One problem lies in the selection of appropriate criteria for evaluating coping effectiveness and in the incompatibility between various criteria, length of survival time vs. quality of life being a popular example of the conflicting values in the study of "successful" coping with severe and chronic disease.

Evidence from the Trier Longitudinal Study of Coping with Chronic Disease[1]

General Aims of the Study

When we started our research project, we concluded from research work done so far, that empirical evidence was still much needed in the realm of coping with chronic disease. As mentioned above, our study is based on the acknowledgement of various research requirements, described in the previous section and repeated here briefly.

Firstly, we attempted to assess coping behaviors based on an a priori classification system of responses. In addition, brief measures of alternatively conceptualized modes of coping (e. g., in terms of comparison processes) were included. Based on these measures, we are looking for temporal variations in modes of coping with cancer using both longitudinal and cross-sectional comparisons. Second, we have related individual differences in coping behaviors as well as in their temporal variations to a set of variables conceived here as being predictive of coping. A variety of medical variables (obtained from the physician as well as from the patient) personality variables and contextual variables are also included. In addition, subjective estimates of illness-related life changes are assessed as "coping tasks" and related to coping behaviors and their changes over time. Assessment of these various predictors is made on at least two occasions in order to allow for more clear-cut causal inferences.

Third, one important aim of our study, of course, is to identify "successful" coping behaviors, both in a short-term and a long-term (two years) perspective. For that purpose we have included a set of multiple criteria such as medical variables (e.g., relapse, tumor growth), psychological variables (e.g., depressive mood), and contextual variables (e.g., return to work, social isolation) for evaluating coping effectiveness.

[1] The research reported here was supported by a grant from the Deutsche Forschungsgemeinschaft (Fi 346/1–3).

This paper will only describe part of the study and will present only some of the evidence we have gained, so far. Besides, we are still involved in collecting data for the last point of measurement from those patients who were enrolled in the study in 1986 and since.

Patient Sample

Our study was conducted in cooperation with several hospitals and institutions for cancer care and rehabilitation in West Germany. All patients had been recruited within these medical settings; data were collected at four occasions of measurement within one year after the initial interview (interval: three months) and at an additional follow-up two years later.

At the first point of measurement, our sample consisted of 332 patients (178 females, 154 males) with a mean age of 51 years. The largest subgroups (range 15–77 years) were patients with carcinoma of the breast ($n=83$), malignancies in the digestive system ($n=63$), in the area of the mouth, the throat, and the larynx ($n=47$), and patients with cancers of the blood or lymphatic system ($n=43$). At the initial interview, 50 percent of the sample has been diagnosed within the previous year and the time elapsed since diagnosis varied between 1 and 840 weeks (mean 112 weeks). 128 patients (38.5 percent) already had a cancer recurrence before participating in the study. The most common types of medical treatment were surgery (79.9 percent of the sample), radiation therapy (48.9 percent), and chemotherapy (27.3 percent).

At the fourth time of measurement 202 patients were still participating in the study; no systematic drop-out effects, so far, are to be observed with respect to gender, age, and time elapsed since diagnosis, which in turn were not correlated with each other at all points of measurement. Since we have rather complete information on deaths in our sample as opposed to patients who refused further participation, we will have to investigate more carefully how drop-out is related to the initial measures after all the data from the last wave are collected .

Measurement of Coping Responses

Besides the assessment of coping behaviors as the main group of variables, a host of other measures had to be collected in order to gain evidence on the determinants of coping responses as well as on their effectiveness. We will refer here only to a few measures to which our brief presentation of results needs to be related to. The assessment of coping behaviors was based on an a priori model comprised of three basic dimensions along which coping responses can be classified. In particular, we selected (1) attentional focus (i.e., behaviors indicating distraction from vs. focus upon the disease), (2) level of coping response (i.e., overt vs. intrapsychic), and (3) degree of sociability (i.e., behaviors reflecting withdrawal from others vs. integrating others into one's coping efforts, such as seeking social affiliation). These dimensions were then cross-classified yielding eight mutually exclusive groups of coping reactions (see Figure 1), each group being represented by eight items describing a particular response. These together 64 items were then included in a questionnaire to be answered by the patient on 6-point scales as to how often within the last weeks he or she exhibited each response (*FEKB*; Klauer & Filipp, 1987).

		Attentional focus			
		Centered on disease		**Distracted from disease**	
		Sociability		Sociability	
		High	*Low*	*High*	*Low*
Level of response	Covert	*"I worried whether physicians can really help me"* (27)	*"I tried to find out whether I did something wrong"* (25)	*I said to myself that there are many people who are worse off compared to me"* (47)	*"I Imagined that things will get better some-times"* (52)
	Overt	*"I shared experiences in managing the illness with other patients"* (01)	*"I looked for information on my illness in books and journals"* (22)	*"I encouraged other people and tried to cheer them up"* (08)	*"I kept busy with things that filled me out"* (06)

Figure 1. A three-dimensional model for the classification of modes of coping with chronic illness including item examples from the *FEKB*

This pattern of eight coping reponses was not confirmed in dimensional analyses of our data. Exploratory and subsequently performed confirmatory factor analyses yielded a structural pattern of five factors (cf. Klauer, Filipp & Ferring, 1989), which, then were used for the construction of the following five scales measuring these five coping modes: (I) *Rumination (RU)*, comprised items that describe intrapsychic behaviors focusing on the disease and implying social withdrawal (e.g., causal reasoning and ruminating on the disease); (II) *Search for affiliation (SA)*, is reflective of highly sociable coping behaviors which imply diversion and attentional distraction from the disease; (III) *Threat minimization (TM)*, describes intrapsychic, presumably emotion-focused coping reactions like self-instructions towards positive thinking and maintaining trust in the medical regimen; (IV) *Search for informaton (SI)* describes overt reactions aimed at gaining knowledge of the disease and its medical treatment, preferrably by joining the company of other cancer patients; (V) *Search for meaning in religion (SR)* comprises attempts to find meaning in the illness experience with special reference to religious issues. Because we used unit weighting instead of factor scores in the calculation of scale values, coping scales *RU* and *SI* as well as *TM* and *SA* are moderately, though significantly, intercorrelated. Without being exhaustive, of course, these scales cover a wide range of coping responses that can also be found in some other studies using a different rationale (e.g., Felton, Revenson & Hinrichsen, 1984; Ray, Lindop & Gibson, 1982; Taylor, 1983; Weisman, 1979). They obviously allow for the description of individual differences which, then, can be related to various predictor variables as well as to various outcome criteria in order to investigate their effectiveness.

Temporal Variations in Coping Behaviors

The issue of temporal variations in coping behaviors is partially related to the question of what determines coping behaviors. As mentioned above, it has been repeatedly claimed that there is a considerable variability in coping responses across time (e.g., due to changing demands or "time healing many wounds"). Evidently, such assumptions necessitate research designs that incorporate more than one point of measurement as well as adequate measurement devices, i.e. measures sensitive for *changes* in coping behaviors over time and/or situations ("process measures"; see Aldwin et al., 1980). These instruments also have been characterized as "episodic" as opposed to "dispositional" measures (Cohen, 1987).

Nevertheless, the construction of most of these measurement instruments is still based on assumptions derived from classical test theory (CTT). These are, however, incompatible with the proposition of coping unfolding as a process over time. Especially, the premise that a test score derived from a particular coping scale is composed of the person-specific true score plus the measurement error inevitably implies that variations observed in test scores across measurement occasions are to be treated as *error* variance.

One first step towards solving this problem (which is, by no means, confined to the stress and coping paradigm) is provided by extensions of the CTT, suggested by Tack (1980) and Steyer (1987). Steyer proposed a class of psychometric models which allow for the decomposition of the variance of the measured variable into one component determined solely by the person, a second one reflecting the influence of occasion-specific situational and/or interactional factors, and the error variance. These "latent state-trait models" are also referred to as "consistency-specificity (CS) models". When having data from at least two occasions of measurement, separate coefficients for consistency and specificity can be estimated which add up to the reliability of the scales.

In order to investigate coping responses across time in our sample, the CS model was applied to the coping measures from those patients who participated at the fourth occasion of measurement ($N=202$).

The CS model was subsequently tested against two other psychometric models which might also be able to account for the observed data structure, i. e., (1) the reliability" model derived from CTT, which, as a latent-trait model, assumes only one true-score variable across all occasions of measurement, and (2) a latent-state model ("stability model") which yields occasion-specific true-score variables which are allowed to be intercorrelated over measurement occasions, thus, indicating different levels of stability.

In order to test these models , the *FEKB* scales (i. e., *rumination, search for affiliation, threat minimization, search for information* and *search for meaning in religion*) each were subdivided into two parallel variables serving as *manifest* indicators of each latent coping variable. With regard to the reliability and stability model, several submodels differing in restrictiveness of the measurement submodel, were analysed (for more detailed description see Ferring, Klauer, Filipp & Steyer, 1988).

Results prove the CS model to be superior to the reliability models in fitting the observed covariances. Some stability models, which are less desirable than the CS models on theoretical grounds (i.e., the latent-state structure does not allow for a decomposition of person and situation as sources of variance), fitted the data equally well.

As can be seen from Table 1, the proportion of true-score variance explained by the "person" (e.g., by coping dispositions) is much higher than the proportion accounted for by the four measurement occasions; nevertheless, the occasion-specific variance proves to be systematic variance and has to be taken into consideration. In sum, the *FEKB* scales obviously are sensitive to change, although they seem to primarily reflect person-specific variations in coping with chronic disease.

Does Coping Help to Maintain Well-Being?

A discussion of "coping effectiveness" in relation to outcome variables is based on the assumption that coping behaviors and "outcomes" are *causally* related in an unidirectional way, thus allowing for inferences of who is coping well and who is coping poorly. However, the test of coping effectiveness needs to be based on more than a significant correlation. It also needs to be shown that the causality assumption is valid in that coping behaviors are causally prior to rather than determined by the respective outcome variable. Yet, empirical evidence on the issue of causal directionality in this realm is rather scarce (for a rare exception, see Felton & Revenson, 1984).

In order to investigate which of the coping modes measured by the FEKB scales might be judged "effective", we used a variety of criteria. Here, we will take only "subjective well-being" as one criterion to illustrate the issue of coping effectiveness.

Well-being as one index of the patient's adjustment status was measured by means of an extensively validated German instrument (*Bf-S'*, von Zerssen, 1976) which comprised 28 bipolar scales describing positive vs. negative affective states. From self-ratings on these scales a single score is derived.

Split-half reliability and internal consistency were high in our sample ($r_{tt}=0.92$; Cronbach's $\alpha=0.94$ at t1; $r_{tt}=0.95$, $\alpha=0.96$ at t4). Compared to the general population, levels of well-being are significantly lower in our sample at all four points of measurement, but also remarkably and significantly higher than within a population inpatients (von Zerssen, 1976). This indicates that, following the diagnosis of cancer, subjective well-being is significantly reduced but not to a level found in psychiatric patients. We used the *FEKB* coping measures and the *BF-S'* measure of subjective well-being to test the plausibility of three hypothetical models, all of which could explain the observed correlation structure, namely that (1) coping determines well-being, (2) well-being is prior to coping, and (3) both interrelate in a reciprocal fashion. Hierarchical regression analyses were performed, in which pretest scores for coping modes and well-being, respectively, were controlled for (i.e., used as "autoregressors") and in which post-test scores for coping and well-being served as criteria. The amount of variance explained by the additional "change

Table 1. *Consistency, specificity, and reliability coefficients for five coping modes and four occasions of measurement*

Coeffic-ient	Measurement occasion			
	1	2	3	4
Rumination				
CON	0.562	0.657	0.698	0.651
SPE	0.271	0.148	0.094	0.155
REL	0.833	0.805	0.792	0.807
Search for Affiliation				
CON	0.564	0.640	0.729	0.594
SPE	0.280	0.183	0.070	0.242
REL	0.845	0.823	0.799	0.836
Threat Minimization				
CON	0.651	0.647	0.628	0.647
SPE	0.106	0.092	0.126	0.150
REL	0.757	0.739	0.754	0.797
Search for Information				
CON	0.720	0.697	0.740	0.671
SPE	0.147	0.174	0.124	0.205
REL	0.867	0.871	0.864	0.876
Search for Meaning in Religion				
CON	0.858	0.895	0.858	0.849
SPE	0.088	0.049	0.082	0.092
REL	0.946	0.944	0.940	0.941

[a]CON: Consistency coefficient;
SPE: Specificity coefficient;
REL: Reliability coefficient

regressor" (i.e., coping when well-being residuals and well-being when coping residuals were the dependent variable) indicates the effect of one variable on pretest-posttest changes in the respective other. Given similar stabilities of the variables under study, a comparison of the relative effect sizes may yield some insight into the relative causal position of each of the variables (cf., Rogosa, 1980).

These analyses are based on data covering two 3-months as well as one 6-month interval (t1–t2; t2–t3; t1–t3). Accordingly, a "proximal" (change regressor measured at the same occasion as the criterion) as well as a "distal" (change regressor measured at t1) prediction model was calculated, using pretest and posttest scores as change regressors, respectively. Table 2 summarizes the most relevant results from these analyses with respect to the 6-month interval and by focusing on those coping modes that proved to be temporally correlated with well-being, i.e., "rumination", "search for affiliation", and "threat minimization" (for a more detailed description, see Filipp, Klauer, Freudenberg & Ferring, 1988).

Table 2 *Hierarchical regression of coping on well-being and well-being on coping controlling for pre-test scores (time lag: six months; N=174 cancer patients)*

Criterion[a]	Change regressor	Regression statistics[b]			
		beta	RSQC	$F_{(1;171)}$	R^2
	Proximal prediction				
WB 3	RU 3	−0.34	0.10	26.41**	0.34
RU 3	WB 3	−0.31	0.09	39.70**	0.62
WB 3	SA 3	0.24	0.05	12.16**	0.29
SA 3	WB3	0.20	0.03	11.79**	0.50
WB 3	TM 3	0.24	0.06	13.73**	0.29
TM 3	WB 3	0.11	0.01	3.48	0.51
	Distal prediction				
WB 3	RU 1	−0.12	0.01	2.94	0.25
RU 3	WB 1	−0.16	0.02	8.40**	0.55
WB 3	SA 1	0.15	0.02	4.64*	0.26
SA 3	WB 1	0.13	0.02	5.20*	0.48
WB 3	TM 1	0.22	0.04	9.87**	0.28
TM 3	WB 1	−0.01	0.00	0.01	0.50

[a]WB, subjective well-being; RU, rumination; SA, search for affiliation; TM, threat minimization; additionally given is the running number of point measurement
[b]Specified are regression coefficients (*beta*), the incremental variance explained by the change regressor (*RSQC*) with the corresponding *F*-value, and the total variance of post-test scores accounted for by pre-test score and change regressor (R^2).
**$p<0.01$ *$p<0.05$

As can be seen, the relation between subjective well-being and *"rumination" (RU)* seems to be characterized by causal predominance of well-being over coping in the distal prediction. While changes in well-being are unrelated to pre-test *RU* scores, changes in rumination can be predicted significantly from pre-test well-being scores. However, in the proximal prediction this pattern is blurred. It seems from these findings that low levels of well-being in cancer patients might be a stronger determinant of dealing with the disease in terms of rumination than the reverse; it is not rumination that lowers well-being, but negative mood that fosters rumination as a coping mode.

An opposite pattern of results can be observed for *"threat minimization"* (TM): In both, distal and proximal, predictions, analyses point to a predominance of *TM* over subjective well-being (i.e., *TM* scores at both times of measurement are predictive of changes in well-being, whereas the effects of well-being on changes in

TM fail to reach statistical significance). These intrapsychic coping behaviors that presumably serve a palliative, emotion-regulatory function, seem to be successful in altering levels of well-being in a positive direction over time.

A third pattern of results, finally, was obtained for the relationship between subjective well-being and *"search for affiliation"* (SA). With regard to both proximal and distal models of prediction, changes in one variable can be predicted from the other. Thus, it is not causal predominance but "reciprocal determinism" which characterizes the relationship between well-being and search for affiliation as a coping mode in the cancer patients. This relationship probably can be described best by referring to the concept of a "positive feedback loop" in which the tendency to socialize and level of subjective well-being mutually enhance each other over time. Alternatively, such a relationship could result in a vicious cycle in terms of low levels of well-being fostering withdrawal from others, which in turn decreases well-being.

Taken these results together, it can be demonstrated that the five coping modes investigated here differ in terms of how they are related to subjective well-being (i. e., one being negatively , two being positively, and two being completely unrelated to levels of well-being). Furthermore, our results show that the assumption of coping behaviors exerting effects on levels of well-being may not be acceptable in general. In particular, in the case of "rumination" coping behaviors (e.g., causal reasoning as to why one has developed cancer) these seem to depend on subjective well-being. Accordingly, it would be incorrect to think of rumination as being maladaptive with regard to well-being. The only clear-cut evidence for coping effectiveness can be reported for "threat minimization" i.e., coping reactions that involve drawing the attentional focus away from one's disease. These are obviously effective in maintaining as well as enhancing well-being, and, therefore, might be a possible "stress buffer" for the cancer patient. However, we will have to await whether they exert equally beneficial effects with regard to other outcome criteria and over a longer time period.

Summary and Conclusions

We have been arguing throughout our chapter that the concept of coping is still rather weakly defined. A few approaches to overcome this weakness have been commented on. In addition, quite a few research agenda in the realm of coping with chronic disease are still in need of empirical clarification. According to our view, this can be accomplished only by using a longitudinal research strategy including various occasions of measurement. Only then should we be able to really prove (instead of simply proposing it) whether or not coping is a process that unfolds over time. Similarly, the question of what determines individual differences in coping, and, how "successful" various coping behaviors prove to be, needs a design that goes beyond "one shot measurements" of coping. A few results from our study with cancer patients have been presented. Whether these results might generalize to how other victims of life crises are coping with their lot, and whether "universals" in the nature of coping may become obvious, will guide our research endeavors for the next years.

References

Abelson, R. P. (1981). Psychological status of the script concept. *American Psychologist, 36*, 715–729.

Aldwin, C. M., Folkman, S., Schaefer, C., Coyne, J. C., and Lazarus, R. S. (1980). *Ways of Coping: A process measure*. Paper presented at the Annual Convention of the American Psychological Association, Montreal 1980.

Bell, P., and Byrne, D. (1978). Repression-sensitization as a dimension of personality. In H. London, and J. Exner (Eds.), *Dimensions of personality* (pp. 449–485). New York: Wiley.

Burgess, C., Morris, T., and Pettingale, K. W. (1988). Psychological response to cancer diagnosis – II. Evidence for coping styles (coping styles and cancer diagnosis). *Journal of Psychosomatic Research, 32*, 263–272.

Callahan, E. J., and McCluskey, K. A. (Eds.) (1983). *Life-span developmental psychology: Nonnormative life events*. New York: Academic Press.

Cohen, F. (1987). Measurement of coping. In S. V. Kasl, and C. L. Cooper (Eds.), *Stress and health: Issues in research methodology* (pp. 283–305). Chichester, U. K.: Wiley.

Feifel, H., Strack, H., and Nagy, V. T. (1987). Degree of life-threat and differential use of coping modes. *Journal of Psychosomatic Research, 31*, 91–99.

Felton, B. J., and Revenson, T. A. (1984). Coping with chronic illness: A study of illness controllability and the influence of coping strategies on psychological adjustment. *Journal of Consulting and Clinical Psychology, 52*, 343–353.

Felton, B. J., and Revenson, T. A. (1987). Age differences in coping with chronic illness. *Psychology and Aging, 2*, 164–170.

Felton, B. J., Revenson, T. A., and Hinrichsen, G. A. (1984). Stress and coping in the explanation of psychological adjustment among chronically ill adults. *Social Science and Medicine, 18*, 889–898.

Ferring, D., Klauer, T., Filipp, S.–H., and Steyer, R. (1988). *Psychometrische Modelle zur Bestimmung von Konsistenz und Spezifität im Bewältigungsverhalten* [Psychometric models for the estimation of consistency and specificity in coping]. Trier: Universität Trier (Unpublished manuscript).

Festinger, L. (1954). A theory of social comparison processes. *Human Relations, 7*, 117–140.

Filipp, S. –H., Klauer, T., Ferring, D., and Freudenberg, E. (1988). *The regulation of subjective well-being in cancer patients: An analysis of coping effectiveness*. Trier: University of Trier (Unpublished manuscript).

Folkman, S., and Lazarus, R. S. (1980). An analysis of coping in a middle-aged community sample. *Journal of Health and Social Behavior, 21*, 219–239.

Folkman, S., and Lazarus, R. S. (1985). If it changes it must be a process: Study of emotion and coping during stages of a college examination. *Journal of Personality and Social Psychology, 48*, 150–170.

Gotay, C. C. (1985). Why me? Attributions and adjustment by cancer patients and their mates at two stages in the disease process. *Social Science and Medicine, 20*, 825–831.

Klauer, T., and Filipp, S. -H. (1987) *Der "Fragebogen zur Erfassung von Formen der Krankheitsbewältigung" (FEKB): I. Kurzbeschreibungf des Verfahrens* [The "Fragebogen zur Erfassung von Formen der Krankheitsbewältigung" (FEKB): I. Short description of the questionnaire]. (Berichte aus dem Forschungsprojekt "Psychologie der Krankheitsbewältigung" Nr.13). Trier: Universität Trier, Fachbereich I – Psychologie.

Klauer, T., Filipp, S.-H., and Ferring, D. (1989). Der "Fragebogen zur Erfassung von Formen der Krankheitsbewältigung" (FEKB): Skalenkonstruktion und erste Befunde zu Reliabilität, Validität, und Stabilität [The "Fragebogen zur Erfassung von Formen der Krankheitsbewältigung" (FEKB): Scale construction and first results on reliability, validity, and stability]. *Diagnostica, 35*, 316–335.

Kneier, A. W., and Temoshok, L. (1984). Repressive coping reactions in patients with malignant melanoma as compared to cardiovascular disease patients. *Journal of Psychosomatic Research, 28*, 145–155.

Maddi, S. R., Bartone, P. T., and Puccetti, M. C. (1987). Stressful events are indeed a factor in physical illness: Reply to Schroeder and Costa (1984). *Journal of Personality and Social Psychology, 52,* 833–843.

Meyerowitz, B. E., Heinrich, R. L., and Schag, C. C. (1983). A competency-based approach to coping with cancer. In T. G. Burish, and L. A. Bradley (Eds.), *Coping with chronic disease: Research and applications* (pp. 137–158). New York: Academic Press.

Miller, S. M., and Mangan, C. E. (1983). Interacting effects of information and coping style in adapting to gynaecologic stress: Should the doctor tell all? *Journal of Personality and Social Psychology, 45,* 223–236.

Moos, R. H., and Schaefer, J. A. (1984). The crisis of physical illness. An overview and conceptual approach. In R. H. Moos (Ed.), *Coping with physical illness. Vol. 2: New perspectives* (pp. 3–25). New York: Plenum.

Pearlin, L. I., and Schooler, C. (1978). The structure of coping. *Journal of Health and Social Behavior, 19,* 2–21.

Pettingale, L. W., Burgess, C., and Greer, S. (1988). Psychological response to cancer diagnosis – I. Correlations with prognostic variables. *Journal of Psychosomatic Research, 32,* 255–261.

Ray, C., Lindop, J., and Gibson, S. (1982). The concept of coping. *Psychological Medicine, 12,* 385–395.

Rogosa, D. (1980). A critique of cross-lagged correlation. *Psychological Bulletin, 88,* 245–258.

Roth, S., and Cohen, L. J. (1986). Approach, avoidance, and coping with stress. *American Psychologist, 41,* 813–819.

Steyer, R. (1987). Konsistenz und Spezifität: Definition zweier zentraler Begriffe der Differentiellen Psychologie und ein einfaches Modell zu ihrer Identifikation [Consistency and specificity: Definition of two central concepts of personality psychology and a simple model for their identification]. *Zeitschrift für Differentielle Psychologie, 8,* 245–258.

Tack, W. (1980). Zur Theorie psychometrischer Verfahren. Formalisierung der Erfassung von Situationsabhängigkeit und Veränderung [On the theory of psychometric procedures. Formalization of the assessment of situational dependency and change]. *Zeitschrift für Differentielle und Diagnostische Psychologie, 1,* 87–106.

Taylor, S. E. (1983). Adjustment to threatening events. A theory of cognitive adaptation. *American Psycholgist, 38,* 1161–1173.

Taylor, S. E., Lichtman, R. R., and Wood, J. V. (1984). Attributions, beliefs about control, and adjustment to breast cancer. *Journal of Personality and Social Psychology, 46,* 489–502.

Turk, D. C., Sobel, H. J., Follick, M., and Youkilis, H. D. (1980). A sequential criterion analysis for assessing coping with chronic illness. *Journal of Human Stress, 6,* 35–40.

Weisman, A. D. (1979). *Coping with cancer.* New York: McGraw-Hill.

Zerssen, D. von (1976). *Die Befindlichkeitsskala* [The Befindlichkeitsskala]. Weinheim: Beltz.

An Analysis of Patterns of Coping in Rheumatoid Arthritis

Stanton Newman, Ray Fitzpatrick, Rosemarie Lamb, and
Michael Shipley

Introduction

The concept of coping has come to play a central role in the armoury of Health
Psychologists attempts to make sense of variable responses and outcomes in the
health and disease process. Some of the earliest work which used the term coping,
considered the variety of responses to normal and abnormal life crisis (Moos, 1986).
In the main, the events considered were discrete in time. Typical of the issues studied
in health psychology has been the emphasis placed upon styles of coping with
stressful medical procedures (Schmidt, 1988). The issues involved in coping with a
discrete event would be likely to differ from a constant stress as in a chronic illness
where the stress, although variable, is constantly present. The response to a chronic
illness raises the possibility of constantly refining and adjusting ones coping skills
according to their perceived efficacy and controllability. It may be expected that the
overall level of stress, in this case the illness, would influence coping (Menaghan,
1982) such that individuals faced with a severe illness would differ in their coping
responses from those with a less severe illness. In addition it would seem
unreasonable to expect coping styles to be static over time. With progressive illness
the individual may learn that particular responses are no longer as effective and
adjust their coping responses accordingly. Time may also act independently of illness
progression and the repertoire of coping skills may increase as the individual learns
new ways of managing their illness.

Some of the earlier research on coping has close parallels to attempts to examine
coping style and chronic illness. Pearlin and Schooler (1978) attempted to study
enduring and widely experienced life strains arising out of social roles that
individuals play. They considered such role as marriage partner, child rearing and
the work role. Their interest was principally on normative responses and as such did
not emphasise individual differences. They found that coping responses were
particularly effective in close personal relationships and tended to be particularly
available to males, the educated and the affluent. The study reported by Pearlin and
Schooler considers problems which are enduring in time but differ from a chronic
illness in that they are experienced by most individuals.

Coping has taken on a number of meanings and it is important to specify the
manner in which it is to be considered in the study reported here. Coping is seen as
a psychological mechanism for managing external stress (Lazarus & Folkman, 1984).
This mechanism may be both action oriented and intrapsychic and is intended
to avoid or mitigate the consequences of a stressor (Cohen, 1987). In this manner
a series of responses may be analysed without presuming any particular outcome.
This approach distinguishes the process of coping from its outcome. In many
studies an individual is defined as 'coping' if they minimise emotional distress

(see for example Pinkerton, Trauer, Duncan, Hodson & Batten, 1985). This approach, by confounding the process of coping and its outcome fails to indicate which individual strategies or combination of strategies leads to a particular outcome.

There are a number of measures that assess coping strategies in response to a specific stressor (Folkman & Lazarus, 1980, 1985; Pearlin & Schooler, 1978). In a number of these the coping styles have been defined by factor analysis but there is little agreement as to the appropriate factor structure even with same measure (Aldwin & Revenson, 1987). More recently attempts have been made to design coping questionnaires specific to a particular problem or event. These are considered to have greater relevance although their reliability is frequently not considered in any detail. Many of the 'off the shelf' measures do not appear appropriate in the consideration of coping with chronic illness.

The analysis of coping responses has differed across studies. In some, individuals have been defined in terms of their dominant coping styles while in others the efficacy of a particular style of coping has been assessed. Consequently individual's have been typed as to whether they used, for example, a problem or emotion focussed coping strategy. The difficulty with this approach is that individual subjects may use one, both, or in fact neither of the defined coping styles specified. There is a need to attempt to specify not only which strategies are being used but also those not being used in order to fully appreciate the pattern of coping and differences in the pattern of responses between individuals. This is particularly pertinent when considering a long term stressor such as a chronic illness where it is possible that some individuals with longstanding disease may not use any particular style of coping. By attempting to consider the overall pattern of responses it is possible to avoid the difficulty of forcing the data to place subjects onto dimensions such as problem or emotion focussed coping styles. In the study to be reported in this chapter an attempt has been made to characterise the overall pattern of coping responses of individuals and to classify them into groups according to this pattern. The analysis, not only considers which coping strategies have been adopted for use by an individual, but also the extent to which they reject possible coping strategies. No categories have been imposed on the responses and therefore no judgment has been made as to the dimension that might result from the data.

One of the outcome measures in any study of coping with chronic illness is psychological well-being. It is important that independent of coping style, the presence of a chronic illness had been seen to result in an increased risk of psychological difficulties and lowered self esteem. In the case of rheumatoid arthritis the combination of pain, joint stiffness, disability and the social restrictions that follow result in significantly raised levels of depressed mood (Newman, Fitzpatrick, Lamb & Shipley, 1987; Anderson, Bradley, Young & McDaniel, 1985; Zaphiropoulos & Burry, 1974). Disability has been found to be the most important variable in determining psychological adaptation in rheumatoid arthritis (Newman, Fitzpatrick, Lamb & Shipley, 1987; Fitzpatrick, Newman, Lamb & Shiply, 1988). In the study reported here three measures of psychological well-being were considered, self esteem, depressed mood and adjustment.

Methods

Patients

The sample consisted of 158 sequential patients attending the outpatient Rheumatology Clinic of the Middlesex Hospital with a diagnosis of rheumatoid arthritis:- all satisfied at least Grade 2 of the NY criteria (Bennett & Wood, 1968) and all had, at some time satisfied the ARA criteria for at least 'probable' RA (American Rheumatism Association, 1959). Patients were in the age range 18–70, of whom 36 (23%) were male and 122 (77%) female were assessed. Mean age was 55 years (sd 10.9) and the mean duration of arthritis was 16 years (sd 11.8). Details of the Functional Grade are shown in the Table 1 (Steinbrocker et al., 1949).

Table 1

	Functional Grade	Frequency	%
Fit For All Activities	1	51	32.3
Moderate Restriction	2	58	36.7
Marked Restriction	3	46	29.1
Incapable of Work	4	3	1.9

Measures

The coping questionnaire developed for this study was constructed from interviews of patients with rheumatoid arthritis, existing questionnaires used to assess coping (e.g., Folkman & Lazarus, 1980), specific strategies suggested to patients by health care staff (e.g. I try to rest as much as possible) and a pilot study. The final questionnaire consisted of 36 items arranged in Likert type format.

Disability was assessed by the Functional Limitation Profile (FLP) which originally derives from the Sickness Impact Profile (Bergner, Bobbitt, Carter & Gilson, 1981) In the form of the FLP it has been standardised for a British population (Patrick, Morgan & Charlton, 1986). The original instrument has previously been used with a rheumatoid arthritis population (Deyo, Inui, Leininger & Overman, 1982) and found to correlate with other measures of functional ability (Bergner, Bobbitt, Carter & Gilson, 1981).

Pain was assessed on both a 6 point scale (thermometer) and a visual analogue scale. Joint stiffness was assessed by obtaining ratings of the severity of joint stiffness on a six point scale (thermometer) and obtaining a measure of the average amount of time joints were stiff in the morning. All measures referred to the past week.

A number of laboratory measures were performed on blood samples taken from the patients at the time of interview. These included measures of haemoglobin level, white blood cell count, platelet count and C-reactive protein. In addition the erythrocyte sedimentation rate (ESR) was measured by the Westergren method to provide an index of the current disease activity.

The consultant rheumatologist (MS) classified the type of onset (slow, rapid and palindromic) and the current level of disease activity at the time of assessment (inactive, moderately active and highly active). Grip strength was assessed in the standard manner, using a bag initially inflated to 30mm Hg:the results were recorded in millimeters of mercury. The extent of joint erosion was assessed by rating X-rays of the hands on a five point scale (modification of Lawrences' method)(Lawrence, 1977). The Ritchie Articular index score was used as a clinical assessment by the clinician. This index involves rating 26 joints for tenderness, each one on a 0–3 scale, the range of possible scores being 0–78.

Social support was measured by the Interview Schedule for Social Interaction (Henderson, Byrne & Duncan-Jones, 1981). This instrument provides measures in four sub-scales reflecting different aspects of an individual's social relationships. Availability (AVAT) and adequacy (ADAT) of close confiding intimate relationships were measured on two sub scales. The availability (AVSI) and adequacy (ADSI) of social contacts with more diffuse relationships were assessed on the remaining two sub scales. The reliability and validity of these measures has been established (Thomas, Gasrry, Goodwin & Goodwin, 1985).

Three measures of deprivation were obtained; the extent to which the person was experiencing financial problems, the quality of their accomodation and whether they had been able to take a holiday in the past year. These measures were combined into a single measure of economic deprivation.

The Beck Depression Inventory was selected as one of the measures to assess psychological well-being as it has been used previously in studies of rheumatoid arthritis patients (Zaphiropoulos & Burry, 1974). Scoring was adjusted to take account of those features which are likely to be due to the physical effects of the disease rather than to psychological factors. There were the items on work problems, fatigue and concern about health (Pincus, Callahan, Bradley, Vaughan & Wolfe, 1986). A second measure of psychological well-being was self esteem which was assessed by means of Rosenberg's (1965) ten item questionnaire. The Arthritis Helplessness Index, an instrument specifically designed to assess patients perception of helplessness in coping with RA, was administered (Nicassio, Wallston, Callahan, Herbert & Pincus 1985). The final measure of psychological well-being was a 15 item questionnaire measuring adjustment which was specifically designed for this study.

Statistical Analysis

The analysis adopted in this paper was to use a Cluster Analysis in order to group the individual subjects according to their responses on the Coping with Rheumatoid Arthritis questionnaire. This technique allocates individuals to groups where their responses on all 36 items are considered. The groups are determined in order to obtain maximum homogeneity within groups and to maximise differences between groups. The technique that was applied to determine which solution, in terms of numbers of groups, was a series of Hierarchical Cluster Analyses and then to consider the point at which the coefficient of the solution shows discontinuity (Blashfield, 1980; Everitt, 1980). Three hierarchical techniques were applied, Complete Linkage (furthest neighbour technique) are both Between and Within Group Average techniques. The analysis of the coefficients of all three hierarchical techniques pointed to a four group solution. The final cluster analysis performed was a k mean iterative solution for four groups. In this technique subjects group allocation is continually reanalysed to ensure that group allocation is closest to the particular group mean. Thus if a more appropriate group is available group allocation is altered and the group means recalculated. This process continues until the optimum four group solution is found. The cluster analytic approach describes the most appropriate groupings of subjects on the data. In order to establish whether these grouping have external validity, further analyses were conducted to the data in which comparisons were made between the groups on other variables in the study. These analyses consisted of Analyses of Variance and Covariance followed, where appropriate, by multiple comparisons. All data analysis was performed on the SPSS X programme (Norusis, 1985).

Results and Discussion

Coping

Cluster analysis was used to analyse the coping strategies of the 158 subjects on the 36 item coping questionnaire. As we have argued above, the value of this statistical technique is that it does not prejudge the performance of coping along preconceived dimensions, rather it analyses the position of individuals by considering the pattern of responses on the whole range of items in the questionnaire and thus takes into consideration both the use and failure to use a specific technique in any individuals repertoire. Furthermore, it is empirical in that the optimum groupings are defined by the statistical process and are uncontaminated by views about outcome. The most important limitation of this and other forms of analysis of coping concerns the nature and extent of the pool of items used in the analysis (Aldwin & Revenson, 1987). In this study the 36 item questionnaire, specific to rheumatoid arthritis, was designed on the basis of other coping questionnaires, open ended questionnaires with RA patients and a pilot study in an attempt to sample the range of coping strategies that patients normally engage in. The hierarchical cluster analysis of the responses yielded an optimum solution of four groups. The k means iterative solution for four groups and the dominant responses of these four groups is shown in Table 2.

One of the features of this analysis is to indicate that the largest group (Group 2) do not show any distinctive coping strategies but rather tend to use a wide range of coping strategies to a moderate extent. One may refer to this group as 'passive copers' as they do not attempt to confront their disease with particular techniques. Group 1, on the other hand, appear to utilise a combination of techniques to cope with their RA. In terms of problem and emotion focussed coping, they appear to use a combination of both these categories and are also distinctive in their use of denial with regard to pain. They at no time use prayer as a strategy to cope with their RA. Overall they may be considered to be a group who use 'mixed strategies and denial'. The third group appear to be active in confronting their disease. When confronted by pain they express it but do not look for support or in contrast to the passive copers (Group 2) use denial as a technique to cope with pain. Group 4 are distinctive in their use of prayer, distraction and alternative forms of treatment. This group also sought support from friends and attempt to confront their RA. Again in terms of problem and emotion focussed coping this group utilised both techniques. Overall the 4 groups do not neatly conform to the categories commonly used to define coping.

Table 2: *Coping characteristics of 4 groups*

Group 1 (n=20):
- moderately seeking information
- moderate exercise
- attempt to be physically active
- use denial as a technique to control pain
- look to friends for support
- fight against the disease
- reorganise routines to accommodate to the illness.
- not use of prayer or religion to assist
- derived no benefits from having RA.
- not buy special foods
- attempts to bear pain alone

Group 2 (n=105):
- not particularly active
- no distinctive coping strategies used or strongly rejected

Group 3 (n=14)
- attempt to be active
- not seek information
- make no adjustment in their routine for RA
- do not seek support or sympathy from others
- do not use prayer, wish fulfilment or distraction
- express feelings and presence of pain to others

Group 4 (n=19)
- engage in activities to distract from RA
- use prayer
- look to friends for support
- rest as much as possible but
- also attempted to exercise joints
- attempt to push against the disease
- selected particular diet
- attempt to control weight.

Moreover this analysis also indicates those strategies which these groups would definitely not engage in.

One of the possible influences on the tendency to use or ignore a particular coping strategy (Pearlin & Schooler, 1978) may be demographic factors such as age and social position. An analysis was made of these factors in relation to the 4 cluster groups. These findings are presented in Table 3.

The only significant finding was the proportion of individuals in families of non-manual occupations (Chi Square = 8.52, p<0.05). Group 1 had the highest percentage of non-manual and group 4 the lowest. Although there was a tendency for Groups 1 & 4 to have a higher percentage of women this did not reach significance. Age and a measure of the extent of economic deprivation were both found not to differ across the 4 groups defined on cluster analysis.

The duration since diagnosis was analysed as an indicator of the time that the person has been required to cope with the illness. Previous research has suggested not only that coping styles may change over time but that time may influence psychological adaptation (Newman, Fitzpatrick, Lamb & Shipley, 1987). Although the results of this analysis indicated no significant difference between the groups

Table 3 *Demographic characteristics and laboratory measures of 4 coping groups derived from cluster analysis*

	Group 1 (n=20)	Group 2 (n=105)	Group 3 (n=14)	Group 4 (n=19)	F^*/CHI^+	p
Sex (% Women)	90% (18)	72% (75)	71% (10)	95% (18)	6.9^+	0.07
Social Class						
% Non Manual	90% (17)	61% (60)	64% (9)	44% (8)	8.5^+	<0.05
Age	53.4	56.5	52.5	54.3	0.9^*	0.42
Deprivation Index						
Low	33% (6)	38% (36)	42% (5)	47% (8)		
Moderate	17% (3)	28% (26)	42% (5)	12% (2)		
High	50% (9)	34% (32)	17% (2)	41% (7)	6.2^+	0.41
Time Since Diagnosis (Years)	14.6	17.9	12.1	12.3	2.1^*	0.09
Haemoglobin Level	12.6	12.7	12.4	11.9	0.8^*	0.52
White Blood Cell Count	745	755	601	786	2.0^*	0.12
Platelet Count	366.1	352.6	874.2	405.9	2.9^*	<0.05
ESR	145	141	136	158	0.7^*	0.53
C-Reactive Protein	154.3	235.5	114	140.5	1.4^*	0.23

*Anova F Ratio
+ Chi Square

(p=0.09) there was tendency for those in Group 2 ('passive copers') to have had the disease the longest. This is consistent with the notion that in the earlier stages of the disease individuals tend to favour the use of particular coping strategies where they attack their illness with a range of techniques. As time progresses individuals tend to adopt a more 'laissez faire' attitude, and use a variety of coping strategies with no particular style predominating.

Laboratory Measures

All the measures on the blood take from the patients at the time of their assessments were performed blind to the psychological and social assessments. Of these measures only the measure of platelets was found to be significantly different between the groups (ANOVA F=2.98, df 3, 152;p<0.04) although some of the other measures did show large differences between the groups (see Table 3).

Rheumatological Measures

Clinical ratings of the current activity of the disease and the nature of the onset were not found to differ significantly across the four groups defined by cluster analysis (Table 4). A similar finding was found for measures of the disease as assessed by Grip Strength (Table 4) and rating of X rays.

The number of times individuals had been hospitalised for RA and the number of concurrent illnesses were found not to differ between groups.

Table 4: *Clinical measures of disease state*

	Group 1	Group 2	Group 3	Group 4	F^*/Chi^+	p
	(n=20)	(n=105)	(n=14)	(n=19)		
1. Inactive	15%(3)	31%(32)	43%(6)	16%(3)		
2. Moderate	45%(9)	35%(37)	29%(4)	42%(8)		
3. High A & B	40%(8)	34%(36)	29%(4)	42%(8)	5.0^+	0.54
Type of Onset						
Slow	60%(12)	60%(63)	50%(7)	68%(13)		
Rapid	37%(7)	37%(39)	43%(6)	26%(5)		
Palindromic	5%(1)	3%(3)	7%(1)	5%(1)	2.0^+	0.92
Grip Strength						
	148.8	145.7	182	119	1.8^*	0.13

* Anova F Ratio
+ Chi Square

In summary both the laboratory and rheumatological measures, with the exception of the platelet count, failed to discriminate between the four groups which were defined on the basis of their patterns of coping.

Social Support

Given that the four groups show relatively little difference on laboratory and rheumatological measures, the question arises as to whether the manifestation of different patterns of coping may be influenced by the amount and type of social supports available. Social supports were assessed by means of Henderson, Byrne and Duncan-Jones (1981) questionnaire which divides the responses into the availability and adequacy of both social contacts (Social Integration) and close confiding relationship. These factors have been found to play an important independent role in the self esteem and depressed mood of patients with RA (Fitzpatrick Newman, Lamb & Shipley, 1988; Newman, Fitzpatrick, Lamb, & Shipley, 1987). An analysis of the four groups with different patterns of coping failed to indicate any significant differences in social support (Table 5). Thus the different patterns of coping cannot be accounted for by differing levels of social support and their perceived adequacy between the groups.

Disability

The measure performed to assess the extent of disability between the subjects in this study was the Functional Limitations Profile (FLP). An analysis of both the full scale and the Physical sub-scale of the FLP is shown in Table 5. An ANOVA was performed to examine whether the groups differed in the extent of their disability on both the full scale and the sub-scale of Physical disability. These both indicated significant differences between the groups with Group 3 scoring at the lowest level on the full FLP (ANOVA F=4.6; df 3, 152;p<0.01) and the Physical sub-scale (ANOVA F=3.15; df 3,152;p<0.03)(see Table 5).

Two possible factors may account for the differences observed between groups on disability. The pattern of coping with RA adopted by Group 3, in comparison to the

Table 5 *Social support, disability, pain and stiffness*

	Group 1 (n=20)	Group 2 (n=105)	Group 3 (n=14)	Group 4 (n=19)	F*/CHI⁺	p
Social Integration						
Availability	7.9	6.5	7.6	6.8	1.01*	0.39
Adequacy	13.4	12.5	14.4	14	1.8*	0.15
Attachment Relationships						
Availability	5.1	6.4	5.9	6	2.23*	0.09
Adequacy	7.6	9.0	8.6	8.5	1.15*	0.33
Disability FLP Total score						
	17.6	18.3	7.5	16.6	4.59*	<0.01
Physical scale	18.1	18.6	8.8	16.4	3.15*	<0.03
Pain						
Visual Analogue	57.6	53.6	21.5	69.9	4.36*	<0.01
Pain Thermometer	2.3	2.2	1.4	2.3	1.97*	0.12
Joint Stiffness						
Thermometer	2.3	1.9	0.8	2.2	6.0*	<0.001
Joint Stiffness (Mins)- 4 categories	Chi=20.6, df=9. p<0.02					

other groups, may have greater efficacy in reducing the impact of the disease on their behaviour and resulting disability. The pattern of coping adopted by this group differed substantially from Groups 2 & 4. and differed less in relation to Group 1. In contrast to Group 1 they did not look to others for support, expressed feelings of pain and did not use denial as a technique for pain. An alternative explanation for these findings would be to suggest that Group 3 may have different demographic, disease or social characteristics in comparison to the 3 other groups. The analysis of these aspects of the four groups, however, failed to show Group 3 as distinctive. This finding therefore may suggest that coping styles may have a direct influence in ameliorating the disabling effects of RA.

Pain and Joint Stiffness

Pain as assessed by means of a visual analogue scale significantly distinguished between the 4 groups (ANOVA F=4.36; df 3, 140; p<0.01). A Duncans Multiple Range Test indicated that Group 3 reported significantly less pain that the three remaining groups (see Table 5). Joint stiffness as assessed by means of a visual analogue rating scale was found to be significantly different in the 4 groups (ANOVA F=5.98; df 3, 151;p<0.001). A Duncans Multiple Range Test indicated Group 3 to report significantly less joint stiffness in comparison to the remaining three groups (see Table 5). A further measure of joint stiffness was obtained by means of a time estimation of early morning joint stiffness (into 4 categories). This also indicated a significant difference between the 4 groups (Chi Square = 20.6, df 9; p<0.02).

One possible account for these findings is to suggest that the less disability experienced by this group is a result of their relatively reduced experience of pain and joint stiffness. The reasons for this reduced experience of the symptoms of

RA may be as a result the pattern of coping strategies that they tend to use. This would suggest that the experience of both pain and joint stiffness are susceptible to modification through psychological (behavioural and cognitive) mechanisms. The evidence that pain experience is susceptible to these modification is overwhelming (Melzack, 1973), little research has, however, been conducted on the influence of psychological factors on the experience of joint stiffness.

Measures of Psychological Well-Being

Table 6. *Psychological well-being*

	Group 1 (n=20)	Group 2 (n=105)	Group 3 (n=14)	Group 4 (n=19)
Depressed Mood*	8.9	7.6	2.6	6.6
		Anova F=2.99, df 3, 151; p‹0.05		
Self Esteem	24.2	24.3	16.5	22.8
		Anova F=4.78. df 3, 154; p‹0.01		
Adjustment	46.2	47.5	62.1	46.8
		Anova F=8.36, df 3, 154; p‹0.0001		
A.H.I.	33.7	35.6	35.3	35.4
		Anova F=0.64. df 3, 142; p=0.589		

*BDI as amended, see text for details

Psychological well-being has frequently been considered the most pertinent dependent variable in research on coping. In this study psychological well-being was analysed by four instruments. In three of these, adjustment, level of depressed mood and self esteem significant differences were found between the four groups (Table 6). In all cases Group 3 showed the most positive scores on these measures. These findings are consistent with Group 3 reporting less pain, joint stiffness and disability.

The findings in this study are consistent with a model where different patterns of coping influence the perception of symptoms and have consequent effects on disability and psychological well-being. In this study no particular effects of demographic factors were found to impinge on the pattern of coping and more importantly the groups were not found to have any major differences in the laboratory measures of their disease and no significant differences on rheumatological measures.

It must however be stressed that the direction of causality in what must be considered a dynamic interplay between coping and other variables used in this study are open to differing interpretation. One important alternative account would be to suggest that the driving force behind different coping styles is level of disability. By this account the pattern of coping styles utilised is dependent upon the level of disability in that particular forms of coping tend to be adopted and rejected at different levels of disability. By this account patterns of coping rather than predicting level of disability would be predicted by them. Different styles of coping may in turn have an influence on psychological well-being. In order to examine whether psychological well-being was influenced by the pattern of coping independent of the level of disability a series of ANCOVA were performed where the score on the Physical sub-scale of the FLP was entered as a covariate. This analysis indicated that a number of the variables remained significant. The visual analogue scale of pain (p‹0.04); joint

Table 7 *Symptoms and psychological well-being of 4 groups with different coping patterns with level of disability controlled*

	Group 1 (n=20)	group 2 (n=105)	Group 3 (n=14)	Group 4 (n=19)
(a) Measures of Pain and Joint stiffness				
Pain Visual analogue	57.6	53.6	21.5	69.9
	Ancova F=3.008, df 3, 138; p<0.05			
Joint Stiffness Thermometer				
	2.3	1.9	0.8	2.2
	Ancova F=4.12, df 3, 150; p<0.01			
(b) Psychological well-being				
Depressed Mood	8.9	7.6	2.6	6.6
	Ancova F=1.03,df 3, 149; p=0.38			
Self Esteem	24.2	24.3	16.5	22.8
	Ancova F=2.25, df 3, 151; p=0.084			
Adjustment	46.2	47.5	62.1	46.8
	Ancova F=5.43, df 3, 151; p<0.001			

stiffness (p<0.01) and adjustment (p<0.001) all significantly discriminated between groups (see Table 7). Of the remaining measures of psychological well-being that were found to be significant by ANOVA, group differences in self esteem approached significance (p = 0.084), the groups were not, however, found to be different on the modified Beck Depression Inventory when disability was controlled. These findings suggest that when a model which considers the disabling consequences of a disease to be the principle determinant of coping, the particular strategies adopted do have an influence on psychological well-being. In order to tease out both the stability of coping strategies and the direction of causality in terms of the models, a longitudinal study is currently being performed.

General Discussion and Conclusions

This study has examined the pattern of coping in a large group of individuals with RA. The analysis performed on the responses classified individuals into groups on the basis of the overall pattern of responses such that both the utilisation and failure to utilise a particular strategy were incorporated in the classification of patterns. By this technique idiosyncratic patterns of coping could be entertained. The results of this analysis yielded 4 distinct groups with different patterns of coping. While these four groups did not show significant difference in their disease as measured by both laboratory and rheumatological measures and were not different in their access to and perceived adequacy of social support, they were found to differ in their level of disability, perception of pain and joint stiffness and psychological well-being. The one group who produced the 'best' findings on these measures appeared to be the group who made the fewest adjustments to their RA and also did not attempt to use denial, seek support or distract themselves from the consequences of their RA. In many ways this group may be considered to be the most independent and reality bound of the four groups identified in the study. When the differences between the groups on symptom perception and psychological well-being were considered while controlling for the different levels of disability between the groups, this group continued to show reduced perception of symptoms and improved psychological well-being.

These findings suggest that when the full pattern of coping strategies adopted and rejected is considered, the individuals may be meaningfully classified into groups. Moreover, the results suggest that the pattern of coping, when analysed comprehensively makes a significant impact on disability, symptom perception and psychological well-being.

Acknowledgments

The authors would like to acknowledge the generous support of the Arthritis and Rheumatism Council. We would also like to thank Dr Michael Snaith for making his patients available to us, the patients for participating in the study, Ms Heather Fields for assisting with the data collection and Dr Tracey Revenson for comments on a draft of the manuscript.

References

Aldwin, C. M., and Revenson, T. A. (1987). Does coping help? A reexamination of the relation between coping and mental health. *Journal of Personality and Social Psychology, 53*, 337–348.

American Rheumatism Association. (1959). Diagnostic criteria for rheumatoid arthritis 1958 revision. *Annals of Rheumatic Disease, 18*, 49–51.

Anderson, K. O., Bradely, L. A., Young, L. D., and McDaniel, L. K. (1985). Rheumatoid arthritis: Review of psychological factors related to etiology, effects, and treatment. *Psychological Bulletin, 98*, 358–387.

Bennett, P. H, and Wood, P. H. N. (1968). Population studies of the rheumatic diseases. *International Congress Series No. 148* (pp. 455–477). Amsterdam: Excerpta Medica Foundation.

Bergner, M., Bobbitt, R. A., Carter, W. B., and Gilson, B. S. (1981). The sickness impact profile: Development and final revision of a health status measure. *Medical Care, 19*, 787–805.

Blashfield, R. (1980). Propositions regarding the use of cluster analysis in clinical research. *Journal of Consulting and Clinical Psychology, 48*, 456–459.

Cohen, F. (1987). Measurement of coping. In S. V. Kasl, and C. L. Cooper (Eds.), *Stress and health: Issues in research methodology* (pp. 283–305). New York: Wiley.

Deyo, R. A., Inui, T. S., Leininger, J., and Overman, S. (1982). Physical and psychosocial function in rheumatoid arthritis. Clinical use of a self-administered health status instrument. *Archives of Internal Medicine, 142*, 879–882.

Everitt, B. (1980). *Cluster analysis*. New York: Halstead.

Fitzpatrick, R., Newman, S., Lamb, R., and Shipley, M. (1988). Social relationships and psychological well-being in rheumatoid arthritis. *Social Science and Medicine, 27*, 399–403.

Folkman, S., and Lazarus, R. S. (1980). An analysis of coping in a middle aged community sample. *Journal of Health and Social Behaviour, 21*, 219–239.

Folkman, S., and Lazarus, R. S. (1985). If it changes it must be a process: A study of emotion and coping during three stages of college examination. *Journal of Personality and Social Psychology, 48*, 150–170.

Henderson, S., Byrne, D., and Duncan-Jones, P. (1981). *Neurosis in the social environment*. London: Academic Press.

Lawrence, J. S. (1977). *Rheumatism in populations*. London: Heinmann.

Lazarus, R. S., and Folkman, S. (1984). Coping and adaptation. In W. Gentry (Ed.), *Handbook of Behavioural Medicine* (pp. 282–325). London: Guilford.

Melzack, R. (1973). *The puzzle of pain*. Harmondworth: Penguin.

Menaghan, E. (1982). Measuring coping effectiveness: A panel analysis of marital problems and coping efforts. *Journal of Health and Social Behaviour, 23*, 220–234.

Moos, R. H. (1986). *Coping with life crises*. New York: Plenum.

Newman, S., Fitzpatrick, R., Lamb, R., and Shipley, M. (1987). Factors precipitating depressed mood in rheumatoid arthritis. *British Journal of Rheumatology, 26*, 121.

Norusis, M. J. (1985). *SPSS X Advanced Statistics Guide*. New York: McGraw Hill.

Nicassio, P., Wallston, K., Callahan, L., Herbert, M., and Pincus, T. (1985). The measurement of helplessness in rheumatoid arthritis: The development of the Arthritis Helplessness Index. *Journal of Rheumatology, 12*, 462–467.

Patrick, D., Morgan, M., and Carlton, J. (1986). Psychosocial support and change in the health status of physically disabled people. *Social Science and Medicine, 22*, 1347–1354.

Pearlin, L. I., and Schooler, C. (1978). The structure of coping. *Journal of Health and Social Behaviour, 19*, 337–356.

Pincus, T., Callahan, L. F., Bradley, L. A., Vaughan, W. K., and Wolfe, F. (1986). Elevated MMPI scores for hypochondriasis, depression, and hysteria in patients with rheumatoid arthritis reflect disease rather than psychological status. *Arthritis and Rheumatism, 29*, 1456–1466.

Pinkerton, P., Trauer, T., Duncan, F., Hodson, M. E., and Batten, J. C. (1985). Cystic fibrosis in adult life: A study of coping patterns. *The Lancet, 2*, 761–763.

Schmidt, L. R. (1988). Coping with surgical stress: some results and some problems. In S. Maes, C. D. Spielberger, P. D. Defares, and I. G. Sarason (Eds.), *Topics in health psychology* (pp. 219–227). Chichester: Wiley.

Steinbroker, O., Traegar, G. H., and Batterman, R. C. (1949). Therapeutic criteria in rheumatoid arthritis. *Journal of the American Medical Association, 140*, 659–662.

Thomas, P., Gasrry, P., Goodwin, J., and Goodwin, J. S. (1985). Social bonds in an elderly sample: characteristics and associated variables. *Social Science and Medicine, 20*, 365–369.

Zaphiropoulos, G., and Burry, H. V. (1974). Depression in rheumatoid disease. *Annals of Rheumatic Disease, 33*, 132–135.

Coping Skills and Perceived Threat: An Examination in Hemodialysis Patients

Peter Schwenkmezger, Jutta Lang, and Willi Landsiedel

According to statistics published in 1986 (in Der Dialysepatient, 1986), approximately 20,000 patients in West Germany are being treated with different forms of hemodialysis or transplantation. There are 2, 500 new patients every year. 4, 000 patients are on a waiting list for transplants; the annual number of transplants is a little more than 1, 300. The average waiting time for transplantation is about two years; in individual cases the waiting time can be as much as 8 years. The number of patients world-wide who are being treated with some type of long-term dialysis is estimated to be about 250, 000 (Wetzels, Coloby & Dittrich, 1986). In the last few years there have been significant improvements in treatment possibilities; however, the most widely-used treatments, such as different forms of dialysis in various settings of kidney transplants, bring about enormous changes in the patients' daily lives. Dialysis patients, for example, are continuously faced with life-threatening situations and because of the many limitations imposed on them they suffer from psychosocial stress. It therefore seemed reasonable to investigate how these patients experience this stress, how they cope with it and what kind of support might benefit them. This, of course, is also an opportunity for coping research with this patient group and, as with other comparable patient groups, one can study short-, middle- and long-term coping processes in a real-life-situation.

Very specifically, we want to focus in this paper on the question of the interaction between perception of coping skills and the threat posed by the disease. Because only patients with chronic renal insufficiency were studied (i.e. those patients who were not suitable for transplantation), we were not concerned with such issues as coping after transplantation. Our work is a continuation of earlier analyses of coping behavior in chronic dialysis patients (e.g., Bierkens & van der Bom, 1982; Koch, Speidel, & Balck, 1982; Muthny, 1985; Balck, Koch, & Speidel, 1985).

For a theoretical basis of our analysis we used Lazarus' transactional stress model (Lazarus & Launier, 1978). One implication of this model is that demands resulting from the illness and treatment can be considered as "stress", which in turn necessitate a range of coping strategies. In addition to analyzing the patient's evaluation of the situation in terms of well-being or threat (primary appraisal), one must also analyze his or her assessment of coping resources (secondary appraisal) and their interaction.

In a process model such as that represented by the transactional stress model, the most important factors under consideration are the conditions that determine the patient's assessment of his/her coping resources and their effectiveness. In particular, we want to analyze the following questions: How stable are coping strategies over the course of the illness? Are the coping strategies that the patients have developed specific to this illness, or are they strategies that they used prior to their illness in other stress situations? Is there any relationship between the

413

perception of coping resources and behavior dispositions such as anxiety and/or locus of control? Are there any relationships between coping strategies and 'objective' parameters of the course of illness?

In addition, we went to take a closer look at the process of confrontation with coping strategies itself. Emotional and cognitive changes that occur during the time it takes a patient to respond to a coping questionnaire have been described in several different ways. Of particular interest is the question whether the contents of these instruments confront patients, particularly those with severe physical disorders, with their limited coping possibilities and thus with a threat situation. This would explain a number of paradoxical results in this field of research. For example, Aldwin and Revenson (1987) found evidence that the perception of coping strategies, as assessed by the Ways-of-Coping-Checklist, can lead to an increase in emotional distress. This is particularly true for emotion-focused strategies. So we investigated this question by examining changes in threat during the time a patient filled out a questionnaire. This point is particularly important if, as predicted by Spielberger's state-trait model of anxiety, interaction effects occur depending upon the person-specific anxiety level.

Method

Subjects: Subjects were 83 hemodialysis patients in different treatment settings. One group (N = 50) were patients of a Limited Care Unit; N = 23 were from a dialysis clinic; another group (N = 12) consisted of patients undergoing home dialysis. The average age of the patients was 51.6 years; 64% of the subjects were male and 36% were female.

Procedure and dependent measures: The investigation was carried out as a combined longitudinal and cross-sectional study.

All of the subjects were given a series of questionnaires following a dialysis treatment. These questionnaires consisted of demographic and medical data, *Trait Anxiety-Scale* (Spielberger, 1983), *Locus of Control* (Krampen, 1981), 10 items from the *State Anxiety-Scale* (Spielberger, 1983), ratings of primary appraisal, *Ways-of-Coping-Checklist* (WCCL)(Lazarus, 1985; modified and translated form).

Assessment of patients at the *Limited Care Unit* (LCU) was repeated twice. Half of the subjects were assessed three times during one week (Monday, Wednesday, Friday) following a dialysis treatment in a short longitudinal study. Reassessment of the other half of the LCU patients was carried out three and six weeks following the first assessment.

Results

Before we go into details about the results pertaining to the different questions, we would like to describe our findings about the structure of the WCCL. For the most part, we used exploratory factor analyses; a summary of the results and a comparison with the factor structure found by Folkman and Lazarus (1985) can be found in Table 1.

In our analyses, the factor problem-focused coping was subdivided into two subfactors, cognitive evaluation and confrontative assessment. Of the six emotion-focused coping factors we were only able to find confirmation for four: wishful thinking, distancing, emphasizing the positive and tension reduction. Quite similar

Table 1. *Factorial Structure of 'Ways-of-Coping-Checklist'*

Folkman & Lazarus (1985)	Hemodialysis patients (N = 83)
– problem- focused coping (11 items)	cognitive evaluation (5 items)
	confrontative evaluation (4 items)
emotion- focused coping:	
– wishful thinking (5 items)	wishful thinking (5 items)
– distancing (6 items)	distancing (3 items)
– emphasizing the positive (4 items)	emphasizing the positive (7 items)
– self-blame	?
– tension reduction	tension reduction (3 items)
– self-isolation (3 items)	?
– seeking social support (7 items)	seeking social support (7 items)
?	religious leaning
?	physical activity (3 items)

results were obtained for the factor seeking social support. In addition, we identified two further dimensions, religious leaning and physical activity.

First, let's consider the question of temporal stability. According to Lazarus, in the coping process there is continual adjustment to new situations, in the sense of a transactional process. As a consequence, there should only be temporal stability and transsituational consistency between measurement occasions, especially if coping mechanisms are assessed over longer intervals.

Table 2. *Stability of coping-factors*

	2-days-intervals			3-weeks-intervals		
	1/2	2/3	1/3	1/2	2/3	1/3
cognitive evaluation	0.77	0.87	0.81	0.53	0.77	0.45
confrontative coping	0.70	0.82	0.56	0.46	0.57	0.63
wishful thinking	0.69	0.84	0.77	0.81	0.83	0.73
distancing	0.18	0.50	−0.13	0.11	0.24	0.20
emphasizing the positive	0.83	0.83	0.62	0.70	0.82	0.55
tension reduction	0.65	0.85	0.81	0.18	0.28	0.15
social support	0.84	0.89	0.86	0.54	0.81	0.56
religious leaning	0.92	0.96	0.93	0.91	0.84	0.90
physical activity	0.58	0.70	0.77	0.80	0.68	0.51

The results in Table 2 show that most coping mechanisms have a very high amount of temporal stability. This isn't really so surprising for the group who filled out the Ways-of-Coping questionnaire at two-days intervals. But the results of the other group, who were given the questionnaire at three-weekly intervals, are very similar.

Exceptions can easily be explained. For example, emotion-focused coping involving tension reduction could be regarded as a very unstable and rapidly fluctuating strategy.

Comparison of means shows that the coping strategies revealed almost no changes during the period studied. Analyses of variance revealed no systematic changes; the few significant effects that were found are probably due to chance.

In order to find out whether there is a relationship with coping strategies used prior to onset of illness in other stress situations, we performed retrospective interviews with a sub-sample of the subjects. The results in Table 3 show that for the most part the patients tended to use coping strategies that they had also used prior to their illness.

Table 3. *Relationship between illness-specific and generally used coping strategies (subsample of N = 42)*

cognitive evaluation	0.49**
confrontative evaluation	0.32*
wishful thinking	0.19
distancing	0.28
emphasizing the positive	0.52**
tension reduction	0.08
seeking social support	0.55**
religious leaning	0.57**
physical activity	0.48**

**p≤0.01; *≤0.05

For example, people who used religious coping strategies during their illness had had a similar attitude prior to their illness. The same is true for physical activity as a coping strategy, and for social support. These results would also help to explain the high temporal stability of the chosen coping strategies.

In contrast, covariations between coping strategy and personality traits such as anxiety or the three questionnaire scales related to locus of control are comparatively small (see Table 4).

Table 4. *Correlations between A-Trait resp. Locus of Control and coping factors (N = 83). Only significant relationships (p≤0.05) are reported*

	A-Trait	Locus of Control		
		I	P	C
cognitive evaluation	0.29			0.37
confrontative coping		0.34		
wishful thinking	0.33		0.34	0.39
distancing				
emphasizing the positive	−0.24	0.35		
tension reduction	0.33			0.32
social support	0.23			0.22

Slight correlations with these other variables were observed primarily with variables of emotion-centered coping. Positive reevaluation and confrontative assessment seemed to correlate with an internal locus of control (I), whereas emotion-centered coping was related more to dependency upon others(P) or to a fatalistic attitude (C).

More interesting is the covariation between coping strategies and the course of illness from a medical point of view. This was studied using a combined rating by doctors and nursing staff based on behavior observations and medical data.

Table 5. *Correlations between coping factors and a combined rating of the course of illness from a medical point of view (N = 83).*

cognitive evaluation	0.31**
confrontative coping	0.08
wishful thinking	−0.01
distancing	0.07
emphasizing the positive	0.22*
tension reduction	−0.39**
social support	0.42**
religious leaning	0.04
physical activity	−0.06
self-blame (single items)	−0.38**

**p≤0.01; *p≤0.05

Table 5 shows that social orientation and problem-centered coping in particular, but to a slight degree also positive reevaluation, correlate with a favorable course of illness. Negative correlations were found with coping factors such as short-term gratification of needs and self-blame.

We mentioned earlier that several investigators have asked whether the act of filling out a coping questionnaire in itself can confront seriously ill patients with the hopelessness of their situation, resulting in an increase in threat. If one also takes into account certain formulations of Spielberger's (1972) state-trait anxiety theory, one would probably expect to find differential effects, depending upon person-specific anxiety level. In our quasi-experimental design, therefore, we gave the patients 10 items of the State-Anxiety Scale (German adaptation; Laux, Glanzmann, Schaffner, & Spielberger, 1981) both before and after they filled out the WCCL. The scale was divided into two half-forms on the basis of item characteristics. High- and low-anxious patients were defined on the basis of a median split on the Trait Anxiety Scale. The results are shown in Figure 1.

The significant main effect for A-Trait, $F(1,50)=22.42$, $p≤0.01$ is of minor importance as compared with the significant main effect for before-and-after measurements, $F(2,50)=30.02$, $p≤0.01$ and the significant interaction effect, $F(1,50)=4.41$, $p≤0.05$. There really is an increase in state anxiety during the time a patient responds to the WCCL; this increase is greater for high-anxious patients at the first and third measurement occasions than for low-anxious patients, in accordance with predictions of the state-trait anxiety model.

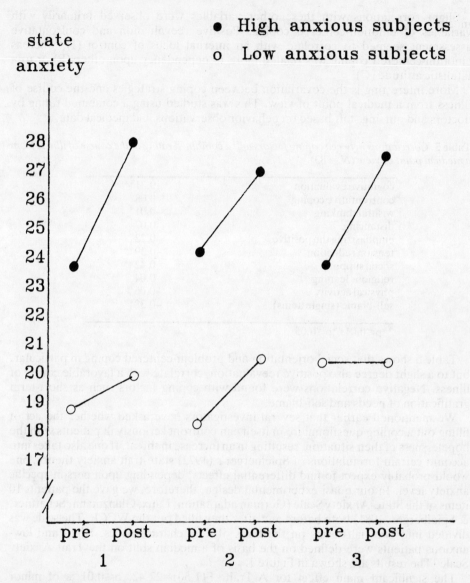

Figure 1. State Anxiety before and after answering the WCCL in three different trials.

Discussion

Surprisingly, almost all of the coping strategies were found to be highly stable over time. We also found evidence confirming that patients used similar coping strategies in stress situations prior to the illness. At first these results seem to contradict the transactional stress model, in which a continual adjustment of coping resources to new situations would lead to a lower temporal consistency and to a lower correlation with behavior dispositions. There are three possible explanations for these findings. First, the groups we studied had already been in dialysis treatment for over four years, on average. Apparently, the patients had developed very stable coping mechanisms during this period of time, which they used over and over again regardless of their effectiveness. Secondly, the relatively high age of the subjects probably resulted in a similar effect. Third, medical reasons make it advisable for dialysis patients to develop relatively rigid behaviors or habits. This is true both for eating and drinking habits and for arranging daily or weekly schedules to incorporate appointments for medical treatment. In a related way it is also true for the construction of a social support system. Insofar as the adaptive process is completed, relatively rigid behaviors probably determine the psychological adaptation to the illness process.

We are also more impressed with the results showing that coping strategies such as short-term gratification of needs (tension reduction) and self-blame tend to be associated with an unfavorable course of illness. The cause-and-effect relationship here, however, remains open. One could speculate that short-term gratification has a detrimental influence on the course of illness (e.g., through deviation in eating and drinking schedules), while self-blame is possibly a result of deviations from behavior styles that favorably influence the course of illness. More specifically, self-blame might be associated with negative mood (i.e., depression) and influence outcome in this way.

In conclusion, we would like to discuss briefly the increase in state anxiety which occurred during the filling-out of the WCCL. Apparently, confrontation with possible coping resources really is capable of contributing to an increase in the threat posed by the disease. It is possible that in this process the patient is also confronted with the inadequacy of his/her own coping strategies, so that this experimental situation takes on the character of a self-evaluation. The observed effect could therefore be explained in the context of Spielberger's state-trait anxiety model.

If our explanation is correct then those patients with more positive coping responses should show less or no increase in state anxiety, as compared with those with poor coping strategies. This hypothesis can be confirmed by considering the results of further correlation analyses. We found negative correlation between state anxiety measured *after* answering the WCCL and unfavorable coping styles like wishful thinking ($r = 0.49$, $p \leq 0.01$), tension reduction ($r = 0.37$, $p \leq 0.01$) and self-blame (aggregation of three single items; $r = 0.53$, $p \leq 0.01$). Additionally, a favorable coping style like emphasizing the positive was negatively correlated with state anxiety after filling out the WCCL ($r = 0.35$, $p \leq 0.01$).

In the meantime we were able to replicate these results in another sample of hemodialysis patients. Applying path-analytic methods Strack (1989) found evidence that the coping factor *rumination* (measured by a coping questionnaire developed by Klauer & Filipp, 1987) has a strong influence on state anxiety. Subjects high in rumination show a high and significant increase in state anxiety immediately after filling out the coping questionnaire. These results are in strong agreement with the study reported in this paper and recently published results concerning other questionnaires (Nebel, Strack, & Schwarz, 1989).

Because these clear effects were found only for state anxiety, we have to discuss the time course of this increase in anxiety, because it might be very transient and therefore of little long-term consequence. This question needs, however, further research. If this findings should prove stable, a major implication would be the need to implement different programs for high and low anxious dialysis patients in training them about different types of coping strategies.

References

Aldwin, C. M., and Revenson, R. A. (1987). Does coping help? A reexamination of the relation between coping and mental health. *Journal of Personality and Social Psychology, 52*, 337–348.

Balck, F., Koch, U., and Speidel, H. (Eds.). (1985). *Psychonephrologie. Psychische Probleme bei Niereninsuffizienz* [Psychonephrology. Psychological problems in nephritic disorders]. Berlin: Springer.

Bierkens, P. B., and van der Bom, J. A. (1982). Psychologische Gesichtspunkte bei Patienten mit terminaler Niereninsuffizienz [Psychological aspects in patients with terminal nephritic disorders]. In W. R. Minsel, and R. Scheller (Eds.), *Brennpunkte der Klinischen Psychologie* (pp. 137–154). München: Kösel.

Folkman, S., and Lazarus, R. S. (1985). If it changes it must be a process: Study of emotion and coping during three stages of a college examination. *Journal of Personality and Social Psychology, 48*, 150–170.

Klauer, T., and Filipp, S.-H. (1987). *Der "Fragebogen zur Erfassung von Formen der Krankheitsbewältigung" (FEBK): I. Kurzbeschreibung des Verfahrens* [Questionnaire for the measurement of dimensions of coping with disease: I. Short description]. Forschungsberichte aus dem Projekt "Psychologie der Krankheitsverarbeitung" Nr. 13. Fachbereich I – Psychologie, Universität Trier.

Koch, U., Speidel, H., and Balck, F. (1982). Psychische Probleme von Hämodialysepatienten und ihren Partnern [Psychological problems of hemodialysis patients and their partners]. In D. Beckmann, and S. Davies–Osterkamp (Eds.), *Medizinische Psychologie* (pp. 310–336). Berlin: Springer.

Krampen, G. (1981). *IPC-Fragebogen zu Kontrollüberzeugungen [Questionnaire of Locus of Control].* Göttingen: Hogrefe.

Laux, L., Glanzmann, P., Schaffner, P., and Spielberger, C. D. (1981). *Das State-Trait-Angstinventar (STAI): Theoretische Grundlagen und Handanweisung* [State-Trait Anxiety Inventory: Theoretical bases and manual]. Weinheim: Beltz.

Lazarus, R.S.(1985). *Ways-of-Coping revised.* Berkely, University of California (unpublished).

Lazarus, R. S., and Launier, R. (1978). Stress-related-transactions between person and environment. In L. R. Pervin, and M. Louis (Eds.), *Perspectives in interactional psychology* (pp. 287–327). New York: Plenum.

Muthny, F. A. (1985). Kausalattribution, Krankheitsverarbeitung und Compliance bei Dialyse-Patienten [Causal attribution, coping of disease and compliance in dialysis patients]. In D. Albert (Ed.), *Bericht über den 34. Kongreß der DGfPs in Wien 1984* (pp. 327–329). Göttingen: Hogrefe.

Nebel, A., Strack, F., and Schwarz, N. (1989). Tests als Treatment. Wie die psychologische Messung ihren Gegenstand verändert [Tests as a treatment. How psychological measurement changes its object]. *Diagnostica, 35*, 191–200.

Spielberger, C. D. (1972). Anxiety as an emotional state, In C. D. Spielberger (Ed.), *Anxiety: Current trends in theory and research* (Vol. 1, pp. 23–49). New York: Academic Press.

Spielberger, C. D. (1983). *Manual for the State-Trait Anxiety Inventory (STAI Form Y).* Palo Alto, CA: Consulting Psychologists Press.

Strack, K. (1989). *Angst und Bewältigungsverhalten bei Dialysepatienten* [Anxiety and coping behavior in hemodialysis patients]. Unpublished master's thesis. Fachbereich I – Psychologie, Universität Trier.

Wetzels, E., Colomby, A., and Dittrich, P. (1986). *Hämodialyse, Peritonealdialyse, Membranplasmapherese und verwandte Verfahren* [Hemodialysis, peritoneal dialysis, membranplasmapheresis and related methods]. Berlin: Springer.

Relations Between Coping Strategies and Presurgical Stress Reactions

Heinz W. Krohne, Peter P. Kleeman, Jochen Hardt,
and Albert Theisen

This study is part of a project which aims at analyzing the interactive effects of person-specific modes of coping with presurgical stress and the psychological and medical preparation of patients facing surgery on indicators of patient stress prior to, during, and after surgery. Patients facing surgery experience, among other stressors, an incapability of instrumentally influencing the essential, threat-relevant elements of this situation. Therefore, such a situation particularly requires the application of coping mechanisms by which a subjective alteration of objective threat elements can be achieved. Central to the study are the following topics: 1. How can the fundamental modes of coping be described and classified? – 2. Which indicators best reflect patient stress prior to surgery? – 3. How are central modes of coping related to indicators of patient stress?

The model of *coping modes* (Krohne, 1986; 1989) distinguishes two main classes of coping strategies by which *a subjective alteration of objective threat elements* can be achieved: *Vigilance* and *cognitive avoidance*. *Vigilance* is characterized by an approach to and an intensified processing of threat-relevant information. Its general objective is to gain control over the main threat-related aspects of a situation, thereby defending the individual against the threat of being confronted with unexpected dangers. Hence, vigilance may be defined as a *defense against the stress of "negative" surprise. Cognitive avoidance* is viewed as a withdrawal from threat-relevant information. Its general aim is to reduce the arousal (at least on the subjective level) engendered by the confrontation with an aversive event. Correspondingly, cognitive avoidance may be defined as a *defense against the stress of "negative" emotional states*.

Both modes are employed to describe actual stress-related actions and cognitive operations as well as interindividual differences in the *dispositional* inclination to employ a certain class of strategies. At the dispositional level, vigilance and cognitive avoidance are considered to *vary independently of each other*.

Method

Subjects and Procedure

Employing 40 patients (19 males, 21 females) awaiting elective maxillofacial surgery as subjects, the study analyzes the influence of (actual and dispositional) vigilant and avoidant coping strategies on self-reported (state anxiety) and biochemical (free fatty acids) stress indicators at different times prior to surgery. (1. After admission to hospital. 2. After the anaesthesiological pre-op visit in the afternoon before surgery. 3. On the morning of surgery. 4. Prior to induction of anaesthesia.)

The influence of coping on stress parameters was tested by means of a series of two-way analyses of variance with repeated measurements. In addition to the four measurement points, dispositional (trait) vigilance (VIG-T) and cognitive avoidance (CAV-T) served as independent variables in a first series of analyses, while actual (state) vigilance (VIG-S) and avoidance (CAV-S) replaced these variables in the second series of analyses. Each coping variable had two levels (defined by median split) and was measured by the "Mainz Coping Inventory" (MCI, cf. Krohne, Rösch & Kürsten, 1989). State anxiety (A-STATE; STAI, Laux, Glanzmann, Schaffner & Spielberger, 1981) and free fatty acids (FFA, analyzed by a gaschromatographic assay) were the dependent variables.

Results

Time Effects

Subjective and objective stress parameters show a significant (each with $p < 0.001$) and almost identical change over time. Both decrease from time 1 to 2 and increase again on the morning of surgery (3). However, while A-STATE remains at his high level until anaesthesia is induced (4), FFAs show a further significant increase from 3 to 4.

Effects of Coping Variables

Patients who employ cognitive avoidance before surgery (CAV-S) report less state anxiety than low avoiders, $F(1, 36) = 3.98$, $p < 0.05$. On the other hand, actual vigilant coping (VIG-S) is associated with a lower level of FFA concentration $F(1,36) = 3.57$, $p < 0.07$.

These two state variables also influence the concentration of FFAs, $F(1,36) = 4.15$, $p < 0.05$. Persons who neither employ vigilant nor avoidant coping show especially high biochemical stress reactions, while employing one or both groups of strategies results in comparatively low levels of stress (see Figure 1).

Actual vigilance and avoidance are also associated with the *discrepancy* between subjective and objective stress reactions (operationalized by transforming the raw data into z-scores and subtracting FFA from A-STATE scores). For subjects who manifest a great amount of cognitive avoidance, both stress components are about equally pronounced, independent of their degree of cognitive avoidance. However, with patients who show the actual coping pattern "high vigilance/low avoidance" the subjective reaction outweighted the physiological one ($z = 1.13$), while in the case of both low vigilance and avoidance, the physiological stress reaction was stronger than the subjective one ($z = -0.67$), $F(1.36) = 9.16$, $p < 0.01$ (see Figure 2).

Considering coping variables and measurement points, a significant interaction between dispositional avoidance and time of FFAs can be observed, $F(3,108) = 3.48$, $p < 0.05$. At time 1 high avoiders show more intense reactions than low avoiders, at time 2 both groups are even, while on the day of surgery (3 an 4) low avoiders show a more marked increase than high avoiders (Figure 3).

The same variables are also associated with the amount of discrepancy between A-State and FFA, $F(3,108) = 3.32$, $p < 0.05$ (see Figure 4). Immediately after admission (1) patients with low avoidance manifest more subjective than objective stress

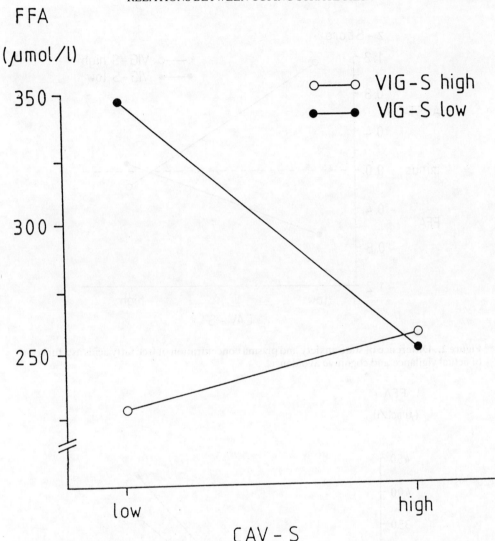

Figure 1. Plasma concentration of free fatty acids as a function of actual vigilance and cognitive avoidance.

reactions, while high avoiders show the reverse pattern. At time 2 the subjective mechanism outbalances the biochemical one for both groups: at time 3 both components are about even, while immediately before surgery (4) the bodily reaction is markedly stronger than the cognitive response, independent of coping mode.

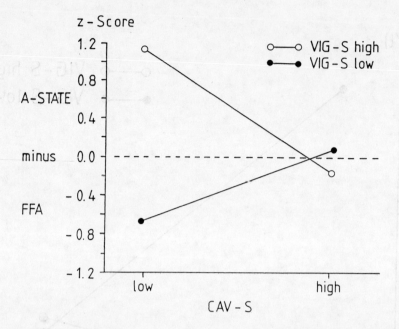

Figure 2. Difference of state anxiety and plasma concentration of free fatty acids as a function of actual vigilance and cognitive avoidance.

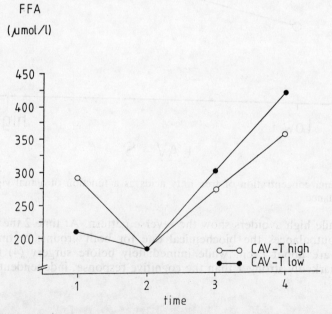

Figure 3. Plasma concentration of free fatty acids as a function of dispositional cognitive avoidance and time.

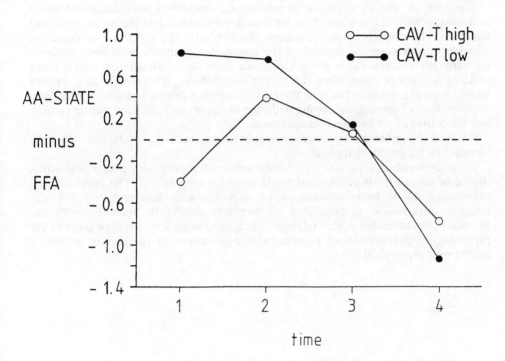

Figure 4. Difference of state anxiety and plasma concentration of free fatty acids as a function of dispositional cognitive avoidance and time.

Discussion and Conclusions

Self-reported anxiety as well as plasma concentration of free fatty acids are sensitive indicators of the course of presurgical stress. Both are comparatively high after admission, then they decrease after the anaesthesist's pre-op visit where reassuring information was received, and increase again on the day of surgery.

Both parameters are also influenced by cognitive coping variables, with state indicators being slightly superior predictors of stress reactions. The most remarkable result is the high somatic reaction of patients who neither manifest vigilant nor avoidant coping. Several interpretations are possible. Firstly, these patients may be "helpless", i.e. have no means of coping with stress in their repertoire. Secondly, they may employ specific, yet in this particular situation insufficient strategies. Thirdly, they may be persons who are defined by our model of coping modes as "non-defensives" (Krohne, 1986; 1989), i.e. they attempt to affect stressful situations primarily by instrumental rather than by cognitive ("intrapsychic") reactions. However, when they are confronted by situations in which instrumental control is practically impossible, then it is to be expected that they will experience (at least initially) a comparatively high degree of helplessness and stress. Further studies should concentrate especially on this group of patients.

Vigilance as well as cognitive avoidance are associated with decreased stress reactions; however, this is only true for specific parameters (subjective or objective) and for certain points of measurement. Particularly, the efficiency of cognitive avoidant coping seems to depend on the imminence of threat, with comparatively high somatic reactions at a greater distance from the confrontation and a more efficient mastery of stress when the danger is imminent. What is needed in further studies is an extension of the time dimension to points during and after surgery and a comparison of presurgical coping with, for example, complication during surgery and the course of postsurgical recuperation.

Results, if confirmed by systematic subsequent studies, imply the following conclusions for practical application:

1. Assessment of a patient's preferred mode of coping with presurgical stress should be part of the psychological preparation for surgery. – 2. This psychological preparation has to be individualized, i.e. a patient's environment (e.g. the way relevant information is presented to him/her) should be matched with the characteristics of his/her preferred mode – 3. Special attention should be given to the psychological preparation of patients with nonexistent or insufficient means of coping with presurgical stress.

References

Krohne, H. W. (1986). Coping with stress: Dispositions, strategies, and the problem of measurement. In M. H. Appley, and R. Trumbull (Eds.), *Dynamics of stress* (pp. 209–234). New York: Plenum.

Krohne, H. W. (1989). The concept of coping modes: Relating cognitive person variables to actual coping behavior. *Advances in Behaviour Research and Therapy, 7,* 11, 235–248.

Krohne, H. W., Rösch, W., and Kürsten, F. (1989). Die Erfassung von Angstbewältigung in physisch bedrohlichen Situationen. [Assessment of coping in physically threatening situations]. *Zeitschrift für Klinische Psychologie, 18,* 230–242.

Laux, L., Glanzmann, P., Schaffner, P., and Spielberger, C. D. (1981). *Das State-Trait-Angstinventar.* [State-Trait Anxiety Inventory]. Weinheim: Beltz.

INDEX

431

434   Index